The Renaissance Diet 2.0

Dr. Mike Israetel | Dr. Melissa Davis
Dr. Jen Case | Dr. James Hoffmann

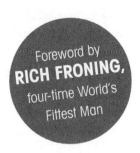

Foreword by
RICH FRONING,
four-time World's
Fittest Man

THE

RENAISSANCE
DIET 2.0

Your Scientific Guide to Fat Loss,
Muscle Gain, and Performance

MEYER & MEYER SPORT

British Library Cataloging in Publication Data

A catalogue record for this book is available from the British Library

The Renaissance Diet 2.0

Maidenhead: Meyer & Meyer Sport (UK) Ltd., 2020

ISBN: 978-1-78255-190-4

© 2020 by Meyer & Meyer Sport (UK) Ltd.
Fifth reprint 2024 of the first edition 2020

Aachen, Auckland, Beirut, Cairo, Cape Town, Dubai, Hägendorf, Hong Kong, Indianapolis, Maidenhead, Manila, New Delhi, Singapore, Sydney, Tehran, Vienna

Member of the World Sports Publisher' Association (WSPA), www.w-s-p-a.org

Printed by Versa Press, East Peoria, IL
Printed in the United States of America

ISBN: 978-1-78255-190-4

Email: info@m-m-sports.com

www.thesportspublisher.com

Contents

Foreword

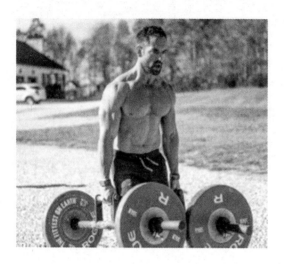

My name is Rich Froning, and I would like to welcome you to the brand-new, revamped *Renaissance Diet 2.0*. I have been competing in fitness sport for nine years, and in those years I have won four individual CrossFit Games Titles, three Affiliate Cup Titles, and a second place in each category as well. Nutrition for performance, recovery, and body composition change has been integral to my success. Whether you are trying to qualify for the CrossFit Games, just shed some body fat or gain some muscle to improve your appearance and health, or anything in between, you are going to want to be aware of the tools available for your fitness journey. As far as such tools go, proper manipulation of diet is one of the most powerful.

Over my many years in sport, I have encountered countless trends, fads, and misconceptions in nutrition. Some pop up for only a short time, others last decades, and some even come and go every few years. Unfortunately, most meant to notably and sustainably change your appearance and performance do not work in the long term. I have seen too many well-meaning, motivated people get ripped off and denied their best results because they invested in a fad diet approach.

The Renaissance Periodization way is different. First of all, as you will soon read, there really is no such thing as "the RP diet." RP has just synthesized all available scientifically derived, research-backed principles of nutrition to create a detailed set of instructions that you can apply to your own diet or to the diets of clients.

This book is the most up-to-date, comprehensive resource on the science and practice of fat loss, muscle gain, and performance-improvement dieting currently available. For those who want the most detailed descriptions of how and why the dieting principles work, RP's team of professors, PhDs, coaches, medical doctors, athletes, and dietitians have provided just that, with a vast reference library for those that want to expand their understanding even more. Each chapter is summarized with the basics you need to know to understand the process, and several chapters are dedicated specifically to helping you design and execute your own diet based on your goals, step by step.

Happy reading,
Rich Froning
Four-Time World's Fittest Man

A Note From the Authors

When we wrote the original *Renaissance Diet*, it was the first comprehensive description of our diet approach based on the most up-to-date nutritional data available and on our experience with hundreds of clients. Our original book was one of the first to synthesize the current literature on nutrition for body composition and performance and to present it in an ordered, logical, and understandable manner. This early version of the *Renaissance Diet* was also the first to identify the most important factors for successful dieting and delineate their practical application.

It has been a few years since the original *Renaissance Diet* was published, and two major things have changed since then: First, the interim years of scientific research have increased and refined our knowledge of how to lose fat, gain muscle, and improve performance. Second, through a combination of one-on-one coaching and digital products, Renaissance Periodization has now helped several *hundred thousand* people with their diets. These people range from those just trying to get in shape for the first time to world champion athletes. This collective coaching experience has refined our strategies and tactics with respect to the application of all our scientific knowledge. The summation of all this data and experience is now available to you, right here in this book.

This newest version of the *Renaissance Diet* is not only updated and refined, but also expanded. Special diet considerations and information on female-specific diet issues have been added along with information on gut health and an extensive section debunking some of the current and pervasive diet fads and fallacies. We put a great deal of effort into making this book bigger and better so that you can use it to become bigger, better, faster, stronger, leaner–whatever your goals call for.

We did this because we hate pseudoscience, scams, and quacks. We did it because we want to give you, our readers, our clients, and our friends in science, the best, most up-to-date information so that you can change your body, your performance, and your health for the better.

We sincerely hope you enjoy this book and will put the knowledge you gain from it to use in reaching your health and fitness goals.

Dr. Mike Israetel
Dr. Melissa Davis
Dr. Jen Case
Dr. James Hoffmann

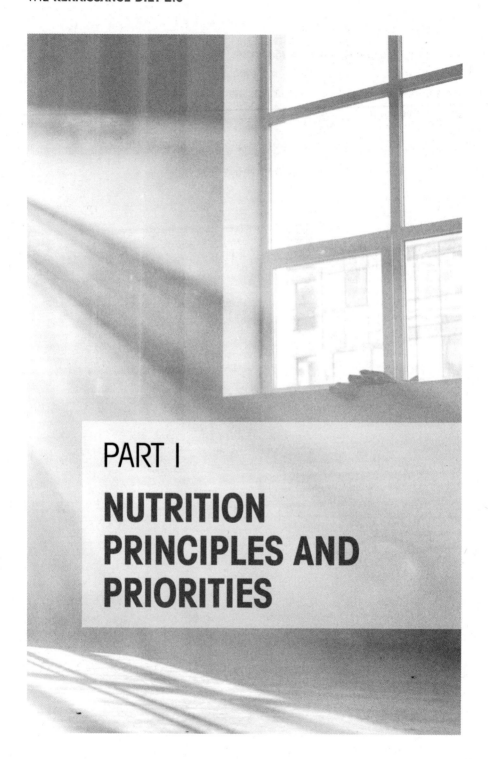

PART I

NUTRITION PRINCIPLES AND PRIORITIES

CHAPTER 1

The Diet Priorities

There are countless diet options available these days. If you would like some evidence to back this statement, try looking up "fat loss diet." New diets that promise to help you lose fat, build muscle, and increase performance pop up online nearly every day. Some diets eliminate entire food groups while others focus on consuming solely those same food groups. In reality, the science of dieting has moved beyond the scope of just controlling food groups; you have likely heard of concepts such as macronutrients, total calorie intake, and meal timing. The scientific basis and reasoning behind the various available dietary regimens are not often made entirely clear. With so many opposing options, just deciding how to diet can be a frustrating and seemingly hopeless endeavor.

The good news is that there are five main principles, along with adherence to those principles, that contribute to any diet's effectiveness. Differences in implementing these principles account for all variations between diets and their outcomes. We can get lost in the superficial aspects of the many diet options available. One diet may require you to eliminate carbohydrates from your meals, whereas another calls for fasting. The intended outcome of each of these is generally weight loss. What might jump out at you is the lack of carbs or the fasting periods, but these are just superficial aspects–both these diet alterations are meant to achieve one goal: a calorie deficit. It is the calorie deficit that results in the weight loss, not the lack of carbs or meal timing.

Calorie balance is the first and most important of the diet principles, and any diet that works well will manipulate calories directly or indirectly. The other four diet principles can also alter superficial aspects of a diet. Once you have learned to see past these superficial aspects and identify each of the five underlying diet principles, you will be able to assess their roles and predict that diet's effectiveness.

Diets vary quantitatively across one or more of the following five principles:

1. **Calorie Balance:** How many calories you eat per day relative to how many you burn.
2. **Macronutrient Amounts:** How many grams of protein, carbohydrate, and fat you eat per day.
3. **Nutrient Timing:** When and how you spread your total food intake across daily meals.
4. **Food Composition:** The sources of macronutrients you consume.
5. **Supplement Use and Hydration:** How much and what type (if any) dietary supplements you consume and your level of hydration.

All these factors contribute to rates of weight loss or weight gain as well as differences in athletic performance. As we will learn, some of these principles are more powerful than others in determining outcome.

Although adherence is not a programmed aspect of a diet, it is critical. If the diet were a race car, adherence would be the driver; without a driver, the car does not race. A good driver can get the best possible performance with any given machine, but a bad driver can crash even the best car. Simply put, you cannot succeed on a diet you do not follow, regardless of how good the diet is.

When we wrote the first edition of this book some years ago, we took an extensive look at the research on dieting for fitness. We assessed effect sizes, which are measurements of how much change in outcome is observed when a specific variable differs between groups. Studies that varied calorie balance alone showed the most significant effects; studies that manipulated macronutrient intake (without altering calories) showed smaller but still significant differences in body composition changes. Altering nutrient timing (without changes to calories or macronutrients) resulted in very small differences in outcome. The effect of changes in food composition or supplement use on fitness outcomes was undetectable in most cases. As a testament to the fact that adherence to any diet is a prerequisite for its success, metabolic ward studies, in which subjects do not leave the research facility and can only eat the food administered by researchers, are the gold standard in nutrition research because of the near perfect adherence that results from these conditions.

We qualitatively consolidated data from these investigations and came up with estimated relative effect sizes for the five principles of dieting:

Calorie Balance: approximately 50%
Macronutrient Amounts: approximately 30%
Nutrient Timing: approximately 10%
Food Composition: approximately 5%
Supplements and Hydration: approximately 5%

Again, these percentages only apply to the extent that an individual adheres to a given diet. A perfectly planned calorie balance, for example, will not have the desired effect if the dieter is not eating those planned calories.

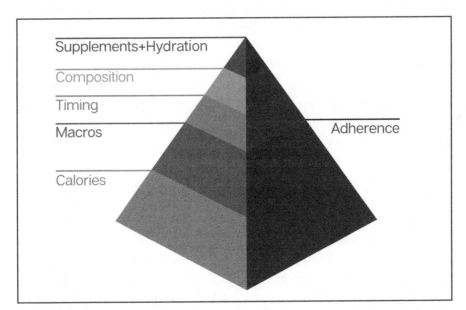

Figure 1.1 *The Diet Priority Pyramid depicts the relative importance of the diet priorities for body composition and performance outcomes.*

If you run a diet based only on calorie balance, you might expect to get about 50% of the potential effect of the diet on body composition and performance. On the other hand, if you based your diet on both calorie balance and proper macronutrient intake, you could get about 80% of the diet's potential results. If you took all the right supplements and ate only healthy food options, but did not worry about macronutrients, timing, or calories, you could not expect more than about 10% of the potential positive outcomes from the diet. We want to make it clear that this analysis is for body composition change and performance outcomes, *not health.* While paying attention to food composition (eating healthy foods most of the time) does not have a huge effect on appearance or performance, it does have a significant effect on health, as detailed in our book *Understanding Healthy Eating.*

AVOIDING PITFALLS AND USING THE DIET PRINCIPLES TO YOUR ADVANTAGE

The differential effects of diet principles provide useful guidelines for programming diets with specific outcomes in mind. Prioritizing the less powerful aspects (such as meal timing and supplements) and taking the powerful principles (such as calorie balance and macronutrient intake) for granted are common mistakes. Someone might eat with exact meal timing and take creatine and whey protein supplements, but if calories and macronutrients vary too much day to day, there simply will not be substantial results. Thousands of people start new fat loss or muscle gain diets every week, and many of them choose diets that are not based on the higher priority diet principles and thus experience minimal results.

Perhaps the most commonly neglected dieting principle is calorie balance. Thousands of people restrict various food types to consume only specific foods—unknowingly prioritizing one of the less important diet principles, food composition. Supplements are the most overemphasized principle. People buy countless bottles of pills and powders and take them religiously, expecting big results. While investing so much time and energy into the minor priorities, many of these well-intentioned dieters do not have the willpower leftover to invest in the big priorities that really matter. In a fat loss phase this can mean eating too much (very healthy) food to create a calorie deficit. In a muscle gain phase this can mean eating exclusively healthy food that is high in fiber and not as appetizing, resulting in a failure to create a calorie surplus for weight gain. Both these failures often occur despite a diet with appropriate food composition, well-planned meal timing, and supplements.

Unfortunately, these mistakes often involve every bit as much effort as a successful diet. Every year, people find their dieting efforts largely wasted on unimpressive results, leading many to assume they are "hard losers," "hard gainers," or otherwise personally flawed. The true underlying problem is simply a mismanagement of dieting principles.

By getting to know the diet principle hierarchy, we can ensure that our hard efforts are being spent where they are most effective. As you read about each of the individual diet principles, please keep their hierarchical organization in mind so that when it comes time to program your diet, you can effectively manage the distribution of these factors to meet your goals.

KEY DEFINITIONS AND CONCEPTS

Some key concepts and definitions that will come up throughout the book are listed below. We will revisit many of these multiple times throughout the coming chapters, so be prepared to return for a refresher as needed throughout your reading:

Set Points
An adult's set point is the bodyweight that they are naturally inclined to maintain. Some people have a high set point and would become obese if they just ate and exercised as they pleased. Others have trouble maintaining sufficient bodyweight for best health when left to their own devices. Set points are genetic predispositions, but your body's preferred weight can be changed.

Settling Points
A settling point is the weight your body is inclined to maintain, taking into account your current *and historical* dietary and activity practices. Your settling point can be very different from your genetic set point. Enough added fat or added muscle maintained for periods of months to years can permanently push your settling point

above your genetic set point. In contrast, there is no convincing evidence as of this book that settling points fall permanently below genetic set points when weight is lost. The good news is that it is often the case that more overweight people have actually pushed their settling point far above their genetic set point as opposed to their having a very high genetic set point.

Muscle mass has its own independent set and settling points—some people are naturally more or less muscular regardless of diet and training, though these points are not affected as easily as those for general body\weight. Once more muscle has been gained and maintained for a year or longer, only a fraction of the original effort is needed to rebuild it if it is lost. Also, muscle takes much less effort to maintain than to build, a fact we can exploit in the construction of nutritional periodization.

Fat-Loss Phase

A period of dieting for the purpose of losing fat. A common secondary goal on such a phase is to minimize muscle loss to the greatest extent possible.

Muscle-Gain Phase

A period of dieting for the purpose of gaining muscle. A common secondary goal on such a phase is to minimize fat gain to the greatest extent possible.

Post-Diet Maintenance Phase

Also known as a "diet recovery phase," this phase occurs after a fat loss or a muscle gain phase, and its purpose is to maintain the changes made to body composition during the preceding diet. This period involves easing back into normal eating, slowly moving out of the deficit or surplus created by the previous phase. The purpose of this phase is also to reset metabolic and psychological homeostasis at a new bodyweight and establish new settling points. Post-diet maintenance begins at the end of a fat loss or muscle gain diet, and its duration will depend on the degree to which bodyweight and metabolism were changed by the previous phase. At the conclusion of post-diet maintenance, you can begin another weight-changing phase or move into long-term maintenance of the current weight.

Long-Term Maintenance/Balance Phase

In this phase of dieting, the individual's physiology and psychology have adapted to the current state of the body. This phase typically starts after the post-diet maintenance phase and can last as long as the individual would like to maintain their results and live a healthy, active, and balanced life.

High-Volume Hypertrophy Training

High-volume hypertrophy training is needed to maintain muscle mass on a fat-loss diet or increase muscle mass on a muscle-gain diet. It consists of resistance training composed of multiple sets of exercises (8-20+ sets per body part per week), mainly in the 6- to 30-repetition range. This resistance training is ideally mainly composed of compound basics like squats, bench presses, rows, and so on–lifts that engage multiple joints and whole muscle groups. For more information, visit renaissanceperiodization. com and check out the eBook, *Scientific Principles of Strength Training*.

Low-Volume Strength Training

Low-volume strength training increases strength and power without changing muscle size. It is composed of fewer sets (5-15 per body part per week), usually in the 1- to 8-repetition range. This type of training is conducive to maintaining muscle during isocaloric periods (post-diet or long-term maintenance phases). It also has the added benefit of making the muscles more sensitive to the muscle growth effects of high-volume hypertrophy training for another fat-loss or muscle-gain diet.

Mesocycle

Mesocycle is a term used to describe training on a month-to-month basis–periods of dedicated training usually lasting between four to eight weeks. The mesocycle is comprised of a series of microcycles, or week-to-week training phases. Mesocycles are strung together to form training macrocycles, which are long-term periods dedicated to progressing toward a particular goal. Mesocycles (or several mesocycles with the same goal sequenced together) are also colloquially known as "blocks" or "phases" of training.

Fractional Synthetic Rate of Muscle Growth (FSR)

FSR generally refers to the rate at which a certain amount of amino acids from dietary protein are incorporated into skeletal muscle. In other words, this describes how much of the protein you eat is used to grow muscle and how fast.

Fractional Breakdown Rate of Muscle Growth (FBR)

FBR generally refers to the rate at which a certain amount of skeletal muscle protein is broken down for use in the body. In other words, this describes how much muscle tissue is lost during periods of insufficient training, insufficient energy availability, or insufficient circulating amino acids and how fast.

Partitioning Ratio

The P-Ratio describes the ratio of fat to muscle gained or lost on a diet. A favorable P-Ratio on a muscle gain phase would mean gaining larger amounts of muscle and very little fat. One of the reasons to periodize diet phases for muscle gain is to maximize the P-Ratio of each gaining phase so that more muscle than fat is gained over the long term.

Beginner, Intermediate, and Advanced Lifters

In this book we will define beginners as having around 0 to 3 years of structured lifting experience, intermediates as having roughly 3 to 6 years of experience, and advanced lifters as having 6+ years of experience. These are not precise timelines, but rather serve as a rough guide to classify lifting experience. In general, beginners gain muscle and lose fat more readily than intermediate and advanced lifters. Advanced lifters need more voluminous training to gain even a small amount of muscle compared to less experienced counterparts. While genetics and other factors play a large role in muscle growth responses, the relative differences between levels of experience are consistent. In other words, there may be outlier individuals who gain more muscle as advanced lifters than less genetically inclined beginners, but on average those early in their lifting career will have better responses to training than their more experienced counterparts.

CHAPTER SUMMARY

- Diets to improve performance and body composition can be evaluated based on how they address the diet principles of calorie balance, macronutrient amounts, nutrient timing, food composition, and supplement use and hydration.
- Individual diet principles do not contribute to success equally, and diets that prioritize the less powerful factors are either less effective or doomed to failure.
- Better adherence increases any diet's effectiveness. Adherence is imperative for success.

CHAPTER 2

Calorie Balance

Any means of achieving a calorie deficit will result in weight loss, and any means of achieving a caloric surplus will result in weight gain. Whether or not that weight change leads to improved body composition depends on other factors, including macronutrient balance, which we will go over in the subsequent chapter. Calorie balance alone can alter weight irrespective of any other diet principles, making it the greatest priority in the diet hierarchy.

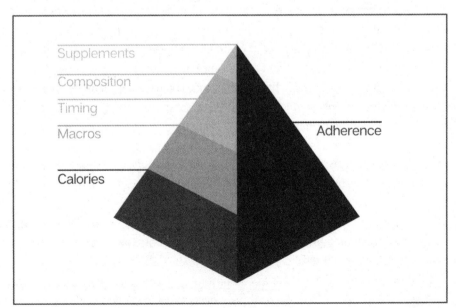

CALORIES

In the simplest terms, a calorie is a unit of measurement for energy. In the strictest sense, a calorie (which actually refers to a kilocalorie) is the amount of heat required to raise the temperature of one kilogram of water from 14.5 to 15.5 degrees Celsius. Interesting, but not very helpful when sitting down and deciding what to eat.

In nutrition, calories measure how much energy we get from food to either use or store in our bodies. Calories can be used to jump, run, operate your brain, recover from hard training, repair broken structures, or simply support the energy requirements of normal body function. An individual might use 2,000 calories a day to meet all of their energy needs, including everything from walking over to pick up the telephone to the firing of neurons in the brain to read this very text.

When someone needs 2,000 calories per day to function, but only consumes 1,700, they do not simply stop breathing or lose the ability to walk or think. The body has a back-up plan for when calories are scarce. Our ancestors did not have local grocery stores or refrigeration, so our bodies are adapted to deal with some periods of calorie deficit without extensive damage to health or function. In the previous example, the body can acquire the additional 300 calories it needs to sustain itself by breaking down some of its own tissues (most commonly fat) to release stored energy. There is a tremendous amount of stored energy in your adipose tissue. While your body does burn fats for fuel in the absence of sufficient food, it can also break down other structures, such as the proteins that compose your muscles. A variety of factors determine which of the body's tissues are broken down for energy and in what amount, but the primary factor deciding whether the body's structures will be accessed at all is calorie balance. When your body is getting enough food per day to meet all of its energy needs, we call this an *isocaloric* or *eucaloric* condition. Isocaloric conditions result in bodyweight maintenance—stable bodyweight over time.

When your body is not getting enough calories per day to meet energy needs, it must break down some of its own tissue for the missing energy. This dietary condition is termed *hypocaloric* and results in weight loss. If you take in more energy than you need, your body stores much of it as carbohydrate, protein, and fat molecules, with fat being the most common. We call this a *hypercaloric* condition, and as you may have already guessed, it results in weight gain.

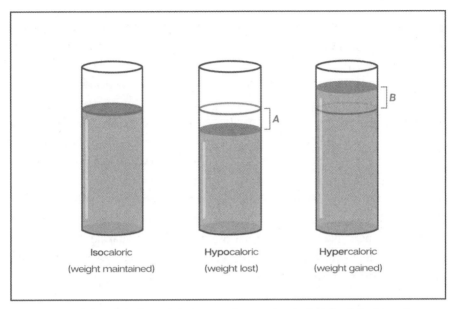

Figure 2.1 *On an isocaloric diet, calorie consumption matches the body's calorie demand. During a hypocaloric diet, fewer calories are being consumed relative to the body's daily demand (designated by bracket A) On a hypercaloric diet, excess calories are being ingested (designated by bracket B).*

CALORIES AND PERFORMANCE

Calorie balance is the most important principle for both body composition change and sport performance. Calorie intake affects sport performance by mediating energy availability, facilitating recovery, and influencing body composition (which indirectly affects performance).

At the onset of exercise, the body accesses a variety of fuel sources. Blood glucose from recent food intake is a readily available fuel source but is tightly regulated (in order to maintain glucose supply to the nervous system and keep you functioning). As exertion continues, non-tissue energy sources (carbohydrate stored as glycogen in your muscles) can continue to provide needed fuel at a rate sufficient to maintain athletic performance. Other glycogen stores in your liver act to moderate blood glucose levels as well. When these liver stores become depleted, blood glucose can drop, leading to bouts of hypoglycemia—clearly not great for sport performance. Glycogen stores are built up in the muscles and liver over time as calories are consumed. If an athlete under-eats for intervals of a week or more, their ability to perform at a high level will degrade substantially, even for less energy-intensive activities.

Both blood glucose and glycogen provide energy more quickly and easily than breaking down your body's tissues. Your fat stores can provide energy for movement as well, but the rate of energy release in this case is much slower and cannot keep up with the energy demands of most sports. To put this in perspective, the breakdown of fat tissue for energy release does not even reach its peak rates until around two hours into an exercise session. Even its peak rates are not as efficient at providing fuel for sport performance as blood glucose and glycogen, making it a much less desirable option. In other words, reducing calories and relying predominantly on fat sources for energy almost always leads to poorer performance.

In addition to providing energy for activity, calories also provide the energy for recovery from training. The process of training for sport is, at least in part, tearing down and rebuilding stronger tissues. Gaining muscle and training for strength both involve induced tissue damage that, under the right conditions, leads to recovery and adaptation to a bigger, stronger state.

Even in cases where an athlete's current sport progress needs are entirely technical, fatigue and tissue damage will arise just from extensive practice and repetition. Many sports also involve contact, such as American football, rugby, and combat sports, which also results in tissue damage or minor injuries. All this damage must be repaired, and this process requires energy. In addition to providing energy for structural repairs, calorie intake can influence how much glycogen stores are refilled. In a hypocaloric state, most available energy is dedicated to basic bodily function. The body will allocate some energy to support repair and recovery processes, but these resources are limited; the process will be slower, and recovery will be incomplete. (If you are severely hypocaloric, you may not be able to rebuild tissue at all.) In a hypercaloric state, repair and recovery will be optimal thanks to a surplus of energy. (For more information about recovery, see *Recovering from Training*, available on our website renaissanceperiodization.com as an ebook or audible file.)

Body size is directly affected by calorie intake and influences performance. Calories, therefore, also indirectly affect performance via their influence on body size. Depending on your sport, your body needs to be within some margin of sizes for best performance. For example, if you are the best gymnast at 130 lb. but you only eat enough calories to support a body weight of 90 lb., your diet will be unable to support your best gymnastic performance. You will not have the energy or raw materials to build muscles big enough to perform at your best. If you are a runner, and you eat enough calories to weigh 210 lb. but your best power-to-weight ratio is at 160 lb., you are dragging around an extra 50 lb., inevitably slowing your running times.

CALORIES AND BODY COMPOSITION

Body composition describes how much muscle and fat makes up your body. Improving body composition usually refers to getting leaner, more muscular, or both. Conversely, poor body composition tends to mean low muscle mass, an unfavorable excess of fat, or both. As you might expect, the vast majority of diets attempt to improve body composition. Calorie balance is the *single biggest tool* for altering body composition.

Your body is primed by millions of years of evolution to prepare itself for impending famine, something that has been a feature of the human (and animal) experience for as far back as biologists can investigate. Millions of years of natural selection have left your body designed to store as much energy as possible to prepare for times of low food availability. When your body is exposed to the hypercaloric condition, it stores most of the excess energy as body fat. This is logical because in ancestral environments, times of plenty were inevitably followed by times of scarcity, and storing excess calories as fat in the former literally saved your life in the latter. If an athlete or dieter is on a hypercaloric diet today, the chances that their body will activate fat-burning pathways over fat-building pathways are quite low. When extra calories are around, fat gain is usually a result.

Muscle growth rates are *much smaller* than fat gain rates. This is again a side effect of our evolution. Muscle mass is metabolically costly; it requires more energy to build and maintain than fat mass. Thus, the body sees adding extra muscle as a survival disadvantage under most circumstances. Only when there is a pressing need (increasingly difficult weight-bearing tasks) and a steady hypercaloric condition will any significant muscle mass be gained and even then to a lesser extent than fat. It is not uncommon for people to lose 15 lb. of fat in three months in a hypocaloric condition, but gaining 15 lb. of muscle in the same timeframe under hypercaloric conditions is virtually impossible. In fact, 15 lb. would be an impressive amount of muscle to build even in your first year of training.

For muscle to grow, there are two fundamental requirements: 1) the energy and raw material (amino acids from protein—the building blocks for muscle) with which to fuel the building of the muscle. Just like a frugal family will not get a new deck added to their home unless there is more money coming in than is needed for food and to pay bills, the body will not activate muscle growth pathways to any large extent until excess calories and plenty of protein are coming in. And 2) the stimulation of muscle growth from proper overload training. For the body to be convinced that metabolically costly muscle mass is worth adding, the consistent need for that muscle mass must be presented in the form of increasingly difficult resistance training.

It might seem obvious that results from concurrent body recomposition—simultaneous fat loss and muscle gain—pale in comparison to losing fat and gaining muscle in separate phases. This is because the most powerful methods for fat loss and muscle gain are diametrically opposed. For fat loss to occur at best rates, a hypocaloric condition is needed. When a hypocaloric condition is detected by body systems, it primes and prepares fat burning precisely to make up the impending deficit. In contrast, for best muscle gain rates, a hypercaloric condition and weight gain are needed. When a surplus of energy is coming in, the body is less resistant to packing on some metabolically costly muscle along with fat for energy storage. An isocaloric diet is the midpoint of the two-principle calorie balance paradigms and is not a powerful stimulator of fat loss nor muscle growth. Because our best tools for each are literal opposites, combining them gives us neither of each. Simply, if your goal is muscle gain, generate a hypercaloric condition. If your goal is fat loss, generate a hypocaloric condition.

There are specific, albeit rare and limited, instances when recomposition does occur. As we discuss these cases, keep in mind impressive social media transformation stories you might have seen in the past, and how one or more of these circumstances may have been at play. Also consider that having recomposition as a goal in your own diet design is likely a fool's errand in most cases, or at the very least not an efficient game plan.

Case 1: New to Dieting

If an individual has been eating poorly for years and dives headfirst into controlling their calories, macros, timing, and food composition, the combined power of all of those novel effects can be quite large—in some cases large enough to build a bit of muscle while simultaneously burning fat under isocaloric conditions. In a hypercaloric condition, individuals new to serious dieting can even gain weight while losing fat. Individuals in hypocaloric conditions can gain muscle and get much stronger while undergoing rapid fat loss. Because these impressive transformations are built on the element of novelty to formal dieting, this ability diminishes after several months as the body adjusts to a state where composition changes occur slowly.

Case 2: New to Training

In the first several months of training, especially if resistance and cardiovascular styles are programmed in high volumes, the demand for muscle growth nutrients and energy can be so high that fat stores are burned in large quantities to meet the need. Those new to the training process can see results very similar to those new to dieting in terms of radical simultaneous muscle gains and fat losses. If someone starts both training and dieting formally for the first time, concurrent recomposition can be achieved for the first several months, seemingly in contradiction with our understanding of physiology. Such abilities will decrease within several months of training. For continued progress, separate hypocaloric and hypercaloric phases will be needed for efficient fat loss and muscle gain.

Case 3: Pharmacological Intervention

Anabolic steroids, growth hormone, and other powerful drugs can facilitate the simultaneous muscle building and fat burning. These drugs come with certain health risks and are very often illegal substances, but this does not mean that they do not play a role in many impressive transformations you may see online. When an individual starts using these types of drugs, they generally achieve rapid, concurrent recomposition. Just like with novel diet and training, the body eventually establishes a "new normal" and concurrent recomposition via drug use diminishes. Increasingly higher doses of drugs or more powerful (with concomitant health risks) drugs are required at that point to continue concurrent recomposition.

Outside of these scenarios, concurrent recomposition is a relatively impractical goal. While concurrent recomposition is appealing on the surface, separate, dedicated periods of muscle gain and fat loss are much more efficient and dependable ways to alter your body composition. We will get into how to sequence such diets in chapter 9, but for now, if you see radical results in before and after photos, be aware that one or more of these exceptions to the rule might be at play. Do not assume whatever diet or training the photos are advertising will work for you or anyone else reliably.

CALORIE DEMAND FACTORS

Calorie needs can vary a great deal from one person to the next. A number of factors contribute to individual variation in daily calorie needs. The following is a list of some of these factors:

Body Size: Larger people have more cells and bigger cells, so it takes more energy to power their bodies.

NEAT: Non-Exercise Activity Thermogenesis, or NEAT, is the amount of calories you expend on daily tasks, including working, studying, walking to the store, moving your hands while you talk, and even fidgeting. Calorie expenditure by NEAT activities can vary from tiny to enormous and, in most cases, account for more daily calorie burning than formal exercise.

Exercise/Training: Any form of working out that you do requires energy, and the more you work out, the more energy you need.

Height and Body Proportions: Taller people usually have more surface area than shorter people of the same weight. It takes quite a few calories to keep body temperature stable with more surface area exposed to the environment. Likewise, any other physical features that increase surface area can increase metabolism.

Stress: Contrary to popular belief, stress actually boosts calorie burning via constant low-level activation of fight-or-flight pathways. It is not at all uncommon for people to gain weight when chronically stressed, but this is generally due to stress-induced excess eating or water retention from stress hormones. Stress on its own usually contributes to weight loss.

Recovery Demands: Not only does hard training burn calories directly, it causes damage to muscle tissues (deliberately) and depletes energy stores. What this means in the grand scheme of things is that your body will require extra calories to perform repairs.

Genetic Metabolic Factors: Some people have very efficient metabolisms and convert more of the energy from the food they eat into other usable forms of energy. Though metabolisms do not vary widely on average, over a long period of time these small variances contribute to the ease or difficulty of weight loss observed across dieters.

Percent Body Fat: Fat is a heat insulator and requires a bit less energy to be maintained than muscle. Thus, individuals who are leaner will have to burn more calories by a small fraction to stay the same weight than similarly sized people with more body fat and less muscle. On the other hand, carrying extra fat can cause movements to become less economical, thus increasing energy expenditure. A surplus of fat can also make thermoregulation in the heat more difficult, requiring additional energy expenditure.

Drug Intake: Stimulants like caffeine boost the metabolic rate to a small extent and burn a tiny amount of extra calories.

Sex: Due mostly to body size, muscle mass, and hormonal differences, men burn more calories than women. If body size and muscle mass differences are obviated, the remaining difference is very small, but still exists.

CHAPTER SUMMARY

- Calories are the single most powerful nutritional variable influencing bodyweight, body composition, and performance.
- The goals of gaining muscle and losing fat are generally antagonistic and should be pursued separately in distinct dieting phases.
- The process of gaining muscle is best achieved with a hypercaloric condition, and the process of losing fat is best achieved with a hypocaloric condition.
- Daily calorie needs can vary significantly from day to day, both between and within individuals.

CHAPTER 3

Macronutrients

Once calories have been accounted for, macronutrient ratios are the next most important diet principle for adjusting body composition and enhancing performance. Macronutrients are made up of the three nutrients that provide most of the calories in a diet; because they are eaten in relatively large (macro) quantities, we refer to them as macronutrients. These macronutrients are protein, carbohydrate, and fat. Alcohol and sugar alcohols also have calories, but for health and performance they should constitute a very small minority of total calorie intake.

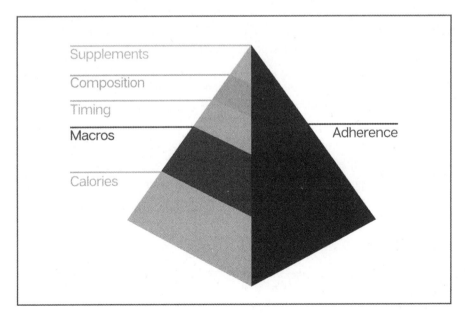

Generally, the macronutrients provide the calories that bodies need to function. While all macronutrients contain calories, each type has unique properties and effects. In selecting which and what quantities of macronutrients to eat, we must consider both the calorie demand of the dieter and the unique effects of each macronutrient on body composition and performance. The ratio of macronutrients used to fill a daily calorie total greatly impacts body composition change and athletic performance. Macronutrient ratios can play an important role in the percent of muscle gained during hypercaloric dieting, the amount of muscle retained during hypocaloric dieting, the amount of energy available during training and competition, and other factors such as baseline hormonal function and health.

Macronutrient considerations should still come only after calorie balance has been addressed. Perfect macronutrient ratios for muscle-loss prevention on a fat-loss diet become moot if there is no calorie deficit. In much the same way, although macronutrient ratios can modify the rates of muscle gained, muscle gain is primarily driven by calorie surpluses (as long as the right kind of training is being done).

If your diet uses appropriate calories and macronutrient ratios, you should get about 80% of the total possible diet effects on body composition and performance. In fact, adjusting only calories and macronutrients sums up the "if it fits your macros" (IIFYM) approach. IIFYM instructs that "if your calories and macronutrients are well established, you will get the majority of potential performance and physique benefits possible from diet." This is a great place to start, especially for those newer to dieting.

Throughout this chapter, all macro recommendations will be given per pound of bodyweight and made with the assumption of a relatively lean individual (under 30% fat). The calculations given subsequently in this book are slightly more precise when done per pound of lean body mass (LBM) rather than pound of bodyweight. However, obtaining an exact LBM is difficult even with sophisticated equipment, so bodyweight can be used as a proxy as long as one is relatively lean. If a person has greater than 30% fat, using a value between bodyweight and estimated LBM might be a bit better.

CALORIE CONTENT OF MACRONUTRIENTS

Calories and macronutrients are not independent variables in nutrition. Calories, as described in the last chapter, are units of energy. All the macronutrients supply energy and, therefore, contain calories. The per gram calorie content of each macro is:

- Protein: **4** calories per gram
- Carbohydrate: **4** calories per gram
- Fat: **9** calories per gram

As you can see, while both protein and carbohydrate carry only 4 calories per gram of macronutrient, fats have more than double, with 9 calories per gram of fat. This information will play a role in your diet construction and in how you allocate amounts of macronutrients to fit within your calorie constraints.

The Caloric Constraint Hypothesis

Since we cannot consume macronutrients without their inherent calorie content, and since calorie considerations are first priority in diet design, all three macros must be manipulated in concert to fit pre-made calorie restrictions or demands. This idea is termed the Caloric Constraint Hypothesis (CCH). Since your dietary goal will begin with a total calorie count, this total will dictate how macronutrients can be distributed within your diet. When one macronutrient amount is raised or lowered, either one or both of the remaining macronutrients must be adjusted as well to keep calories constant. Since all of the macronutrients have an effect on diet outcomes, it would be incorrect to simply say "eat more protein to grow muscle" without considering what the effect will be on carbohydrate and fat intakes. Thus, in assigning macronutrient totals, you should determine the total calories needed for the goal, determine optimal ranges of macronutrient totals, and then adjust those macronutrients to both meet minimum values and fit within the caloric constraints. There may be a few possibilities within the constraints and macro ranges where trade-offs can be made for desired outcomes or preferences. In chapter 10 we will go into exactly how to make the decisions and calculations for macronutrient ratios within a caloric constraint.

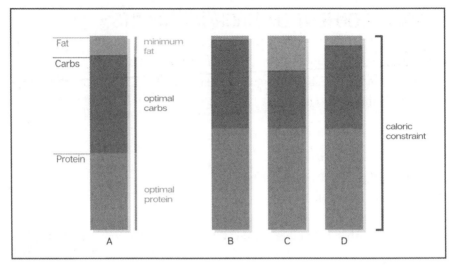

Figure 3.1. *A depicts protein, carb, and fat ratios when protein is set at its optimum. B, C, and D illustrate the relative carb and fat deficiencies that can result from overeating protein within a given caloric constraint.*

PROTEIN

Protein is made of large molecules which are made of other, smaller molecules called amino acids. Protein makes up many of the tissues in the human body and comprises enzymes that govern reactions and underlie most bodily functions at some level. Human proteins are comprised of 20 amino acids, of which our bodies can produce 11 endogenously. The other nine amino acids must be ingested via food sources.

There is a balance between protein degradation and protein synthesis in the body, termed "protein turnover." Some of the amino acids that are liberated when protein is degraded are lost in urine, sweat, and other bodily fluids. Cells full of protein are lost constantly in skin, hair, and intestinal lining. Other amino acids are burned for energy, especially when carbohydrates and fats are not available in sufficient quantities to meet immediate energy demand. In order to address this net loss, amino acids must be consumed regularly via protein consumption.

Protein is critical to survival and health, but it also plays an important role in performance and body composition. Muscle mass is predominantly constructed from protein. Actin, myosin, titin, nebulin, and many other protein compose the contractile apparatus. Protein from the diet supports replenishment of skeletal muscle as it is broken down to support important bodily functions–this helps keep your muscles from shrinking over time. Thus, protein consumption is anti-catabolic as it helps maintain muscle tissue equilibrium. When muscle growth is the goal, there must be a positive net balance of amino acids. Building new tissue is termed "anabolism." Constructing new muscle with an amino acid surplus is an example of an anabolic process.

In terms of performance, enzymes (made of protein), mediate all energy-liberating and movement-producing activity in the human body. Protein also makes up a huge percentage of connective tissues such as tendons, ligaments, and bones. Under-eating protein not only shrinks the muscles that drive performance, but it can also reduce the amount of hemoglobin (the unit that helps blood carry oxygen to the muscles) that supports endurance, weaken joints and bones, and degrade functions supporting health–the base upon which performance is built.

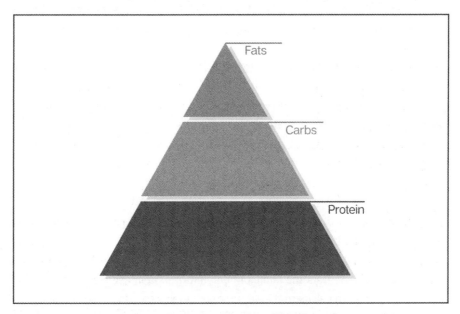

Figure 3.2 *Protein has the largest impact on body composition and performance of the macronutrients and thus must be a priority in a structured diet.*

Because amino acids literally are the building blocks of most of our body's functional and structural machinery and because new amino acids are mostly sourced from diet, protein is the most important macronutrient for body composition and health. Research on performance and body composition shows that although variations in fat and carb intake significantly impact outcomes, variation in protein availability also does so to a much greater extent.

Minimum, Maximum, and Recommended Daily Protein Intake

We have two means of establishing maximum protein intake. The first is to ask whether some amount of dietary protein can be toxic. Protein needs to be broken down into the constituent molecules, and many of the by-products are processed by the kidneys. Though an important consideration, both theoretical supposition (what volumes of protein breakdown would be required to overtax the kidneys) and direct evidence from carefully controlled research point to the same conclusion: There appears to be no realistic protein amount that is dangerous for human consumption (this, of course, excludes individuals with kidney disease or other conditions requiring restricted protein intake). Recent research tested outcomes of up to 2.0 g per pound of bodyweight per day and found no ill health effects. This amount is probably more than most people would realistically eat on any diet that accounted for macronutrients anyway, so not the most useful figure in determining protein maxima.

The second means of establishing a top end for protein intake comes from caloric constraint and the need for minimum intake of other macronutrients. It is from the CCH that a more applicable maximum protein amount comes. Very simply, if you eat *all* your daily calories in protein, you will not be able to get sufficient fats or carbohydrates, and your health, sport performance, and recovery will suffer. Maximum protein intake is as much protein as can be eaten within the caloric constraint while still allowing the minimum amounts of fat and carbohydrate for health.

Somewhere between this and the minimum protein needed lies an optimal range of intakes. It would be great if we could recommend one minimum protein intake amount that would fit all dietary needs. Unfortunately, the minimum protein to support health differs from the minimum amount of protein needed to gain muscle and so on. In order to calculate the appropriate range, assessing protein minima for various purposes (health and various specific sports) is required.

Protein Needs for General Health

The minimum amount of daily protein needed for health is about 0.3 g of protein per pound of bodyweight. Note that this minimum is not a recommendation for physique or performance, it is the minimum needed *just* for health.

Current research cannot agree on a specific value of protein intake for best health. Some studies have suggested that better health comes from a lower protein diet, but these conclusions were probably not the best interpretation of the data. When variables such as saturated fat intake or overly processed food consumption are accounted for in literature reviews, it appears that individuals who eat mostly whole food diets that include high protein are just as healthy as their low-protein counterparts (and likely have better physiques). It does seem that the consumption of a minimum of 0.3 g of protein per pound of bodyweight per day can support good health, at least for non-athletes and relatively sedentary individuals.

On the other hand, higher protein intakes support greater muscle masses, which can potentiate higher activity levels, greater resistance to injury, and better long-term health. Eating more protein has also been shown to enhance satiety (the feeling of fullness) for longer than carbs or fat in calorically equivalent amounts. Obesity has negative health effects that can lead to diabetes, cardiovascular disease, and other comorbidities that can be prevented or ameliorated by weight loss. Raising protein intake may therefore make dieting easier and enhance weight loss in obese individuals, indirectly improving health. Increased protein consumption can also increase lean body mass in old age, which is positively correlated with longevity, the ability to exercise later in life, and resistance to injury in older age—all relevant to long-term health.

These indirect benefits are extremely valuable and should be taken into consideration in the big picture of health choices. Even if one can get by acutely on lower protein diets, long-term health is likely benefited by the daily consumption of more than 0.3 g protein per pound of bodyweight.

At this time, the data suggest a range of between 0.3 and 2.0 g of protein per pound of bodyweight per day as best for health—though we suspect that the low end of this range may not be ideal for long-term health and independence in old age. Athletes should likely lean toward a range of 0.8 to 2.0 g of protein per pound of bodyweight per day to support lean body mass maintenance for sport performance.

Protein in Performance and Body Composition Enhancement

As discussed, protein is the building block for muscle, and the rigors of sport require more muscle mass than the activities of everyday life. The processes of sport training and competition also tear down muscle via exertion and contact damage, so this larger muscle mass requires more maintenance as well. Even for aesthetic-based body composition goals, additional muscle mass and training are required for a firm, athletic look. Most people can survive on the previously recommended 0.3 g minimum of protein per pound of bodyweight per day, but this amount is unlikely to support an athletic physique or best sport performance. Next we will discuss the various ranges of protein needs for different types of sports and dietary circumstances.

Protein Needs for Endurance Sports

Optimal protein intakes for endurance athletes is likely around 0.5-1.0 g protein per pound of bodyweight per day, with the lower end approached only during special circumstances.

Although endurance sports such as marathon and triathlon do not require large muscle masses, the extremely high volume and heavy energy demands of these sports often exceeds immediate availability of carbohydrate and fat stores. Protein must be burned for some fraction of training energy, and these fractions can add up over time, requiring a larger protein intake to keep muscle mass in equilibrium. Because such voluminous training stresses muscle fibers often and for long duration, protein turnover rates are elevated, which means even more protein must be eaten to compensate. The CCH is a prominent player in protein intake determination for endurance athletes because they rely on relatively high intakes of carbohydrates to enhance their training and recovery.

The minimum protein intake for endurance athletes (around 0.5 g per pound of bodyweight per day) is probably best approached only for short periods of time (weeks) during very high-volume training phases when carbohydrate intakes are maxed out. Higher protein intake during other periods of lower training volume and lower carbohydrate intake is likely beneficial for muscle maintenance.

The CCH caps maximum protein intake for endurance athletes at around 1 g per pound of bodyweight per day to allow for adequate carbohydrate intake to support training. Our best recommendation for endurance athletes is to average around 0.7 g protein per pound of bodyweight per day, making occasional, temporary drops to 0.5 g per pound per day during periods of heavy training that require increased carbohydrate intake and occasional increases to 1.0 g during periods of lower training volume. This provides additional protein to deal with energy needs and wear and tear without taking too much of the daily caloric allotment away from critical carbohydrates.

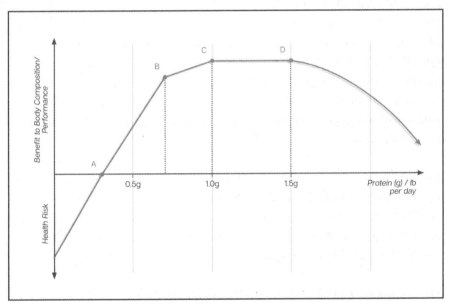

Figure 3.3 *A graph of the relative benefits of varying protein consumption rates (in grams per pound of bodyweight per day) is shown from point A (minimum protein needed for health) through point D (the point at which protein amounts force a reduction in other macronutrients to below recommended levels via the CCH).*

Protein Needs for Team Sports

The daily protein needs per pound of bodyweight per day for team sport athletes is likely around 0.8 g on average, with 0.6 g per pound of bodyweight per day as a minimum and 1.5 g as a maximum. In team sports like soccer, basketball, and rugby, high energy use in practice and competition increases need for protein to prevent net muscle loss. In contrast to endurance sports, most team sports require greater muscularity for optimal performance and have a lower total demand for energy. Since the carbohydrate needs of team sport athletes are much lower than endurance sport athletes and the benefit from added protein is higher, their optimal protein range is higher than that of endurance athletes.

Protein Needs for Strength and Power Sports

Strength and power sport athletes need around 1.0 g of protein per pound of bodyweight per day on average. Strength and power sports include weightlifting, powerlifting, fitness sport, American football, short-distance sprinting, jumping events, throwing events, and strongman and have a considerably different set of protein constraints and demands than other sports. Athletes in these sports require substantially more muscle mass for performance and more frequent weight training. Strength and power athlete protein intakes have been well researched, and the minimum recommendation is 0.7 g of protein per pound of bodyweight per day. This minimum is an amount of protein that can nearly guarantee no muscle loss from regular hard training on an isocaloric diet and can provide a reasonable amount of anabolic substrate.

Because strength and power athletes have still lower average energy demands per day than both endurance and team sport athletes, their carbohydrate needs are lower, and their CCH-derived protein maximum is higher. Depending on their training phase, strength and power athletes can consume up to around 2.0 g of protein per pound of bodyweight per day without pushing fats or carbs too low.

A recommended optimal intake for strength and power athletes is likely around 0.9 g per pound of bodyweight per day on average. Rounding up to 1 g per pound per day can make calculations a bit easier and is well under the maximum protein intake, so probably poses no risk to reducing other macronutrients to minimum levels via the CCH.

Protein Needs on a Hypocaloric Diet

The rate of catabolism is higher under hypocaloric conditions, so protein needs are elevated. A minimum of around 0.8 g of protein per pound of bodyweight is needed per day under hypocaloric conditions. On longer and stricter fat-loss diets, an argument for a higher minimum protein intake can be made as the propensity for muscle loss increases across longer term, more aggressive hypocaloric phases.

In most cases, 1 g of protein per pound of bodyweight per day is optimal to prevent catabolism on a hypocaloric diet while leaving enough room for carbohydrates. However, because protein is so effective at reducing hunger overall, diet outcomes might be improved with slightly increased protein intake. Research on lean, drug-free bodybuilders shows the potential for added anti-catabolic benefits up to around 1.2 g per pound of bodyweight per day—suggesting more extreme diets and leaner individuals might need slightly more than 1 g per pound per day for optimal outcomes. Though the effect is likely small, protein is also very filling and can help with adherence, so increases can indirectly benefit fat-loss diets. On the other hand, too much protein intake can eat into calories allotted for carbohydrates, which have an anti-catabolic effect and fuel high-volume, high-intensity training which helps prevent muscle loss. To prevent an excessive CCH-derived reduction in carbohydrates, hypocaloric diets should generally cap their protein intakes at a maximum of around 1.5 g per pound of bodyweight per day. Anything higher will start requiring such big carb reductions that training volume and intensity may suffer, and risk of muscle loss will increase.

Our recommendation for hypocaloric protein intake is a baseline of 1 g per pound of bodyweight per day, with potential increases up to around 1.5 g per pound per day for more extreme dieting or satiety effects.

Protein Needs on a Hypercaloric Diet

Hypercaloric diet conditions reduce anti-catabolic-based protein needs. This effect is so powerful that the protein minimum for anabolism on a hypercaloric diet is actually a bit lower than the hypocaloric diet minimum and sits right around 0.7 g per pound of bodyweight per day. While this amount of protein might be sufficient, it is unlikely that optimal gains in muscle mass will be obtained.

Protein is unlikely to offer any special benefits (to added muscle mass) beyond optimal consumption, but because carbohydrates lead to insulin secretion and because insulin is highly anabolic over time and when paired with resistance training, eating as much carbohydrate as possible within constraints is practical for muscle gain. Carbohydrates are so valuable for muscle gain that the recommendation for maximum protein on a hypercaloric diet should likely be capped at around 1.5 g of protein per pound of bodyweight per day so that a greater caloric value of carbs can be programmed.

Data have consistently shown that consumption above about 0.9 g of protein per pound of bodyweight per day does not enhance muscle gain. Since carbs do not have quite as low a cap for their anabolic effects, any extra protein consumed is going to risk pushing out carbs within the constraint of calories, and thus net anabolism could suffer. Our recommendation for optimal muscle growth is therefore around 1.0 g of protein per pound of bodyweight per day.

CARBOHYDRATES

Carbohydrates are large molecules that come in several main categories:

- Monosaccharides

Single-molecule carbohydrates. These include glucose, fructose, and galactose.

- Disaccharides

Two-molecule combinations of monosaccharides used to form a single, large molecule. These include sucrose (a glucose and a fructose bonded), lactose (a glucose and a galactose bonded), and maltose (two glucoses bonded).

- Polysaccharides

Longer strings of monosaccharides chained together. These include starch (a digestible form of many glucoses linked together), cellulose (fiber which is mostly indigestible by humans and made up of glucose molecules), and glycogen (an irregular matrix of connected glucose molecules which is the most common form for carbohydrate stored in muscle tissue and the liver).

All the listed carbohydrates (aside from fiber) can be converted into glucose and used for the following, usually in this order of priority:

- Transported to cells and broken down for immediate energy use.

- Transported to the blood to circulate and provide glucose to needy cells, such as neuronal cells that do not store much fuel of their own and prefer glucose.
- Transported to the liver to be assembled as glycogen for storage. Liver glycogen can be broken down to release glucose into the blood when blood glucose levels fall too low.
- Transported to skeletal muscles to be assembled as glycogen for storage. When skeletal muscles are working at higher effort intensities (anything as hard as a jog or harder), they rely heavily on this stored glycogen to provide the energy to power contractions.

Energy-needy cells get first priority for incoming glucose. Not until most cells are energy-satiated will carb consumption result in increased blood glucose. Once blood glucose is at an appropriate level, liver glycogen synthesis becomes priority. Only when all the above carbohydrate needs are attended to will muscle glycogen start to be synthesized in any meaningful amount.

Originally, "simple" carbs were defined as monosaccharides and disaccharides and "complex" carbs were meant to denote polysaccharides. It was previously thought that simple carbs digested quickly, tasted sweet, were more addicting, and were worse for health whereas complex carbs were opposite in every respect. Unfortunately, this model for carbohydrates was fundamentally flawed. For example, fructose is a simple carbohydrate, but is incredibly slow digesting. In contrast, starch is a complex carbohydrate that, in its pure form, is digested and absorbed even faster than glucose. Furthermore, simple carbs are no more addicting than starches. When consumed appropriately, simple sugars are no worse for health than starches and can have some distinct timing-related benefits for training. There is no reason to assign "good" or "bad" monikers to different carb sources based on their molecular complexity alone.

As you may have already inferred, the primary role of carbs in the human diet is for use as an energy source. Proteins are mainly used as building blocks for tissue and only used for energy on occasion (when carbohydrates and fats are lacking). Carbohydrates are the raw materials for energy metabolism and are used only in limited forms as structural components. In other words, the body's primary use for carbs is to power cells, and carbs are particularly important in powering the operation and contraction of muscle cells. As energy substrates, carbohydrates have no equal–they easily and rapidly provide energy, especially for high-volume users like nervous system cells and muscle cells.

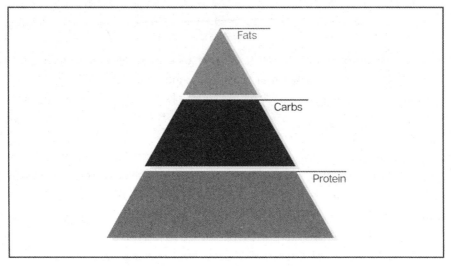

Figure 3.4 *Carbohydrate have the second largest impact on body composition and performance compared to the other macronutrients and thus must be prioritized after protein in a structured diet.*

Minimum, Maximum, and Recommended Daily Carbohydrate Intake

Glucose can be obtained from other macronutrients, albeit less efficiently. The human body does not actually need any carbohydrates from the diet for basic survival and health. So the minimum carbohydrate intake could be set at zero. The most abundant sources of needed vitamins, minerals, phytochemicals, and fiber, however, are vegetables, fruits, and whole grains, all of which contain carbs. While most of these micronutrients can be supplemented, many are absorbed more efficiently when consumed via whole foods, so eliminating carbs entirely presents some risk to health.

How much plant-based food must be consumed to meet micronutrient needs for health depends on which foods are consumed. If a high diversity of colorful veggies and fruits are eaten regularly, the micronutrients they contain will satisfy health requirements with relatively low-carb intakes. On the other hand, if more processed grains are the primary source, a considerably higher amount of carb-rich food must be eaten to ensure adequate micronutrient intake.

The ceiling for carbohydrate intake is best set by using CCH to dictate carb amounts once protein and fat at are their respective minima. Within this constraint, there is no notable downside to very high carb consumption. These recommendations are fairly vague, so we will outline some specifics for carb intake here.

Carbohydrate Needs for Health

In our estimate, if the predominant carb sources in the diet are vegetables and fruit, a minimum of around 0.3 g of carbs per pound of bodyweight per day is sensible for vitamin and micronutrient intake needs. Though currently popular, ketogenic diets are not ideally healthy.

Many of the conclusions regarding the benefits of ketogenic diets have been determined in studies using obese subjects for whom any means of weight loss leads to improved health. Better studies are needed in healthy but sedentary individuals for a full assessment of the benefits and downsides to low-carb eating. For short periods of time (months), ketogenic diets might be safe, but they are not recommended for health in the long term (years). This is different for people who eat a ketogenic diet for medical reasons, a topic that is being widely researched.

Direct study of the subject and decades of research on individuals who eat vegan or otherwise highly plant-based diets have shown that relatively high carb consumption has no negative health effects on its own. Remember, though, that we are viewing all these statements through the lens of the CCH. If you are eating so many carbs that you begin to violate your calorie needs and gain excessive fat, negative health effects will almost certainly follow. On the other hand, if you displace too much fat and protein with carb calories, you will also likely suffer negative health effects. Within these CCH-based constraints, even the maximum amount of carbohydrate consumption in no way interferes with health. For example, many vegans regularly consume upwards of 80% of their calories from carbohydrates, and as a group, they tend to be just about as healthy as any group ever studied.

The important exceptions to this rule are, of course, individuals who have conditions related to blood sugar regulation, such as diabetics, individuals with thyroid issues or Polycystic Ovary Syndrome (PCOS), and many people with chronic digestive illnesses and other metabolic disorders. For any diet change they wish to make, a consultation with their medical doctor or clinical nutritionist (registered dietician in the United States) is essential.

Because vegetable, fruit, and whole-grain consumption is so supportive of optimal health, we do not recommend carbohydrate intakes of much less than 0.5 g per pound of bodyweight per day for most people in the long term. This minimum can be dropped to 0.3 g per pound of bodyweight per day if carb sources are all whole food fruits and vegetables–to get enough micronutrients for best health. Remember that these relatively low needs for health are not adequately supportive of sport performance or muscle retention and that carb levels must be increased for best fitness outcomes.

Carbohydrate in Performance and Body Composition Enhancement

The nervous system relies heavily on glucose; so much so that large rapid drops in blood glucose can cause failures in brain function and even death. The nervous system can use other fuel sources, like the ketones that are produced from fat and protein during times of low carbohydrate intake, but this is your body's "emergency only" back-up.

Normal blood glucose levels sustain mental acuity, force production, and fatigue prevention. Brain cells are well fed and very responsive when glucose is readily available in the blood. This means that reaction times are quicker, decision-making is sharper, and motivation is higher.

When blood glucose is too low, nervous system operation can falter, leading to fewer motor units (parts of a muscle all connected to one nerve), contributing to a muscle contraction. This in turn leads to lower contractile force and less strength, speed, power, and endurance.

Falling blood glucose levels have been consistently shown to correlate with rising levels of fatigue. Tough competitions lead to mental and physical fatigue naturally, but low blood sugar hastens this fatigue. Maintaining blood glucose levels through carbohydrate consumption during sport training or competition can therefore delay the onset of fatigue.

Glucose is also the preferred fuel for high-intensity or voluminous physical exertion. Repetitive exertions of over 30% of the muscle's maximum contraction force rely primarily on carbohydrates, particularly muscle glycogen. Nearly all sports require high levels of force exertion. While many sports are characterized in part by lower intensity exertions, it is often the magnitude of the high-intensity components that determines positive performance. This is particularly true for any style of weight training. There is an argument that singles (sets of 1 repetition) do not require much carbohydrate, and this is true at the acute level. Singles and doubles rely on stored ATP and creatine phosphate for energy. These contractions are still initiated by the nervous system, and thus dietary carbohydrate still benefits them even if high glycogen stores specifically do not. In addition, the recovery of ATP and creatine phosphate stores after each set relies on carbohydrate. In any case, repeated sets and any repetitions over 3 get a significant proportion of their energy needs via glycogen, so almost all weight-training styles, in addition to almost all sports, rely on carbohydrate for maximum performance.

Consuming carbohydrate is an extremely powerful means of preventing muscle loss. Carbs provide an energy source that prevents the breakdown of tissue for fuel. In addition, anabolism is achieved via both glycogen- and insulin-mediated pathways, both of which are directly affected by carb intake. Elevations in blood glucose resulting from carbohydrate consumption lead to the secretion of insulin, a highly anabolic hormone. Although insulin is anabolic to both muscle *and* fat tissue, for leaner individuals doing resistance training, the net effect of insulin is biased toward building muscle tissue more than fat tissue. Like many other hormones (be it testosterone, growth hormone, estrogen, etc.), insulin exerts most of its power when its concentration is chronically elevated. If insulin is high post workout for an hour but very low during the rest of the day, the total exposure of the muscles to insulin is relatively insignificant. If insulin is instead elevated for a large portion of each day, its anabolic and anti-catabolic signaling effects can add up to make substantial differences in muscularity over the long term (months).

While protein elevates insulin to some extent, fat does not elevate insulin much or at all. Carbohydrate consumption, on the other hand, has a predictable, consistent effect on blood insulin levels. If elevating insulin for muscle growth is the goal, then eating carbs is the easiest and most effective path.

Glycogen-mediated anabolism is perhaps even more important to muscle gain and retention. Eating carbs allows you to train harder, which grows more muscle and diverts more calories toward muscle repair and upkeep. When this is done on a hypocaloric diet, it has the potential to cancel the catabolism stimulated by insufficient calorie intake. Additionally, it has been repeatedly shown that training under low-glycogen conditions (resulting from low-carb eating) leads to more muscle loss than training under high-glycogen conditions. Multiple molecular pathways for these effects have also been elucidated, so both the effect and mechanism have been well studied. In other words, if you chronically under-eat carbs you will almost certainly gain less muscle on hypercaloric diets and lose more during hypocaloric phases.

Carbohydrate Needs for Endurance Sports

High levels of performance in conventional endurance training require carbohydrate intake. Energy production, nervous system demands, and recovery for endurance training is best addressed through carbohydrate consumption. For performance and recovery, minimum carbohydrate intake recommendation is around 1.5 g per pound of bodyweight per day. In most cases, 1.5 g per pound per day is only appropriate for light- or low-volume days. This means that low-carb diets are relative non-starters for endurance sports.

Because of the numerous benefits of carbs to endurance training, the lack of downsides of maximal consumption, and the ineffectual result of increasing fat intake past minimum levels, endurance trainers will likely see optimal results by maxing out their carb intake within the CCH. That being said, anything past about 3.0 g of carbs per pound of bodyweight per day is not likely to have any additional benefit for most training days. Targeting that value and eating the remaining calories in extra fat and protein is a good approach for an endurance athlete. On days when training volumes are extremely high, a temporary increase can be beneficial. For example, a cyclist doing a 12-hour bike ride or an ultrarunner doing a 50-mile race might benefit from 5.0 g or more per pound of bodyweight per day on those days. Because calorie consumption will be so high on days with such extensive output, increasing carbs this much is unlikely to even violate CCH constraints for an isocaloric diet and will allow for better performance and recovery.

Carbohydrate Needs for Team Sports

A rough minimum of about 1.5 g of carbs per pound of bodyweight per day is a reasonable dose across team sports. Athletes who train on the lower end of this category and lead very sedentary lifestyles outside of sport can make do with less. Others training on the higher end of the potential range who are otherwise more active might need a slightly higher minimum carb intake.

For most team sports, optimal carbohydrate intakes range between 1.5 to 3.0 g of carbs per pound of bodyweight per day. Similar to endurance recommendations, if a particularly grueling event or training day occurs, an acute increase in carbohydrates from the upper limit of this range can improve performance and recovery.

When determining these ranges, we are referencing the competitive pursuit of sport, not merely recreational involvement. If you participate in sports mostly for recreation and not competition, you can have fewer carbs (leaving more room via CCH) in your diet and probably make meal planning easier. Higher carbs for competition come at the cost of fats in diet design.

Carbohydrate Needs for Strength and Power Sports

During periods of high-volume hypertrophy or work capacity training, up to 2.5 g of carbs per pound of bodyweight per day might be needed. In contrast, for strength, power, and speed work phases, most athletes can meet their minimum needs with about 1.0 g of carbs per pound of bodyweight per day. In the context of the average sport diet and the average western diet, this is quite a low number, but it makes sense for many strength and power sports.

While heavily dependent on differences in training volumes and daily activity levels, an average intake of 1.5 g of carbs per pound of bodyweight per day is a good rough start for a strength or power athlete. This baseline intake can be modified from between 1.0 to 2.5 g per pound per day based on activity levels and training types.

Carbohydrate Needs on a Hypocaloric Diet

Carbs have powerful anti-catabolic properties, so dropping them very low on a fat-loss diet can result in muscle loss. Assuming a dieter is engaging in hypertrophy training and some form of sport training or cardio to help stave off muscle loss, around 1.0 g of carbs per pound of bodyweight per day is our minimum carb recommendation. Anything below this recommendation would lead to glycogen depletion in most major muscles, chronically low blood glucose levels, decreases in the chemical milieu that supports muscle size, and would hamper high-volume and high-intensity training that also contributes to muscle retention. Lower intakes can be handled for shorter periods (e.g., on rest days). As glycogen becomes severely depleted, it must be refilled in order to prevent muscle loss.

During fat-loss diets, the CCH plays a larger and larger role as calories are decreased. With less calories to work with, the options for various macronutrient ratio combinations begin to shrink–all macros might need to be at or near their minima by the end of a hard fat-loss diet.

Thus, the optimal amount of carbohydrates recommended on a fat-loss diet becomes the maximum amount of carbohydrates that fit within the CCH constraint when protein and fats are brought to their minimum.

Carbohydrate Needs on a Hypercaloric Diet

A minimum of 1.0 g of carbs per pound of bodyweight per day is recommended to support muscle gain on a hypercaloric diet. Anything much lower would reduce insulin secretion and necessitate such a high fat and protein intake that muscle gain would be much more difficult and much less effective. Gaining muscle on lower carb intake is possible, but less probable. As we have discussed, the performance and especially glycogen- and insulin-mediated potentiation of anabolism that carbs promote lead us to recommend their maximal consumption (within CCH) for optimal muscle growth on a hypercaloric diet.

FATS

There are four main classes of dietary fats:

•   Monounsaturated fats

Fatty acids with only one double bond in their fatty acid chain. These molecules can exist in *cis* or *trans* configurations, the latter of which is the fourth class.

•   Polyunsaturated fats

Fatty acids with multiple carbon–carbon double bonds in their fatty acid chain. These molecules can also exist in *cis* or *trans* configurations.

•   Saturated fats

In saturated fat, no double bonds between carbons exist, allowing maximum hydrogen bonds so that the molecule is "saturated" with hydrogen.

- Trans fats

Trans describes the configuration of an unsaturated fat. In unsaturated fat, double bonds between carbons exist, preventing hydrogens from bonding and thus preventing "saturation" with hydrogen. Due to this, the carbon chain extends from a double bond in only two directions and can either extend from the same side (*cis*) or from opposite sides (*trans*) of the double bond.

Essential fats, much like essential amino acids, are fats that are critical to survival and health, but that cannot be made by the body and so must be consumed. The two types of essential fats in the human diet are Omega-6 and Omega-3 polyunsaturated fatty acids. Both occur in a wide variety of foods and can also be supplemented. Very low-fat diets can risk deficiencies, especially for Omega-3s. Further, some vitamins cannot be absorbed in the gastrointestinal tract without the presence of fat, so extremely low-fat diets also risk vitamin deficiencies. Hormone dysregulation can also occur when fats are under-eaten as fats supply some of the raw materials for hormone production.

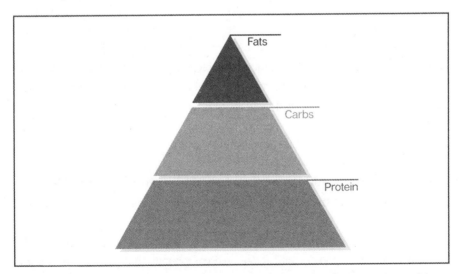

Figure 3.5 *Fats have the smallest impact on body composition and performance compared to other macronutrients.*

Minimum, Maximum, and Recommended Daily Fat Intake

Fat Needs for Health

Minimum fat requirements are uniform irrespective of activity level and are matched for health and sport outcomes. The minimum recommendation is around 0.3g per pound of body weight per day—this amount makes it very likely that enough essential fats (Omega-3 and Omega-6 fats) will be consumed to meet minimum needs. In addition, this minimum value ensures enough fat intake to support sufficient testosterone, estrogen, and prostaglandin production for best body composition and performance outcomes. As with other nutrients, there is some variance in this value based on the individual; 0.3g per pound of body weight per day figure covers almost all individuals in most circumstances. In terms of maximum fat intake, current science suggests that as long as fats are not so high as to violate the CCH for carbs, proteins, and calories, the amounts eaten within these constraints can be considered healthy. There is some evidence to suggest that keeping calorie contribution from fat under 40% of total daily calories might be better for gut health and body composition, so this is a sensible maximum to consider within caloric constraints. What types of fats and in what ratios they are consumed can alter health and body composition outcomes. (See chapter 5.)

It must be noted that some individuals will have slightly better bloodwork at lower or higher fat intake levels. If health is your number one priority, trying different ranges and assessing your health with a medical professional via bloodwork is likely a good idea. This means that some people might be able to have a diet that meets minimum carb, protein, and micronutrient needs and is relatively high in fat and still be very healthy. Some prerequisites in quality of food sources would have to be met on such a diet, but it is within the realm of possibility. Unfortunately, such a diet is not optimal for performance or body composition changes.

Fats in Performance and Body Composition Enhancement

The production of testosterone and estrogen relies, in part, on fat intake, and both these hormones are critical to muscle gain, muscle retention, and nearly all performance adaptations. In addition, fat intake supplies essential fatty acids for the production of physiologically active lipid compounds that play key roles in the regulation of muscle growth and repair, particularly through their mediation of inflammatory processes.

Some have argued for fats as a primary fuel source for athletic performance, most recently for ultra-endurance performance. Proponents of this often argue that such performance benefits are not truly realized until an individual becomes "fat adapted" by staying away from carbohydrates almost entirely for weeks on end. As of this publication, there is very little evidence that fat is a high-performance fuel and a wealth of evidence that carbohydrates are the better performance fuel source. As important as fats are, they are not the best performance fuel, so recommendations for fat consumption ranges for sport are very similar to those for general health. CCH based on sport and recommendations for compliance on particular diet phases do alter these recommendations slightly, and these are discussed next.

Fat Needs for Endurance Sports, Team Sports, and Strength and Power Sports

Due to carbohydrate needs and the CCH constraint, the fat intake recommendation for endurance athletes is very close to the minimum 0.3 g per pound of bodyweight per day. For team sports and strength and power sports, the recommended range of fat intake is anything between minimum fat intake and CCH maximum, assuming that adequate amounts of proteins and carbs are already being consumed. The only difference here is that team sport and strength and power athletes, depending on training phases, may have periods when carbohydrate intakes can be dropped to allow room for more fat without any detriment.

Fat Needs on a Hypocaloric Diet

On one hand, keeping fat intake higher on a hypocaloric diet can mean a higher flexibility in food choices. This can result in better adherence and thus success. On the other hand, the lower the calorie "ceiling" in your diet, the more necessary carbohydrate becomes to prevent catabolism and drive training energy, and the more sense it makes to preferentially cut fat for calorie reductions. We recommend that calorie reductions be achieved via reductions in fat to the minimum level needed for health.

Fat Needs on a Hypercaloric Diet

Maximizing carbohydrate intake on a diet geared toward muscle gain is optimal. Keeping fats at or near minimum to allow more room for carbohydrates is beneficial here; however, in practical terms we know that the caloric surplus in a hypercaloric diet is of greater importance than macronutrient amounts for muscle gain. Fats have distinct practical advantages that help a dieter get in the needed calories to maintain a surplus. Fats are tasty and easy to add to food, making eating more food easier and more fun. Additionally, fats occupy less space in the stomach, so that eating more calories from fat can make a hypercaloric diet more comfortable. For beginners and intermediates, we recommend generating a calorie surplus with any of the three macros (proteins, fats, or carbs) as long as protein and carb requirements are being met. For individuals who struggle with eating enough food to gain weight, more fat might make gaining easier. For more advanced trainers and those without problems eating, keeping fat close to their minimum values (0.3 g per pound of bodyweight per day) and achieving the hypercaloric condition with carbohydrate might be best practice.

Recommended Macronutrients (in grams per pound of body weight per day)		
Protein	Carbs	Fats
Best Health 0.3g (0.8g for athletes) - 2.0g (or CCH max)	0.3g - 5.0g -	0.3g - 40% daily calories -
Endurance Sports 0.5g - 1.0g	1.5g - 5.0g	0.3g - CCH max
Team Sports 0.6g - 1.5g	1.5g - 3.0g	0.3g - CCH max
Strength/Power Sports 0.7g - 2.0g	1.0g - 2.5g	0.3g - CCH max
Hypocaloric Diets 1.0g - 1.5g	1.0g (0.3g for rest days) - CCH max	0.3g - CCH max
Hypercaloric Diets ~1.0g	1.0g - 5.0g	0.3g - CCH max

Figure 3.6 *Best recommended ranges of macronutrient intake for body composition or performance under various sport and dietary circumstances.*

Keep in mind that running a hypocaloric or hypercaloric diet while training in a specific sport might require trade-offs in performance for diet progress or vice versa, so choose the range appropriate to your prioritized goal. Optimal macronutrient amounts might change across training phases in a specific sport. For example, endurance sport will lean toward the higher end of the recommended carbohydrate range during peak training and competition, and team and strength and power sport recommendations will lean toward the lower range during more low-volume training phases and so on.

HIERARCHY OF MACRONUTRIENTS

Protein > Carbohydrate

In most cases, the accrual and maintenance of muscle mass is the most important goal. In this respect, protein is simply more determinative than carbs. While carbs are anti-catabolic and provide anabolic signaling, protein is literally the building block for muscle—carbs just work as supporters and facilitators, albeit effective ones. After calories, protein should be first priority in most cases. There are some exceptional situations in which carbs are temporarily just as important or more important than protein intake in the diet.

Instances When Carbohydrate > Protein

The most clear-cut case in which carb intake outranks protein intake is in endurance athletics. In high-volume endurance training, glycogen and blood glucose are depleted so fully and rapidly that eating enough carbs to counterbalance this is an intense uphill battle. If protein is under-consumed, while the effects will be negative, they will mostly manifest over weeks and months as muscle mass declines. If insufficient carbs are consumed, there will be an immediate negative effect on training quality and performance. As an endurance athlete, you should be concerned with protein intakes being above the minimal recommended values on average in the long term, but for hard training periods and races, temporarily prioritizing carbohydrates can be beneficial for optimum performance. Additionally, when recovery from intense competitions or training sessions is paramount, such as during a team's competitive season, carbohydrates may take a priority over protein.

Carbohydrate > Fat

Fats are a very poor source of fuel for high-intensity athletic performance. Fats can be a fuel for very low-intensity movements, such as walking or slow jogging, explaining why ketogenic (low-carb) diets have fared better in ultra-endurance sports than they have in most every other sport. Performances even in these extreme endurance

THE **RENAISSANCE DIET 2.0**

races, however, still greatly rely on endogenous carbohydrate stores and benefit from high carbohydrate dietary conditions. Since most sport activity is best powered by carbs, consuming them is more determinative of performance (both in training and competition) and is thus a priority over fat. In addition, carbohydrate is a better fuel source for the nervous system, which governs mental aspects of performance in sport. Carbs exert more beneficial effects on the body in abundant quantities than do fats and for that reason are ranked higher in priority within the macros.

CHAPTER SUMMARY

- Protein, carbohydrate, and fat comprise the macronutrients that contribute to the vast majority of daily calories.
- Macronutrients need to be consumed in large amounts (on the order of grams) daily for survival.
- Protein is the most important macronutrient for body composition change and performance, followed by carbohydrate, and then fat.
- Protein provides the raw materials for muscle growth and repair and is essential to virtually all physiological systems.
- Recommended protein intake can range between 0.5 to 1.5 g per pound of bodyweight per day, with 1.0 g per pound per day on average, covering a large spectrum of athletic scenarios.
- Carbohydrate is the primary source of energy for all exercise and sporting endeavors, as well as the preferred source of energy for the nervous system.
- Carbohydrate is essential to both enhancing the performance of exercise and stimulating anabolism.
- Carbohydrate intake is directly proportional to training workload and can range from virtually no intake to over 5.0 g per pound of bodyweight per day.
- Most athletic endeavors will have carbohydrate intakes ranging from 1.0 to 3.0 g per pound of bodyweight per day, outside of very low or very high activity days.
- Fat is essential to health, but also plays a limited role in enhancing body composition and sport performance.
- Aside from hitting a minimum of 0.3 g per pound of bodyweight per day, fats are very malleable within the CCH and can be increased or decreased to meet individual wants and needs.

CHAPTER 4

Nutrient Timing

Nutrient timing has a small but significant effect on physique and performance outcomes. While 10% might seem inconsequential, consider that differences of much less than 10% in performance separate top athletes in the rankings. A difference of 1% or smaller in performance can determine whether you medal (or not) in the Olympics. Even in amateur sport competition, it is rare to see large differences in performance between athletes on the podium. A 10% difference per diet phase can also add up across years to make a more significant impact on long-term outcomes. For competitive athletes and fitness enthusiasts, especially those who are more experienced at training and dieting, meal timing is an important factor for optimizing progress. This chapter will cover the theoretical aspect of this principle. Practical application will be addressed in chapter 10.

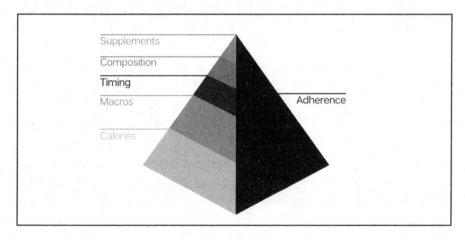

Nutrient timing has six distinct components:

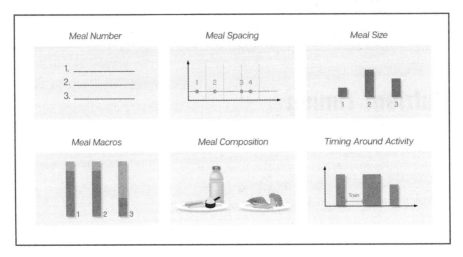

Meal number describes the number of meals an individual consumes per day. A meal is defined as *any amount of food ingested in a single bolus (i.e., one ball of food and saliva)*. If you take a few bites of a sandwich at 1:00 pm and then take a few more at 1:30 pm, by sports nutrition standards, you have eaten two meals.

Meal spacing describes the timing of meals relative to each other. Choosing appropriate lengths of time between meals can depend on digestion time and hourly bodily needs. That being said, eating six, evenly sized, evenly spaced meals per day is not identical to eating three large and three small evenly spaced meals per day, even though by meal number and spacing they are the same; these differ in the third component: meal size.

Meal size is simply the amount of food eaten per meal and is measured in *calories per meal*.

Meal macros describe how much of each macronutrient is present in a meal and can differ between meals even when calories are held constant. For example, while two meals might each have 500 calories, one could contain 50 g of protein, 25 g of carbs, and 22 g of fat, and the other 25 g of protein, 50 g of carbs, and 22 g of fat. The *size* of each meals is the same in terms of calories, but they differ in macronutrient content.

Meal food composition describes the types of foods comprising the calories and macronutrients in each meal. The type of food within the meal can influence digestion rates, absorption rates, the satiety the meal provides, whether the meal causes gastrointestinal distress, and other factors worth consideration. Even when matched for calories and macronutrients, some food choices may be advantageous at certain times and not others. For instance, 30 g of protein is the same amount of protein whether it comes from a chicken breast or a whey protein shake, but one can be preferable to the other depending on when it is consumed. Whey protein digests very quickly and does not take up much stomach space, so it can be useful when trying to gain weight and feel full. In contrast, chicken digests slowly and has a higher volume, and therefore might be a better choice when you are feeling hungry and would like to feel satiated longer after a meal.

Meal timing around activity is the last of the nutrient timing components, but certainly not the least important. This component refers to structuring meals and macronutrients around training times to best support physique and performance outcomes. Of particular interest are the meals before, during, and immediately following training bouts.

NUTRIENT TIMING EFFECTS

Manipulation of the components of nutrient timing has well-studied effects that dictate the recommended optimal nutrient timing structure within diet design, which we will outline in the following sections. The various components of nutrient timing are very intertwined, however, and manipulation of one often affects the other. We will discuss the components according to effect and then summarize the resulting recommendations.

Meal Timing and Sizes for Satiety Levels and Adherence

According to the hierarchy of diet principles, poor nutrient timing schemes can result in 10% loss in performance and body composition results. Poor meal timing can also lead to issues with diet adherence, at further detriment to results. For example, if your muscle-gain diet requires 4,000+ calories per day, and you choose to eat two meals per day, those are 2,000-calorie meals. This might sound fun at the tail end of a fat-loss phase, but after several weeks of eating at a surplus, taking in meals of this size will become extremely difficult. Splitting the eating burden into four or five

800- to 1,000-calorie meals is much more sustainable. On the opposite end of the calorie spectrum, hypocaloric diets make people feel hungry. Outside of risking breaks in adherence (cheating on the diet), prolonged hunger can add to stress and fatigue levels that impact performance and decrease muscle retention. There are two kinds of timing extremes that needlessly increase hunger on a fat-loss diet. First is the very low frequency approach in which you spend most of your day starving and then indulge in a few large meals. Pulses of food-mediated pleasure can promote food craving and unhealthy relationships with food that last beyond the diet phase. On the other end, very high frequencies of feeding (10+ tiny meals per day) can result in never feeling that you have eaten a real meal and increase likelihood of off-diet eating.

The best recommendation for timing with relation to hunger *and* fullness is to eat four to eight evenly spaced meals of similar calorie content per day and avoid extremes outside of those boundaries. Biasing meal size a bit according to intermeal interval can be a good idea if schedules prevent evenly spaced meals (figure 4.1). Conveniently, these recommendations fit with protein frequency and proportion recommendations, which we will discuss shortly.

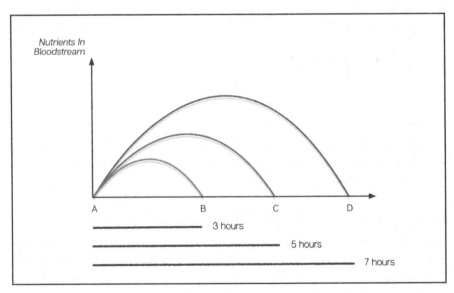

Figure 4.1 *Point A marks your first meal of the day. Points B, C, and D mark when you would eat your second meal if (B) your first meal were smaller (absorbed in around 3 hours), (C) moderately sized (absorbed in around 5 hours), or (D) very large (absorbed in around 7 hours). In all these cases, a steady stream of nutrients is delivered across intermeal periods thanks to appropriate meal sizing.*

Digestion Rates and Meal Timing

The GI tract takes longer to digest larger amounts of food, but only to a certain extent. This is one of the reasons that four meals per day is the lowest recommended frequency. Three or fewer meals per day on a hypocaloric diet might seem logical for fat loss. The trouble is that this meal structure leaves stretches of time between meals when food is fully absorbed, but no new nutrients are coming in. This is a problem for muscle retention. During the time between meals when you have digested and used the previous meal's protein, your body will begin to break down muscle tissue for amino acids. If you instead ate the same number of calories distributed over six evenly sized meals, fat would still be lost (because of the hypocaloric aspect), but due to the continuous input of amino acids, muscle would be spared.

Meal composition can also alter digestion time, playing an important role in meal-timing choices. Different protein and carb sources digest and absorb at different rates. For example, while whey protein digests and absorbs within the hour if taken alone in small doses, a chicken breast of equivalent protein content can take two to four hours to absorb. Casein protein can take longer than seven hours to fully absorb. Similarly, carb sources like dextrose powder (pure glucose) are absorbed in minutes, whole-grain breads in several hours, and some fruits take even longer.

Fats slow the digestion of other nutrients and decrease their rate of delivery to muscles. If you consume a large amount of fat but very little protein in a meal, protein delivery to muscles will be delayed. Higher fat meals are best eaten with additional protein so that per-hour amino acid availability is sufficient during the lengthened digestion and absorption period.

You can choose nutrient sources to fit your schedule. If you eat four times a day, your typical food sources should be moderately or slowly digesting protein and carbs that will gradually release nutrients into your bloodstream for the entire meal interval (figure 4.2). Since added fats slow down the digestion of all nutrients, they can make these differences moot, but individuals on lower fat diets should pay more careful attention to meal composition.

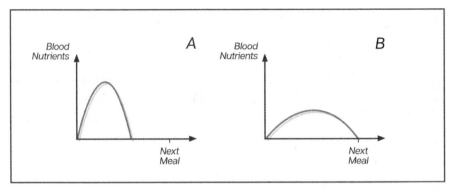

Figure 4.2 *Graph A depicts the absorption time of a meal made up of fast-digesting carbs and proteins that is digested and absorbed prior to the next meal, a poor timing strategy. Graph B depicts the absorption time of another meal with the same macro content as graph A, but composed of slower digesting carbs and proteins that provide nutrients for the entire intermeal interval, a better timing strategy.*

Protein Timing and Portioning for Anabolism and Anti-catabolism

Protein intake supports homeostasis as the body constantly breaks down and rebuilds its structural and functional proteins. The protein needed for this turnover can come from the diet or, if the diet is insufficient, muscle tissue. Generally, under hypercaloric conditions, sufficient protein intake supports muscle growth. Under isocaloric or hypocaloric conditions, sufficient intake helps prevent muscle loss.

Interestingly, the human body can only use so much protein at a time to build or maintain muscle. The literature shows roughly four evenly spaced meals, each containing one-fourth of your daily protein needs, supplies sufficient protein at a usable rate. A 200-lb. athlete who needs around 200 g of protein per day should therefore consume meals of no more than 50 g of protein at a time for maximum protein utilization. Any additional protein per meal will just be burned for energy. Although there are no direct drawbacks to eating extra protein per meal, if one is constrained by calories on a fat-loss diet, eating more than one-fourth of one's daily protein per meal will mean protein will be insufficient in later meals. This is often misunderstood to mean that protein will not be digested or used at all after a certain per meal threshold; however, this upper limit pertains only to skeletal muscle protein synthesis. If you eat all your daily protein in one meal, the protein will still be digested and used for other various bodily functions, but only about one-fourth will go toward skeletal muscle growth or maintenance.

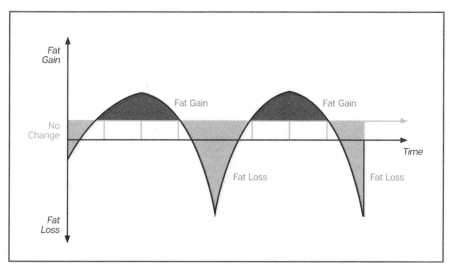

Figure 4.3 *A theoretical graph illustrating the concept that meals themselves will cause some fat gain (dark areas), and spaces between meals will case some fat loss (light areas), resulting in no net fat gain if the diet is isocaloric.*

There are mechanistic reasons to expect that uneven protein distribution across meals is suboptimal. Research has yet to confirm exact numbers, but approximately one-eighth of daily recommended protein intake per meal is a safe minimum to set for muscle maintenance. For a diet with 200 g of protein recommended per day, less than 25 g might not be enough protein per meal, and more than 50 g per meal will leave other meals without protein. Thus, eating between one-eighth and one-fourth of daily intake per meal is recommended (figure 4.4). There is some flexibility here: If you under-eat protein a bit at one meal and overeat at the other, some compensation occurs. This is a relatively narrow margin, though; when some meals are overly heavy with protein or smaller protein consumptions are followed by long stretches without eating, you run the risk of muscle loss.

It is particularly important to supply sufficient protein at timely intervals during hypocaloric diets when much of the ingested protein is burned for energy and only a fraction is used for muscle-specific functions. In fact, because of the general energy surplus on a hypercaloric diet, protein needs are lower (as low as 0.7 g per pound per day) than they are during a hypocaloric diet (up to 1.2 g per pound per day to prevent muscle loss). Meal timing choices are still relevant on a hypercaloric diet, as amino acids are in constant demand in order to supply FSR curves for muscle growth (figure 4.5).

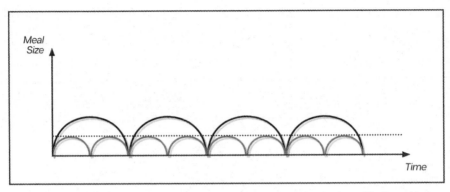

Figure 4.4 *Eight smaller meals (depicted by the smaller waves under the dotted line) provide a faster initial rise, as well as a more rapid drop in blood nutrients. Four larger meals (depicted by the larger waves above the dotted line) provide a slower rise and drop in blood nutrients. The dotted horizontal line depicts average nutrient amounts in the blood.*

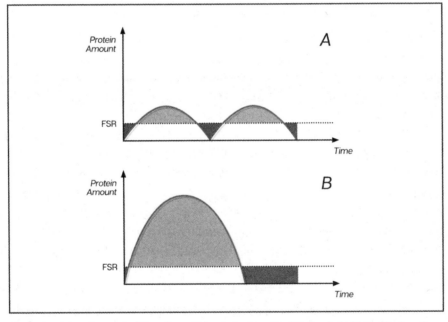

Figure 4.5 *When the graphed line of protein intake is above the FSR threshold (dotted line), amino acids are available in the bloodstream for maximal muscle growth. Periods in which not enough amino acids are available are indicated by the shaded areas below the dotted line. A. Depicts smaller protein amounts eaten more frequently, supplying amino acids for maximal FSR for most of the time shown. B. Depicts a large amount of protein eaten at one time, followed by a long period without protein consumption. Because FSRs are limited, even though the total protein eaten in A and B is equivalent, option B (one large protein meal) facilitates less total muscle growth.*

Though it is likely unnecessarily tedious, we can also examine per-hour protein needs. The actual process of muscle growth is measured by the FSR of muscle tissue. Right after weight training, these rates rise for up to 24 hours. Once the FSR peaks, it can take days to fall back to baseline. Therefore, the real "post-workout anabolic window" is between one to three days post training. Because most people are training multiple times a week, the demand for amino acids to supply FSR is rather stable as another workout is always pushing them back up before they can fall to baseline again (figure 4.6). This means that our bodies need a certain amount of protein hourly, no matter what time of the day we worked out, slept, or whatever else. We can also divide our daily protein dose by the 24 hours in a day to get our per hour protein needs, though this may be best suited for thought experiments and not practical dieting.

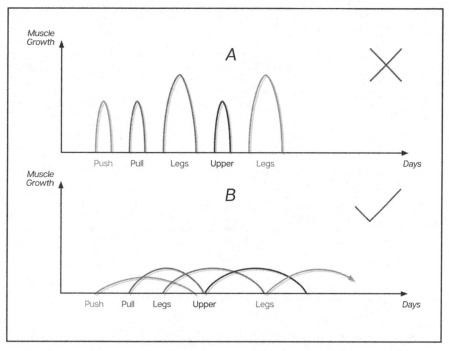

Figure 4.6 *A. An incorrect representation of FSR curves following lifting sessions. B. An accurate representation of FSR curves following lifting sessions. FSR rises slowly for many hours and stays elevated for days.*

For example, an athlete who weighs 240 lb. needs 10 g of protein per hour of the day (240 g/24 hr.). If our athlete wanted to eat two meals at three hours apart, they would need to eat about 30 g of protein at meal one to supply amino acid needs across those three hours between meals. If meals were separated by five hours, the first meal should have around 50 g of protein to supply amino acids across that five-hour period. This becomes problematic when we factor sleep into the equation. If this 240-lb. athlete is awake for 16 hours and eats according to hourly protein needs, they will consume just 160 g protein during their waking day. That leaves 80 g to consume before bed, which is more than one-fourth of their daily protein and therefore more than their body can use for muscle production when consumed at one meal. In reality, the one-eighth to one-fourth daily protein total per meal across four to eight meals is sufficiently precise and more practical a recommendation. Hourly calculations might come in handy for those working 24-hour shifts or dealing with other odd schedules in which prolonged periods without sleep occur.

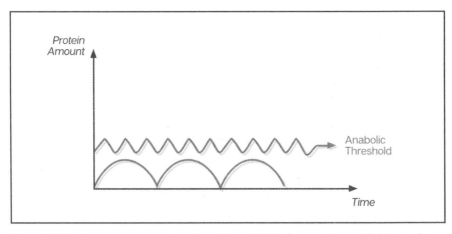

Figure 4.7 *The lower curves represent amino acid availability from smaller protein boluses that do not reach the anabolic threshold, represented by the upper wave.*

For anti-catabolism, splitting up protein feedings evenly is sufficient. The situation with *anabolism* might be a bit more complicated, but the consensus in the literature is not quite established on this topic yet. From molecular research, it seems possible that leucine, an amino acid component of most food proteins, is one of the central regulators and activators of muscle growth. If the leucine content of a meal is below some value, the musculature may engage only in anti-catabolism. This hypothetical threshold for anabolism is termed the "leucine threshold" or "anabolic threshold".

What this means is that consuming more protein per meal, even over fewer meals (less than six) might be more effective for muscle gain. There has, as yet, been no evidence from long-term human studies confirming the effect of this threshold, but the molecular evidence is notable. To be on the safe side, consider eating no less than one-sixth daily protein per meal when trying to gain muscle (figure 4.7).

Carbohydrate Timing and Portioning

Carbohydrate support immediate energy needs and glycogen synthesis up to its maximum rate. (Once you exceed immediate energy needs and glycogen synthesis rates, remaining carbs are converted to fat tissue.) Although laboratory glycogen synthesis studies have reported rates up to around 0.8 g per pound per hour (g/lb/hr), these are unlikely outside of laboratory conditions. Intakes over 0.4 g/lb/hr have been shown to exceed intestinal absorption rates. In reality, the upper limit for glycogen replenishment in individuals is probably around 0.3 g/lb/h. This means that a 150-lb. individual should not exceed approximately 50 g of carbohydrate per hour, even when doing their hardest training. If this person eats every 4 hours, 200 g of carbs per meal should be their absolute maximum. Not the most relevant limit, as that is much more carbohydrate than most people need or would eat per meal, but pertinent for timing extremes. For example, in some intermittent fasting diets, people might eat all their daily carbohydrates in one meal.

Maximum glycogen synthesis rate becomes relevant here because if you weigh 150 lb. and your daily carb allotment is 500 g of carbs and you only eat one meal, as many as 300 g of those carbs may go toward fat storage.

Because carbs are significantly anti-catabolic, their consumption in most meals is recommended in order to prevent muscle loss (figure 4.8). This is especially true on a hypocaloric diet; if smaller meals are composed of only protein, most of that will be burned for energy with little left to go toward muscle retention. Carbs are ideal as a fuel source to spare protein, and in fact your body will tend to use them preferentially for that purpose if they are co-ingested with protein.

The benefit of increasing carbohydrate intake for anti-catabolism is non-linear, however, and probably loses potency above values of 0.1 g/lb/hr. This means that our 150-lb. athlete does not likely need more than 60 g of carbs per meal for this purpose when eating every 4 hours. In contrast to protein intake, lower carbs in one meal make the musculature more sensitive to absorbing higher amounts of carbs in the next meal, so under-eating carbs in one meal can be compensated with overeating carbs in the next to a greater extent. Maximum carbohydrate intake recommendations are therefore in the range of 0.1 to 0.2 g/lb/hr, which translates to around 3.0 to 5.0 g per pound of bodyweight per day. This is the maximum amount of carbohydrates that most individuals would be able to absorb under heavy training conditions. General daily recommendations for normal training and for non-training days will be substantially lower.

Details for appropriately assigning carbs will be discussed in depth in chapter 10.

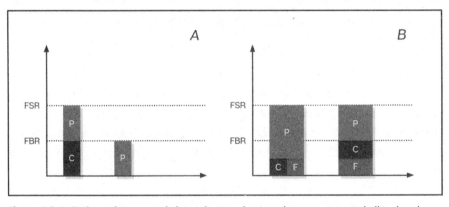

Figure 4.8 *A. Eating only your needed protein at a given meal can prevent catabolism (reaches the threshold to prevent FBR; fractional breakdown rate of muscle tissue), but leaves no protein to support anabolism (reach the threshold to support FSR; fractional synthetic rate of muscle tissue). Adding carbs allows the meal to reach the needed protein and total calories to reach the FSR threshold. B. Different ratios of macronutrients in addition to protein can be consumed to reach the FSR threshold.*

STRUCTURING MEALS AROUND PHYSICAL ACTIVITY

Carbohydrate also plays a very important role in meal timing around activity—an important component of nutrient timing. Your body has different nutritional needs depending on recent, present, or upcoming physical activity. We can outline six general periods, each with unique nutritional needs:

1. Pre-training window
2. Intra-training window
3. Post-training window
4. High-activity, non-training periods
5. Low-activity periods
6. Bedtime

Pre-Training Window

The pre-training window refers to the 30 minutes to 4 hours before training begins. During this window, carbohydrate is needed to top off muscle glycogen stores and help regulate blood glucose levels in preparation for the high-energy demands of training. A state where muscle glycogen stores are full has two interesting benefits. The better known of these is to energetically support high-intensity muscular activity. A lesser known benefit is that full muscle glycogen stores *directly* signal the muscle to become more anabolic, which enhances muscle retention or growth (depending on calorie intake).

Pre-training window meal restrictions include limiting meal size and avoiding slow-digesting foods when the meal is eaten closer to training. Most blood will leave the GI tract during high physical exertion in order to circulate between the working muscles, heart, and lungs. Without blood to pull nutrients out of the intestines, undigested food in the GI tract can lead to discomfort, nausea, or even vomiting. If an individual is too full to perform well after a large meal, training will be impaired, ultimately defeating the purpose of the pre-training meal. Likewise, having insufficient energy for training from fasting all morning can have equivalently detrimental effects.

The size of the pre-training meal and digestion time of its contents should be scaled to the time between this meal and training (figure 4.9). Larger, slower digesting meals can be an option if the pre-training meal comes three to four hours before training. In contrast, a very small amount of quickly digesting protein and carbs (with minimal fat and fiber) should be consumed if one is eating around 30 minutes before training. In the latter case, some intra-workout carbohydrate ingestion may be advisable to prevent sudden changes in blood sugar due to the fast absorbing carbs and their rapid use during training. Maintaining stable blood sugar is preferable for best performances.

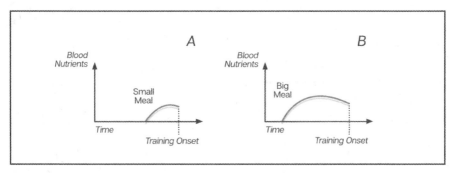

Figure 4.9 *A. Smaller meals can be eaten closer to training time and still provide sufficient nutrient availability to support training. B. Larger meals should be eaten if the pre-training meal will occur earlier so that there is still sufficient nutrient availability by the time training occurs.*

Intra-Training Window

Most workouts, especially those that last less than an hour, rely almost exclusively on stored glycogen and pre-workout nutrients. Intra-workout nutrition becomes more useful for longer workouts (more than 60 minutes). Fast-digesting carbohydrates can be combined with small doses of fast-digesting protein to supply the working muscles with an anti-catabolic mix. In addition, fast-digesting carbs can help maintain blood glucose levels through the workout, which is both anti-catabolic and supports performance. The top end recommendation for intra-training nutrition is about 5 to 10% of daily protein per hour up to the maximum carbohydrate depending on the workout. This protein amount is reasonable for most, but the carb amount should be decreased from the maximum for all but super-high-volume workouts like endurance cycling.

Post-Training Window

Training engages a catabolic hormonal and intracellular condition that persists for some time post-training unless a more anabolic state is attained by the introduction of nutrients. Recently trained muscles are also very sensitive to carbohydrate intake and primed to replenish glycogen during the post-training window. This effect decreases slowly over the subsequent three to six hours following training. Thus, carbohydrate intake during the six hours post training will have the greatest anabolic effects. Because the uptake of carbs into the muscle for glycogen storage is so high during this time, conversion to fat is much lower, a twofold benefit. It has also been found that fat cells are less sensitive to nutrients in the post-training window, which magnifies the post-workout nutrient consumption benefit even more. Studies suggest significant muscle glycogen resynthesis at consumption rates of 30 to 60 g per hour post exercise for the average 150-lb. person. Maximal resynthesis was seen at intakes of around 84 g per hour, but this level of intake is likely unnecessary for most individuals under most training circumstances.

If you happen to be training twice or more in one day, replenishing glycogen in the post-workout window is critical to being able to maintain glycogen levels for all training sessions that day.

There is no special role for protein in the post-workout window, aside from maintaining adequate hourly protein consumption. Fats should be kept to a minimum in the first post-workout meal as they delay digestion of carbohydrates (figure 4.10). The post-training meal should be consumed as soon as the athlete feels comfortable taking in food. Consuming mainly fast-digesting proteins and carbs in the post-workout meal supplies carbohydrates for glycogen storage and anabolism the fastest and keeps the risk of gastrointestinal distress low.

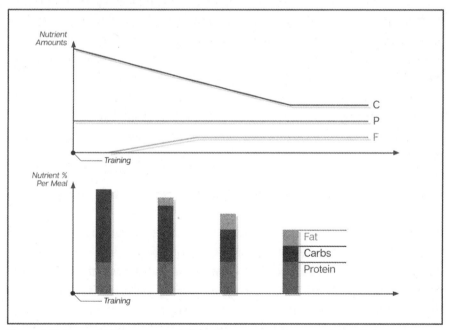

Figure 4.10 *Macronutrient recommendations change across the post-training window. Upper graph: In the hours after a workout, carb needs decline while fat allowances go up. Protein needs are relatively unchanged mostly due to the smooth and stable nature of FSR curves. Lower bar graph: Bars indicate best qualitative ratios of macros for post-training meals across time.*

High-Activity, Non-Training Periods

Examples of high-activity, non-training periods include hiking for leisure, running around shopping with your children all day, or physically intensive jobs like construction or professional dancing. These activities require more energy than sitting at a desk or relaxing on the couch on your day off. Carbohydrate intakes should be increased to reflect energy expenditure rates compared to low-activity periods.

Low-Activity Periods

Being sedentary does not require any special nutrition other than the consistent intake of protein. Because the immediate energy demand of such times is low, the amount of carbs and fats needed to offset potential protein burning is also lower.

Bedtime

Bedtime meals have very similar constraints to meals that precede other low-activity periods, but there are some unique considerations for this meal. Ideally the pre-bedtime meal should be *right before* bed for maximum amino acid titration overnight. Eating too close to bed can, however, cause gastrointestinal distress or interfere with sleep quality for some. Similarly, fat slows protein absorption, so it offers us the ability to extend an anabolic and anti-catabolic environment longer into the night, but some research has indicated that eating large amounts of fat in the pre-bedtime meal may interfere with sleep as well. Thus, although eating closer to bedtime and adding fats to the bedtime meal is advantageous, some individuals may have to experiment with bedtime meal timing and fat content and make trade-offs of maximum results for quality sleep.

There have been proponents of waking during the night to eat a meal in order to minimize muscle loss risk further. The detrimental effects to sleep quality which impact recovery and muscle growth, however, likely make any benefits of this practice moot. There is also some evidence that for best intestinal health, periods without nutrient ingestion might be needed. It is possible that nutrient sensitivity is improved by the lack of nutrient intake during sleep, but it is unlikely that this means that we should fast for any duration longer than the sleeping period.

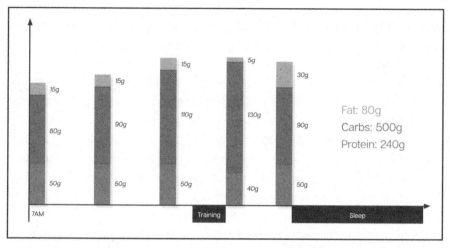

Figure 4.11 *A sample diet across a training day for a 240-lb. athlete. Daily macros are split into five meals, with protein held steady meal to meal, carbs heavier around the workout, and fats kept lower near the workout.*

A NOTE ON PRACTICAL APPLICATION

There is a range of recommended number of meals (around 4-8 per day) and meal intervals (around 3-6 hours between meals). There is also some flexibility for how long before training (30 minutes to 4 hours) and how soon after training (immediately to about an hour after) it is best to eat. Some degree of undereating in one meal and overeating in another can make up for each other. This is all to say that overly religious dedication to the tenants of good meal timing is not necessary. Tedious meal scheduling can deter diet adherence and make your life overly stressful. Take advantage of the flexibility and range of options in order to improve your diet with nutrient timing, but avoid overemphasizing this principle. Chapter 10 will cover more precise practical details for applying this principle in the design of your own diet.

CHAPTER SUMMARY

- Nutrient timing describes how calories and macronutrients are assigned relative to time throughout the day. Factors of nutrient timing include meal number, meal spacing, meal size, meal macro content, meal food composition, and timing around physical activity.
- Nutrient timing manipulations may not be nearly as powerful as calorie or macronutrient manipulations, but they still provide a tangible and practical benefit to enhancing body composition and performance.
- Daily protein intake should be divided into four to eight meals across the day, each containing one-eighth to one-fourth total daily protein.
- Meals should be larger and more slowly digesting the longer the following intermeal interval will be, but extremely large or small meals should be avoided.
- Daily carbohydrate intake should be biased toward activity periods, with the largest doses generally occurring in the pre-, intra-, and post-training periods.
- Daily fat intake should be biased away from activity periods and instead biased toward longer periods without regular meals, such as sleep or while at work.
- Slow-digesting protein should be the core of your bedtime meal.
- Extreme timing manipulations that sacrifice your daily calories, macros, or sleep quality are not recommended. The latter variables are more impactful to your physique and performance.

CHAPTER 5

Food Composition

Food composition refers to a food's quality. It describes what other nutrition is obtained along with the desired macronutrient and how the food is digested and utilized by the body. Food composition is measured by things like digestibility and digestion time as well as by vitamin, mineral, phytochemical, and fiber content. Food composition is a lower priority, contributing to around 5% of body composition and performance outcomes. For health outcomes, food composition plays a much larger role, so paying attention to this principle can pay off in the long term despite its small contribution to immediate fitness outcomes.

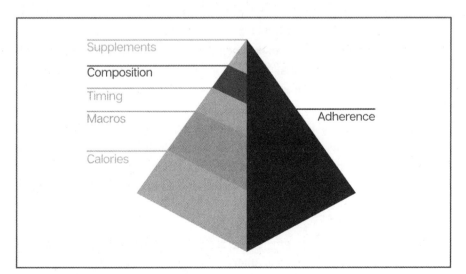

PROTEIN COMPOSITION

Protein sources vary across three main food composition aspects: digestibility, protein quality, and to a lesser extent the presence of other micronutrients.

Protein Source Digestibility

Protein sources can be ranked by their digestibility. Digestibility refers to how much of ingested protein is absorbed and utilized by the body. Animal protein sources tend to be among the best digested protein sources. Dairy, eggs, and isolated protein powders tend to be the most completely digested protein sources. After these, meat and soy products are a close second.

On average, plant-sourced protein is much less efficiently digested in part due to cellulose—a component of plant cell walls that cannot be broken down by the human gut. Processed plant protein sources can be healthier than non-processed whole food options because of this; the processing of plant protein can break down cellulose and make the amino acid contents more accessible. Some exceptions are mycoprotein (a fungus-based protein) and nutritional yeast. Because fungus and yeast do not contain cellulose, they are much better digested and absorbed.

Protein Quality

Sources of protein can also be ranked based on the types and ratios of amino acids they provide. A food source containing all the essential amino acids is termed *complete*. Sometimes, particularly in the case of vegan diets, two or more protein sources are needed to get all the essential amino acids in adequate amounts. Multiple protein sources that together contain all essential amino acids are called *complementary*. While all animal sources are complete, most plant sources are not. Consumption of complete protein at every meal is not likely to have a large effect on health so long as the needed amino acids are consumed on average in the appropriate daily amounts. For body composition and performance concerns, however, getting enough of all essential amino acids at every meal is valuable and recommended for best muscle growth or retention.

Protein Digestibility-Corrected Amino Acid Score (PDCAAS) is the gold standard for evaluating the quality of a protein source. This method takes into account both the essential amino acid content and the digestibility of the protein. A score of 1 is the highest possible score and means that the protein source contains all the essential amino acids and can be fully digested such that all of the amino acids can be absorbed when that source is eaten. Quality of protein decreases with PDCAA score down to 0. A food with a score of 0 would provide no accessible essential amino acids. Table 5.1 is a list of some protein sources and their PDCAA scores.

Table 5.1 *A list of some example protein sources and their PDCAA scores*

Protein Digestibility-Corrected Amino Acid Scores (PDCAAS)	
Milk proteins (casein, whey)	1.00
Egg protein	1.00
Soy protein isolate	0.99
Mycoprotein (fungus-based vegan protein)	0.99
Beef	0.92
Chickpeas	0.78
Black beans	0.75
Peanuts	0.52
Rice	0.50
Whole wheat	0.42
Wheat gluten	0.25

Protein Source Micronutrient Density

Vitamins, minerals, and fiber are known as micronutrients because they are required by the body, but in only very small amounts (usually measured in milligrams) relative to macronutrients (usually measured in grams) for body composition, performance, and health. Phytochemicals are biologically active compounds found in plants, and although they are *not essential* to health or performance, evidence suggests that some types might improve both by a small amount. In addition to providing high-quality protein, animal products are also rich in a number of vitamins and minerals which plants tend to lack or have in much smaller quantities. Examples include some of the B vitamins (in particular B12) and iron. In contrast, although plant-based protein sources are often lower quality and harder to digest, they tend to be higher in fiber and phytochemicals and lower in less healthy classes of fats.

CARBOHYDRATE COMPOSITION

Two primary factors determine the quality of a carbohydrate source: its digestion time and its nutrient density.

Carbohydrate Source Digestion Time and the Glycemic Index

The glycemic index measures how quickly a source of carbohydrate is digested and absorbed into the bloodstream. Glycemic indices can be determined in a lab setting by measuring the blood sugar concentrations of study participants over hours after having consumed a particular carb source; values are ranked on a scale of 0 (lowest) to 100 (highest). Quickly digested carbohydrate sources cause a rapid spike in blood sugar resulting in a high glycemic index value. Slowly digested carbohydrate sources cause more gradual and sustained elevations in blood sugar and therefore have lower glycemic indices. Table 5.2 lists some example glycemic index values.

Table 5.2 *A list of some example carbohydrate sources and their glycemic index values.*

Glycemic Index Values	
Pure dextrose (glucose) powder	100
Gatorade	90
Plain white potato (average of all cooking methods)	85
Cocoa Puffs cereal	75
White bagel	70
White rice	65
Sweet potato	60
Quinoa	55
Oatmeal	55
Whole-grain bread	50
Brown rice	50
All-Bran cereal	45
Pasta (higher glycemic index the longer you boil it)	30-50
Oranges, peaches, pears, apples, carrots	40

Kidney beans	35
Skim milk and low-fat yogurt	30
Grapefruit	25
Soybeans, chickpeas	15
Hummus dip	5
Pure insoluble fiber	0

Processed carbohydrate sources often have a higher glycemic index value compared to whole food counterparts because the processing of food can break it down, making it more quickly and easily digested. On the other hand, glycemic index values are lower in the presence of fat, protein, or fiber, which can slow digestion. For this reason, hummus, the processed version of chickpeas with added fats, has a lower glycemic index than chickpeas themselves. It is also important to note that eating other food sources along with a particular carbohydrate source can effectively alter its glycemic index by slowing digestion. Glycemic index values affect nutritional recommendations for body composition and performance in several ways, as detailed in the following.

Pre-Training Meal

Pre-training or pre-competition meals should ideally digest quickly enough to prevent gastrointestinal distress and be able to restock muscle glycogen in time to support the activity. In addition, a good pre-training or pre-competition meal should provide a stable stream of blood glucose throughout the activity. Types of carb sources that are ideal for pre-training depend on the timing of the meal. The further from training onset the meal is eaten, the lower its glycemic index should be. A sugary sport drink can be a great pre-training meal if it is consumed 30 minutes prior to training or competing—sports drinks have a very high glycemic index, no fat or fiber, and their liquid consistency allows them to be digested quickly. If the meal is eaten much earlier, a slower-digesting whole food meal like a turkey sandwich on whole-grain bread is a better option. The pre-training meal should always contain enough carbs for basic function in addition to carbs for training. A pre-training meal eaten further in advance of training requires more total carbs than a meal eaten immediately before training to support basic function in the hours before training along with energy for the training itself.

Intra-Training Meal

Intra-training meals should provide immediately available energy during the workout itself. Lower glycemic index carbohydrate sources increase chances of gastrointestinal discomfort and cause more blood to be allocated to the digestive tract and away from working muscles, so should be avoided entirely. Quickly digested liquids are easier to consume during training than solids, so the best recommendation for intra-workout is a high glycemic index liquid such as a sugary sports drink.

Post-Training Meal

In hours immediately following training, the body is particularly efficient in its ability to resynthesize glycogen from ingested carbohydrates. This is notable not only for single training sessions, but particularly when dealing with multiple training sessions per day, as glycogen resynthesis can be a rate-limiting step in subsequent exercise performance. For this reason, it is beneficial to bias post-training carbs toward higher glycemic index sources with minimal fiber and fat. Kids' cereal in whey protein or fat-free milk is a great option here. Thanks to the training stimulus after a workout, your body can utilize more carbs in a shorter time span to refill glycogen stores. In this instance there is little concern about fat storage—as there might be if you were slamming Lucky Charms after spending a day sedentary on the couch. As the post-workout window stretches out, the sensitivity of the muscles to carbs declines, and previous meals have already done much of the glycogen filling. The rate of glycogen filling is no longer an immediate concern. Thus, the later it is after training, the food sources should have a lower glycemic index and the more added fiber and fats they can contain.

Meal Interval Considerations

Lower glycemic index foods and the additions of fiber, protein, and fat sources can slow digestion and better provide energy across longer intervals between meals. If you have a five-hour window between meals and need to concentrate at work, a meal of chicken, veggies, whole-grain bread, and nut butter would provide the sustained energy needed before your next meal, whereas gummy worms and whey protein shakes would likely leave you hypoglycemic after just a couple hours. Adjusting food composition for slower digestion is like creating a sustained release system for energy and should be considered when designing meals with different inter-meal intervals.

Glycemic Index Values and Real-World Eating

Popular opinion would have you believe that highly glycemic foods cause excessive insulin secretion thereby making you fatter. While there is a seed of truth to this claim, it is not consistently true, and unwanted fat gain is not always the result. Some foods with low glycemic index values cause high amounts of insulin to be secreted. A perfect example is skim milk and lean yogurt products; despite inducing significant insulin secretion, heavy consumption of these products is inversely associated with obesity. This means that people who eat lean dairy products are less likely to be obese. Carrots are another example; they have a relatively high glycemic index value, but their consumption is not generally associated with obesity. While high glycemic foods can make people want to eat more, cravings are actually more dependent on how satiating a food is, irrespective of glycemic index values. White potatoes are very glycemic but are extremely filling and so do not tend to increase cravings. Glycemic indices are not of themselves a measure of how healthy a given food item is or is not. Carb sources are generally consumed within a meal containing other foods; estimating glycemic index values for mixed meals is very difficult, and the value for any given mixed meal will be lower than any of its ingredients alone. Author Mike Israetel's middle school physical education teacher, with the best of intentions, instructed students not to eat candy bars before sports games because the sugar would "burn up quickly and have them crashing" midway through the event. In reality, Snickers bars or any other chocolate-based candy bar have glycemic indices of around 50, similar to whole grains. The fructose in high fructose corn syrup is extremely slow digesting, and the high fat content of such candy decreases its glycemic index even more. When protein, fat, and fiber are involved in real meals people actually eat, the glycemic index value becomes just a very small factor in a bigger equation in which macro amounts, calories, and actual digestion times play a more dominant role. That being said, high glycemic carbs, eaten alone without other foods to slow their digestion, serve a valuable purpose in intra- and post-training meals, improving health and fitness outcomes in that context.

Carbohydrate Source Micronutrient Density

Along with factors affecting digestion time, the density of micronutrients within a carbohydrate source also define its compositional quality. Carbohydrate sources vary greatly in their micronutrient and phytochemical content. For example, dextrose powder can provide all needed carbs, but without any vitamins, minerals, phytochemicals, or fiber. Extreme diets that cut carbs very low for long periods (e.g., ketogenic diets) might elevate the risk of nutrient deficiencies. Getting carbs from a wide range of veggies, fruits, whole grains along with less nutrient-dense sources as needed allows you to get all the carbs you need and consume digestion speed-appropriate carbs without missing out on any nutrients.

FAT COMPOSITION

The quality of a fat source is determined based on the class of fat. Each of the four main classes of dietary fat has its own effects on body composition, performance, and general long-term health.

Monounsaturated Fats

Monounsaturated fats are found in plant sources, such as olive oil, canola oil, avocados, and a variety of nuts. This fat type not only promotes better health than others, but also, to some extent, supports leaner, more muscular physiques. Fat in any diet focused on health, performance or body composition should come primarily from monounsaturated sources.

Polyunsaturated Fats

Polyunsaturated fats can be found in certain vegetable oils, such as canola oil and safflower oil; walnuts; many fatty seeds; and some animal products like fatty fish and grass-fed animal meat. The most nutritionally relevant are the essential fats, Omega-6 and Omega-3 fatty acids. In most modern diets, Omega-6 fats are consumed in sufficient quantities, but Omega-3 fats are often under-eaten. This means that those training for high levels of fitness might need to supplement Omega-3 fats or tailor their diet especially for these fats. A diet relatively high in polyunsaturated fats supports performance well and is relatively neutral for general health.

Saturated Fats

Saturated fats come mainly from animal sources, such as dairy, eggs, meats, and coconut oils. Opinion on saturated fat has swung from recommended consumption of steak and eggs prior to marathons in the 1970s, to its demonization in the 80s and 90s, and back to an overemphasis on its consumption in the 2000s with bacon-and-heavy-cream-based, low-carb diets. Today, if we look at the data on saturated fat and health as a whole, they suggest that too much saturated fat can have a negative impact on health. On the other hand, saturated fat might have a positive effect on anabolic hormone levels for those interested in physique and sport performance. More data is needed for saturated fat recommendations in terms of potential physique benefits, but health detriments currently support limiting saturated fat intake.

Trans Unsaturated Fats

Trans fats are unsaturated fatty acids—as described briefly in chapter 3, *trans* or its counterpart *cis*, refer to the configuration of the fat molecules' functional groups. Different configurations have different biological and chemical properties. Trans fats occur only rarely in nature and in small quantities. This class of fats is mainly produced during the chemical manipulation of naturally occurring fats. These manipulations are made to achieve distinct advantages for food production and distribution. Some of these alterations of molecular structure allow fats that would normally be solid to remain liquid at room temperature. This makes them appealing as cooking oils and for use in baked or fried foods that have to be stored at room temperature.

Also, in part because of their unique chemical nature, trans fats are not nearly as likely to go rancid or be consumed by bacteria, increasing safety for the consumer and extending the shelf life of the product. This means that foods can be shipped farther and stored longer, which can be critical in emergency aid situations and in places where refrigeration and access to food are limited.

As big a boon as trans fats are for preserving food and reducing foodborne illness, they also have a substantial downside. Most studies show that high levels of trans fat consumption results in increased likelihood of negative health effects such as higher rates of cardiovascular and other systemic diseases. One primate study suggested that diets high in trans fats might also lead to decreased muscularity and increased fat mass, suggesting a potential contribution to changes in body composition. Avoiding trans fats as much as possible is therefore likely the best advice from both health and fitness standpoints. That being said, it is unlikely that the occasional indulgence within an otherwise healthy diet will have significant effect.

Fat Source Micronutrient Density

Many fat sources do not contain other nutrients, so micronutrient density contributes far less to the compositional quality of fats than it does for other macronutrients. Fat is the only way to transport fat soluble vitamins, but the vitamins come from other food sources in most cases and are merely facilitated by proximal fat consumption. The way the different types of fat are digested and stored constitute the most meaningful differences in composition.

In table 5.3, we have parsed fat class information into estimated percentage recommendations for the daily intake of each type of fat. Bear in mind that these are estimates, not exact numbers to hit daily. In general, acquire most of your daily fats from monounsaturated sources, take in enough Omega-3s, be moderate with saturated fats, and avoid most trans fats in your regular diet.

Table 5.3 *Suggested range of intake as percentage of total daily fat intake for the four types of dietary fat.*

Fat Intake Recommendations	
Fat Type	**Recommended % of Daily Fat Intake**
Monounsaturated	45 - 60%
Polyunsaturated	35 - 50%
Saturated	5 - 20%
Trans fats	< 1%

THE MICRONUTRIENTS

Vitamins

Vitamins are a class of micronutrients composed of vitamins C, A, D, E, K, and the B-complex vitamins. Water-soluble vitamin C and B-complex vitamins are found in most fruits, vegetables, and some grains, with the exception of B12, which is found in seafood, meat, dairy, and eggs. The fat-soluble vitamins A, D, E, and K are found in vegetable oils and dairy products. Most vitamins are converted to an active form upon entering the bloodstream at which point they regulate numerous body processes from vision to energy metabolism to bone formation.

Water-soluble vitamins bind to water molecules in the digestive tract and freely move into the bloodstream. Fat-soluble vitamins, on the other hand, must bind to dietary fat in the digestive tract in order to be absorbed and used. Diets that are chronically low in fat can result in a fat-soluble vitamin deficiencies.

When consuming a balanced diet, vitamin deficiencies are rare, but possible. Eating multiple servings of fruits and vegetables per day and consuming adequate amounts of grains, proteins, dairy, and healthy fats can decrease the chance of developing these deficiencies. Food variation across the week can also help as vitamin levels vary between different fruits, vegetables, and grains. For best health and fitness make sure your food choices contain adequate vitamins. Vitamin supplements are an effective option, though you should not program your diet such that you are relying entirely on supplements for your vitamin intake over long-term periods. When on a hypocaloric diet, it can be a good idea to take a once-a-day multivitamin as an insurance policy, though this is not a substitute for making generally healthy choices.

Minerals

Dietary minerals are naturally occurring chemical elements required by the body for basic function and health. Essential minerals include calcium, phosphorus, magnesium, and iron. Trace minerals—those needed in very small amounts, but potentially toxic in large amounts—include zinc, copper, manganese, iodine, selenium, molybdenum, and chromium.

Although all essential minerals are necessary for health purposes, for body composition and performance considerations, a subgroup of minerals called electrolytes are probably the most important. Electrolytes such as sodium, potassium, chloride, calcium, iron, and magnesium carry a positive or negative charge. This charge can impact cell function by altering cell membrane permeability. Such changes are responsible for neuronal firing in the central nervous system and muscle contractions in cardiac, smooth, and skeletal muscle tissue. Electrolyte balance also mediates hydration and blood pH—though only very severe imbalances can disturb blood pH as it is very tightly regulated.

It is important to replace electrolytes and fluids during activity, particularly if the activity is sweat-inducing: high intensity, prolonged duration, or occurring in a hot and humid environment. During and after such activity, electrolytes can help the body return to a homeostatic state. Consuming additional electrolyte beverages during such training is recommended.

Daily electrolyte needs for rest or light training are usually achieved with normal food consumption. Most people meet daily requirements of sodium and chloride easily as these two minerals are what make up table salt and are found in many foods and other seasonings.

Magnesium is also found in a variety of food products, such as spinach, beans, shellfish, and milk. The primary dietary source of calcium is usually dairy, but almond and soy milk as well as dark green leafy vegetables contain small amounts as well. Potassium can be found in most fruits and vegetables, with white potatoes and bananas having the highest amounts. Dietary sources of iron are divided into two categories, heme and non-heme iron. Non-heme iron is present in an oxidized form that must be reduced before it can be absorbed. Because it does not have this need for reduction, heme iron is absorbed at a much greater rate than non-heme iron. Heme iron comes mainly from meat, fish, and poultry. Non-heme iron can be found in plant sources, such as whole wheat and dark green vegetables.

Many people do not consume adequate amounts of iron; this is particularly true of vegans, vegetarians, and females of childbearing age, particularly if they experience heavy menstrual bleeding. For athletes this can be especially problematic. Chronically inadequate iron intake or absorption results in iron-deficiency anemia, which is a decrease in the number of healthy red blood cells able to carry oxygen. This means a decrease in the blood's ability to deliver oxygen to working tissue where it is needed to produce energy for muscle contractions. Anemia can hinder high-volume weight training and cardio, as well as recovery from physical activity. A dietary supplement of iron may be needed for those limiting or avoiding the consumption of animal products, under-eating heme-iron for any reason, or those prone to iron deficiency.

Fiber

Dietary fiber is not digestible by humans, but some types can be fermented in the human gut by the microbiome. Because the absence of fiber does not result in a nutritional deficiency, it is not technically an essential nutrient, but it is an important part of a healthy diet and has many health-, fitness-, and diet-related benefits. In addition to possible heart health benefits and bowel movement regularity, fiber increases feelings of satiety. This can be helpful on a fat-loss diet.

Further, fiber slows digestion, which can help maintain steady blood glucose by decreasing the glycemic index of faster digesting carbohydrates during periods of lower activity.

Phytochemicals

Phytochemicals are chemicals found in plants. Although no phytochemical has been identified as an essential nutrient, some have potential health and fitness benefits. While research is still actively determining potential effects of many phytochemicals, there is strong evidence that many contribute to lower rates of cancer and heart disease and some suggestion that they can promote improved overall bodily function. While recommended intakes for most have yet to be agreed upon or set, you can likely get most beneficial phytochemicals by consuming multiple servings (a serving is generally defined as 1 cup cooked or 2 cups raw) per day of fruits and vegetables. Varying the types of fruits and veggies and being sure to include an assortment of brightly colored options as well as leafy greens will help ensure consumption of an array of phytochemical nutrients and their potential health benefits.

HOW FOOD COMPOSITION FITS INTO THE DIET PRIORITIES

The combined effects of all food composition choices contribute only 5% of potential fitness outcomes. This means food composition choices for any one macronutrient source will make only a percent or two of difference. Transitioning from terrible carbohydrate composition choices to perfect ones would probably result in barely notable physique and performance changes even over the course of months. That being said, the effects on long-term health of such a switch are much larger. Your long-term ability to pursue and cultivate fitness rests on the foundation of your overall health. Across a lifetime, the indirect effects of good food composition choices on physique and performance might add up to well over 5%. In other words, you can get in shape eating pop tarts and potato chips for carbs, but if you want to stay in great shape for decades, switching to mostly veggies, fruits, and whole grains is likely a better strategy.

In most cases, you can reap the full benefit of good food composition as long as you get around three-fourths or more of your intake from recommended sources of protein, carbs, and fats. Getting the rest from processed junk food will come at little or no detriment to your training and physique goals. This is because the value of good food composition is in getting *enough* of certain nutrients.

Once the required values of these nutrients have been met, more of them do not necessarily provide additional benefit. For example, if your fat intake is predominantly monounsaturated fats and you meet your essential fat needs regularly, some saturated fats and even a bit of trans fat intake from junk food occasionally has not been shown to negatively impact health, performance, or body composition. The downside of junk food is that it lacks these healthy micronutrients, so adding some junk once you have the minimum of all these micronutrients has no significant downside if properly moderated. Having some leniency in your diet regimen can relieve some of the stress of diet discipline and improve adherence.

Finally, when reviewing your diet program for food composition, it is important in any case to be wary of macro extremes. If an entire macro category is very low, perhaps at the tail end of a fat-loss diet when fats have been dropped to their minima, the food composition of the fat source begins to matter to a greater extent. At this point, it might be wise to supplement Omega-3 fats to ensure that at least essential fat needs are met. In more extreme cases, when fats are at their lowest and carb cuts are needed to continue fat loss in the final weeks of a hypocaloric diet, it is probably time to exchange the workout carb powders and white rice for more veggies and fruits so that your micronutrient intake remains at a healthy level. Vitamin supplements at this point might also be warranted.

CHAPTER SUMMARY

- Food composition describes the quality of food in terms of its digestibility, digestion rate, and the micronutrients and fiber content.
- The quality of protein is largely determined by the essential amino acid profile and its digestibility and, to a smaller extent, by its micronutrient content.

- The quality of carbohydrate is primarily determined by the digestion rate, or how quickly it can be absorbed into the bloodstream, and its micronutrient and fiber content.
- The quality of fat is primarily determined by the class of fat, and diets should generally prioritize monounsaturated fats, polyunsaturated fats, and saturated fats, in that order, while keeping trans fat consumption to a minimum.
- A well-balanced diet will generally meet all the daily micronutrient requirements; however, during hypocaloric periods and periods where certain macronutrients are deprioritized, a vitamin supplement can help ensure micronutrient values are met.

CHAPTER 6

Supplements and Hydration

The final 5% of dietary outcomes comes from a combination of supplement consumption and hydration management. You might be wondering why water intake, which is necessary for life itself, would be ranked so low in the nutritional hierarchy. Fortunately, hydration levels for best performance and body composition are very similar to those needed for health; most people fulfill these requirements intuitively. In other words, drinking when you are thirsty will hydrate you adequately for health and get you very close to your best fitness hydration needs. The degree of muscle gain or fat loss anyone attains on a diet has almost nothing to do with how hydrated they are (outside of extreme circumstances). Performance can be affected by inappropriate hydration, but the effects are only substantial with more extreme or consistent dehydration or hyperhydration.

Supplements share the 5% improvement margin with hydration because they have a similarly small effect on fitness outcomes. Many available supplements have no effect at all, and even the most effective ones have been shown to have an extremely small impact on performance and body composition. Using the verified supplement options appropriately can give you an edge that may absolutely add up to a significant difference in the long term (even a less than 1% improvement on each diet phase can lead to measurable differences across a decade). Because of their small effect size however, supplements should be considered only after you have thoroughly implemented the main diet principles and only if adding supplement use does not over stress you and decrease your adherence.

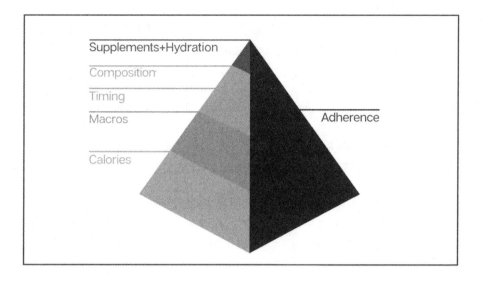

HYDRATION

Hydration is the degree to which the compartments of the body are supplied with water. *Dehydration*, *euhydration*, and *hyperhydration* are the states of having too little, normal ranges, or too much fluid in the body's compartments, respectively. Many trainers and nutritionists unnecessarily emphasize hydration as a top priority. Performance can be very negatively impacted if an athlete is dehydrated from a water cut prior to competition or a failure to hydrate before an extremely hard workout in a very hot environment. Under normal conditions, it takes fairly extreme mistakes in hydration to negatively impact performance, and even more to affect body composition. As mentioned, most people stay in a fairly euhydrated state just by drinking to thirst.

Preventing Dehydration

If an average person is carrying water bottles around and timing and measuring their intake precisely (not to mention using the bathroom hourly), they are not making the most of their time and focus. If you get your calories, macros, and timing in order and drink when you are thirsty, meticulously measuring water intake will not get you any additional body composition results. For those competing in sport or training under circumstances where a great deal of water is lost via sweat, thinking a bit more about hydration is warranted. By the time you feel thirsty, you are already slightly dehydrated; when water will be lost across a long, intense training session or during competition in hot weather, for example, drinking when thirsty might leave you increasingly behind in your hydration. In lab settings, testing urinary specific gravity can give a precise measure of hydration, but most people do not have a refractometer lying around. For the average person who happens to train in a way that results in substantial water loss through sweat, following are some options for the assessment and maintenance of euhydration:

Consume 1.5 ml of water per calorie eaten per day

Again, this is very specific and probably only necessary if one needs to be prepared to be perfectly hydrated for performance during hard training or competition. If you take in 2,000 calories per day, this recommendation means you would consume 3,000 ml (3 liters) of water per day. To put this in perspective for our readers in the United States, this means you should get about 5 oz of fluids per 100 daily calories. This is an average recommendation for individuals training hard under isocaloric conditions. If you are training hard while cutting calories, or in extremely hot environments, you might need more fluids. Using bodyweight and urine color assessments can help dial in these values.

Monitor Urine Color

When you are euhydrated, your urine should be light yellow like lemonade. Certain circumstances can make urine color a poor indicator of hydration such as rapid intake of large amounts of fluid or alcohol consumption. The best way to use urine color to assess hydration is to consider the average color over multiple hours and days. If you consistently see dark yellow urine, you need to drink more fluids daily. In contrast, if your urine is consistently clear, you are likely overhydrating.

Track Bodyweight

If you track your bodyweight regularly and are in an isocaloric phase, bodyweight can be an especially helpful tool in assessing hydration levels. Most daily fluctuations in bodyweight are from fluid balance. If you undertake a very high volume of training during any particular day, you can assess water loss by weighing yourself before and after that training and rehydrate accordingly.

Determining Degree of Dehydration

Dehydration levels can be classified by percentage of bodyweight change from fluid loss. Reductions in performance and increases in health risks are seen as dehydration gets more extreme.

1-2% = Mild dehydrations
2-4% = Moderate dehydration
5-6% = Severe dehydration
7%+ = Extremely severe dehydration

Following are the symptoms and effects of these dehydration classifications:

Mild Dehydration
- Thirst
- Difficulty focusing
- Mild fatigue
- Small reductions in strength and athletic performance

Moderate Dehydration
- Further difficulty focusing
- Further reductions in strength and athletic performance
- Increased risk of overheating
- Decreased sweat volume

Severe Dehydration
- Cramping
- Increased respiratory rate
- Decreased cardiac output
- Chills
- Rapid pulse
- Possible heat exhaustion (weakness, nausea, dizziness)

Extremely Severe Dehydration
- Dizziness
- Muscle spasms
- Poor balance

- Fainting
- Hallucinations
- Possible heat stroke
- Extreme body temperature
- Possible loss of consciousness
- Possible shock and coma
- Possible death

Though you may have heard of weight-class athletes in MMA and other sports pushing the limits of water weight cuts, we limit our weight cut recommendations to losses of 5% total bodyweight or less due to the dangers of severe dehydration. Above 10% bodyweight loss from water death becomes a realistic risk. For those of you dieting for other sports or for more practical reasons, techniques and supplements used to cut water weight should generally be avoided.

Chapter 15 will go over safe practices for water weight cutting up to 5% bodyweight.

Hydration Protocols

Pre-Training Hydration

Some degree of dehydration during intense activity is nearly inevitable because the average person can sweat out roughly double the amount of fluid that the gastrointestinal tract can absorb per hour. If you show up to hard training or competition a little dehydrated, you are already behind. Before training or competition, make sure you are taking in regular fluids and monitoring your weight and urine color to stay well hydrated. When daily bodyweight varies during fat-loss or muscle-gain phases, urine color becomes your best tool to monitor pre-training hydration.

Intra-Training Hydration

Around 5 fl. oz. per 20 minutes of hard exertion is a baseline recommendation for hydration during training or competition. This can be lower in cooler and less difficult training scenarios and higher in hotter and more strenuous ones. Consuming electrolytes with this fluid is highly recommended. This can be done using sports drinks or by adding electrolyte tablets or powders to water.

Post-Training Hydration

As we mentioned earlier, your GI tract does not absorb all the fluid you drink; about one-third is lost in urine. This means that if you lose 2 lb. of sweat during your training session, you actually need to consume 3 lb. of fluids after training to fully rehydrate. Rehydration should occur somewhat gradually for comfort and best fluid absorption. A general guideline is about 8 oz of fluid every 15 minutes after training until the required total is met. If the fluid has electrolytes or is consumed with food, euhydration will be reached more quickly as electrolytes facilitate water absorption. Drinking large amounts of water without electrolytes, especially over a short period of time, can cause a dangerous electrolyte deficiency called hyponatremia.

Preventing Hyponatremia

Hyperhydration with fluid that contains electrolytes will mainly cause bloating and excessive urination—uncomfortable, but not dangerous or extremely impactful for performance in most cases. Excessive intake of fluid with little to no electrolytes (pure water) can result in hyponatremia, a potentially life-threatening condition wherein you lose electrolytes as you urinate. Because the hydrating fluid in this case does not contain enough electrolytes to replace those lost with frequent urination, electrolyte concentrations in your body can become too low. This leads to problems in the basic functions of the skeletal muscles, heart, and nervous system and can ultimately lead to death.

The most common cause of hyponatremia for athletes in sport and exercise is hydration during or after hard training (where lots of sweating occurs and electrolytes are lost) by using only water. The probability of hyponatremia is increased with rapid consumption of water (think drinking 3-4 liters in one go). There is a greater risk for hyponatremia on a hypocaloric diet because less food is being eaten and therefore fewer electrolytes are taken in. This problem can be exacerbated by low-salt dieting—unless you are a salt-sensitive hypertensive or have another health condition calling for limited salt, there is probably no benefit to this type of diet. Unfortunately, the early symptoms of hyponatremia are similar to many other conditions.

Nausea and vomiting are common, as are low energy, mental fatigue, headache, muscle weakness, cramping, or spasming. Loss of consciousness and death can also occur. The best way to prevent hyponatremia is to drink electrolyte beverages during and after hard training and competition. If you drink plain water after training, keep the volume under around 32 oz (one liter) at a time, drink it slowly, and with food.

SUPPLEMENTS

Finding Effective Supplements

Supplements are diet additives consumed on top of regular food intake. They are taken with the explicit intention of enhancing body composition, performance, or health beyond what can be done with food. *The vast majority of supplements available today do not do anything to improve performance or body composition.* Many supplements claiming to enhance body composition and performance do not even have a plausible biological mechanism. In other words, given their chemical structure and human physiology, there is no hypothetical way in which they could exact their purported effects. It is, of course, possible that these supplements operate via mechanisms that are yet unknown, so testing for outcome even in the absence of mechanistic understanding is warranted. Randomized controlled studies can confirm whether supplements have any real effect. Many of the supplements (especially herbal and naturopathic varieties) on the market have never been tested in this way and thus have no evidence for their claims. Of the hundreds of supplements that have been tested, *only a handful* have been reliably shown to affect performance and body composition. Unfounded claims about performance and health benefits abound and entice dieters to spend money on unnecessary products. Though companies are legally permitted to make such unfounded claims, the food label on the packaging (at least in the United States) will bear the disclaimer: "This statement has not been evaluated by the Food and Drug Administration."

Because so few supplements have any effect at all, it is important to know how to choose the verified ones. The conclusions, history, and volume of research on a supplement should be considered. The more studies that agree on a supplement's effects, the less likely effects are due to chance or error. The presence of review articles summarizing data on a supplement with clear conclusions is a good sign as well. Repeated studies also have a better chance at representing the responses of more diverse groups of people—some supplements might have a larger effect on older people or one effect on males and a different effect on females. The more independent labs have tested a supplement and agree on its effects, the better. Longitudinal, or long-term, studies also lend credibility to results. Supplements often get more scrutiny over time and later research can be more careful and critical than initial, hopeful, published results. We recommend a research history of more than five years, the longer the better. Consensus is also important. Even if a supplement has a long history and many studies observing the same effects, a few well-designed studies with opposing results is enough to cast doubt on the former claims.

Another relevant factor in making supplement choices is real-world feedback. Lab tests are critical for confirming that something works, but long-term use by real athletes can provide equally important information about the practicality of the supplement. For example, sodium bicarbonate was lab-vetted, but real-world athletes stayed away from it because the doses needed to enhance performance ran a significant risk of causing volatile diarrhea. In order for us to consider a supplement effective, it must meet all four of the selection criteria: sufficient data, sufficient data history, consensus of results within that data, and real-world positive feedback.

Supplements That Actually Work

There are seven supplements on the market at the writing of this book that meet all four of our selection criteria:

- Caffeine
- Whey protein
- Casein protein
- Creatine
- Carbohydrate formulas
- Multivitamin and mineral supplements
- Omega-3 fat supplements

Caffeine

Caffeine is a sympathomimetic, which means it activates your sympathetic ("fight or flight") nervous system. This has some predictable effects, such as:

- Increased alertness and focus
- Increased pain tolerance
- Improved repetition performance and endurance
- Increased motivation
- Decreased hunger

Caffeine is from a family of stimulants that all carry roughly the same physiological effects. Though there are other food products and supplements on the market that contain other stimulants, the overall content is not great enough to have a significant effect. Furthermore, many alternative stimulants are controlled substances. Caffeine is available, time-tested, and FDA approved for your use. Caffeine in general allows you to train slightly harder in any given session, making it useful in particularly hard workouts, very long workouts, or workouts you are attempting when you are tired or hypocaloric.

Whey Protein

Whey protein is one of the naturally occurring proteins found in milk. It is one of the fastest digesting protein sources available and also one of the highest quality proteins ever studied. In fact, older scales of protein quality used egg protein as the reference value of 100 for "highest quality protein," until isolated whey protein came along and scored *over 100*. Whey's quick digestion rate makes it an excellent intra-training protein source. There are three main categories of whey sold commercially: whey concentrate (the least pure), whey isolate (intermediately pure), and whey hydrolysate (the purest). Whey concentrate is the cheapest by far and still very effective, so unless you have gastrointestinal sensitivities or cash to burn, it is your top choice. Isolate rarely causes gastrointestinal distress and is of incredibly high purity, but it is costly compared to whey concentrate. If you are very sensitive to dairy, whey hydrolysate can be used; however, the price of the supplement is often prohibitive.

Casein Protein

Casein is the other main protein (along with whey) that makes up milk protein. Casein is the exact opposite of whey protein in terms of digestion time. Even without any added foods, casein can take up to seven hours to fully digest and absorb. This means that delivery of amino acids to the blood is gradual and steady across many hours after consuming casein, making it a perfect bedtime protein option and a good protein source before any long period without a meal.

Carbohydrate Formulas

Liquid carb sources such as Dextrose, Gatorade, or Powerade are processed and therefore faster and easier to digest. There are also some very slow-digesting carb powders, such as Waximaize. Carbohydrate powders are usually very low in other nutrients, so they should not make up a large percentage of your carb allotment per day, especially during fat-loss dieting when fulfilling micronutrient requirements is more difficult. Fast-digesting options are excellent for intra-workout intake, however, and the data on the benefits of fast-digesting carbohydrates during training is extensive. Slow-digesting options can be combined with casein protein to act as easy on-the-go meal replacements as well.

Creatine

Creatine occurs naturally in the human body. In muscle tissue, it acts as a buffer for ATP (adenosine triphosphate). ATP is a molecule that stores energy derived from food and fuels nearly every cellular reaction, including muscle contraction. As powerful as ATP is, humans only have enough of it to fuel around one to three seconds worth of maximal muscle contraction at any time. Maximal exertion beyond one to three seconds–as is required by most training–requires ATP levels to be restored. The creatine phosphate system is the most immediate mechanism for this restoration (figure 6.1). The more creatine you have in the cell, the longer near-maximal efforts can be made in training. If you can curl 50 lb. for 10 reps, more creatine might mean you can manage 12 reps, and so on.

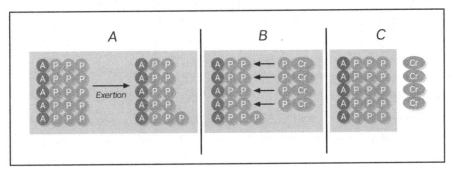

Figure 6.1 *A. Hard training depletes phosphates, releasing energy for training by turning ATP (adenosine triphosphate) to ADP (adenosine diphosphate). This process is indicated in the figure by the transition of APPP to APP. B. Phosphocreatine donates phosphates to the depleted ADP, and they become energy-providing ATP again. This process is indicated in the figure by the transition of APP to APPP as PCr (Phosphocreatine) donates its P. C. Creatine-lacking phosphate can then attract more phosphates to donate to ADP and repeat the process. More creatine in the muscle means more readily available energy from ATP.*

Creatine has been very consistently shown to improve performance as well as muscle retention and growth. Although the benefits of creatine are well supported, the mechanism for its actions is still unclear. The muscle growth and retention benefits of creatine may be related to cell swelling (which has been independently shown to result in hypertrophy) or workout performance increases, such as training at slightly higher volumes and intensities. Regardless of the mechanism, creatine consistently supports significant improvements in performance and physique outcomes. Individuals with more fast-twitch fibers (muscle fibers that lend themselves to power and strength sport performance) tend to benefit more from creatine supplementation. Vegans and vegetarians can also usually benefit more from creatine than meat-eaters, as food sources of creatine include animal protein, especially red meats.

Weight gain during the first week or two of creatine supplementation is very common. Weight gain can be as much as 3% of bodyweight. The increase in bodyweight comes from retained *intramuscular* water. Water added to muscle tissue tends to make people look more muscular rather than bloated—so nothing to worry about in terms of aesthetics, but something to consider for weight-class athletes. Water weight will fall away across a week or so after creatine supplementation is ceased. For some people, creatine can cause gastrointestinal distress. A proposed solution to this has been to deliver the creatine in chemically bound forms such as creatine ethyl ester. Unfortunately, many such exotic creatines do not seem to work as well as creatine monohydrate. Sticking to creatine monohydrate for the time being is our recommendation. If creatine gives you gastrointestinal distress, consider whether the trade-off is worth the small improvement in fitness outcomes.

Multivitamins

If a balanced diet rich in lean proteins, veggies, fruits, whole grains, and healthy fats is consumed, most nutrient needs will be met. At times when healthy eating is not as easy to pull off or calories are restricted, taking a daily multivitamin can ensure that you are not missing any nutrients. Essential vitamin and mineral needs are well established, and multivitamins can provide these whenever there is a risk that whole foods are not.

Omega-3 Fat Supplements

In the typical western diet, Omega-3 consumption is often low. Unless food sources of Omega-3 are eaten often (fatty fish being the main one), this mild deficiency can persist in otherwise very healthy diets. The direct research on Omega-3 supplementation shows health and cognitive benefits (though may not be correlated with improved cardiovascular outcomes as previously thought).

If you are curious about in-depth studies on other specific supplements, please visit Examine.com for continually updated, industry-standard research on all things supplement related.

CHAPTER SUMMARY

- Drinking to thirst is sufficient to meet most people's hydration needs, though circumstances involving high sweat output or exercising in the heat may require more deliberate hydration routines.
- Urine color and bodyweight changes are simple tools that can be used to assess degrees of dehydration.
- Excessive water intake, particularly without electrolytes, can lead to hyponatremia.
- The vast majority of dietary supplements have no supported effects, and even the most effective contribute minimally to fitness outcomes.
- The supplements with the most support for body composition, performance, and health are caffeine, whey protein, casein protein, creatine, carbohydrate formulas, multivitamins, and Omega-3s.

CHAPTER 7

Diet Adherence

Flawless diet adherence is not required to get results, but the more precise and consistent you are, the closer to maximum results you can achieve. Adherence can mean slightly different things depending on the type of diet you're attempting. On a fat-loss diet, adherence means staying within the allotted per-meal calorie and macro amounts, eating at assigned mealtimes, making healthy food composition choices, and taking any planned supplements. It also means skipping snacks and avoiding any off-diet eating. On a muscle-gain diet, the former list also applies, but some extra snacks, "cheat" meals, and less healthy food composition choices can be helpful in this case for maintaining adherence to the critical hypercaloric aspect of the diet with no detriment to results. Once you have a logical diet plan laid out according to your goals, adhering to that plan will make or break the final outcome.

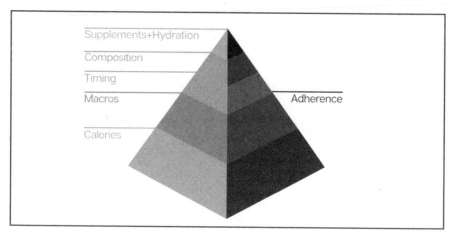

CHOOSING DIET PHASE TIMING

Diet Interruptions

It is important to consider the timing of your diet as this will influence the likelihood of adherence. If you have the freedom to choose your diet timing and are not constrained by sport competition, choosing periods free of social or travel obstacles is your best bet. In other words, do not plan your fat-loss phase during a period when you have weddings to attend and vacations to enjoy, and do not plan your muscle-gain phases when you will have little control over your meals or meal timing.

Sleep and Stress

When choosing to run a fat-loss or muscle-gain diet, maximizing muscle retention or growth respectively is critical. Lack of sleep and stress not only directly impact recovery and therefore your ability to retain or grow muscle, but they also affect your capacity to adhere strictly to a program. Dieting to alter your body composition is inherently stressful and difficult to do. Lack of sleep or additional stressors will sap your willpower. Choosing periods of low stress when you will be able to get regular sleep will greatly increase chances of adherence and diet success.

INDIVIDUAL TOLERANCES

Weight Change Rates and Durations

Precise recommendations will be discussed in chapter 9, but there are ranges of safe and effective weight-change rates and durations for both fat loss and muscle gain. The rate at which you choose to lose or gain will be based on personal preference for the most part. When making decisions about rate and duration of diets, the likelihood that you will adhere to this plan should be the deciding variable.

How Long and How Much to Gain on a Muscle-Gain Diet

Examining your willingness to gain fat before starting a muscle-gain phase is crucial. Set realistic limits that you will be able to tolerate. Some people are confident enough to handle months of being less lean for the sake more muscle growth. Others will break down once they have lost a certain amount of definition, end the diet, and disrupt their long-term body composition diet and training plans entirely. Knowing or honestly estimating what you can handle in terms of fat gain before you begin will help with both short- and long-term adherence to goal-directed diet plans.

How Long and How Much to Lose on a Fat-Loss Diet

You should honestly assess how much hunger and discomfort you can handle and for how long when preparing to run a fat-loss diet. Maximal results are always appealing, but maximum deficits can very easily lead to lapses in adherence, eliminating even minimal results.

Determining your limits may take some trial and error, but tracking your experiences at different weight-loss rates and durations can help you find your ideal parameters for maximum adherence.

A SIX-CONSTRUCT MODEL OF ADHERENCE

Any diet phase will have a beginning, a middle, and an end, and each interval will have its own challenges. Ideally, healthy and scientifically sound diet habits will continue beyond any single fat-loss or muscle-gain diet phase, so the "end" might be defined as both the final days of diet and the return to isocaloric weight maintenance and healthy living. The promotion of adherence can be broken down into six aspects that characterize distinct stages of the diet process.

The six promoters of diet adherence are as follows, in chronological order of their typical presentation during a diet:

1. Inspiration
2. Motivation
3. Intention
4. Discipline
5. Habit
6. Passion

We will define each of these and recommend behaviors that will maximize chances of success at each phase.

Inspiration

Inspiration is the feeling that first pushes you to start a diet. It can be positive, like being inspired by an impressive transformation photo on social media and wanting a similar result for yourself. It can also be negative, like seeing a recent picture of yourself and realizing how far out of your ideal shape you have gotten. Inspiration is what initiates the decision to make a change and begin a diet. This is a strong, emotional promoter of adherence at first, but it does not last very long.

If you are trying to use inspiration to spur yourself or someone else into dieting, it helps to understand that positive inspiration is more likely to result in effective adherence than negative. Similar to what has been found in child psychology, inciting behavioral change via hopes of a positive reward is often more effective in the long term than shaming someone into behavioral change. If you are trying to inspire others, leading by example is a good place to start. Even if using positive inspiration with others, it is best to be subtle. People should (and likely will only) change because they want to, not because you want them to.

Motivation

Motivation drives you to accomplish a goal and is a strong promoter for adherence in the early weeks of a diet phase. You might be inspired to "get in shape," but the motivation phase can only begin when you define what "in shape" means. Once you have defined your goal, keeping that goal in mind will promote adherence, especially once the initial rush of inspiration wears off.

Motivation is powerful, but can wax and wane, especially on a fat-loss diet when energy is low. Your morning coffee might have your motivation sky high, while an afternoon after a long day at work might leave it in the gutter. Keeping your goal realistic, yet challenging, with attention to individual tolerance (as described previously) can help keep the motivation to struggle ratio high enough for good adherence. Once a goal is set, giving yourself daily or weekly reminders of what you want out of your diet can go a long way toward maintaining motivation in the early weeks of the diet. This can include a written reminder stuck to your refrigerator, trying on a pair of pants you want to fit in, or occasionally peaking at a future competition roster and remembering why you set the goal in the first place.

Intention

Motivation works by giving you a clear goal to aim for, but aiming alone does not get you anywhere, just as knowing your destination on the map does not put you in that place. In order to get there, you have to get in the car and drive, and in order to reach your diet goals, you have to *create a diet plan and stick to it*. Intention is the application of inspiration and motivation to create a plan; you can think of it like the driving instructions on your directions app; it tells you what you need to do in order to reach your destination. If you have all the motivation in the world but no plan or no intention of following a plan, you will not see results.

Because intention supports commitment to a plan, the first and most important action you can take to support intention is to develop a plan. It is nice to think of losing 15 lb. in the next three months, but getting there requires that you determine exactly what meals you will eat tomorrow and the next day and so on.

Discipline

You must set your intentions to follow your diet plan, but your motivation and intention will not always be powerful enough to guarantee that you will adhere to it. To fill the occasional gaps between the high tide of your intentions and the low tides of your motivation you need discipline.

Discipline is the use of willpower to get things done. Willpower is finite, so you cannot use it all the time, but when your motivation is temporarily low, it must kick in. This promoter of adherence involves following the plan even though you may no longer want to.

Knowing when going into the diet that you will face times when you want to quit can help prepare you to be disciplined. Expecting things to get rough and expecting to have to be disciplined and use willpower on occasion is one of the best ways to prevent falling off the wagon.

Habit

Because willpower is finite, you cannot use discipline all the time without risking burnout. At some point deep into the diet, when inspiration has gotten you started, motivation has allowed you to define a goal, intention has helped you make a concrete plan, assuming you have been disciplined throughout, your diet practices will have become a habit. Weeks and months into a diet, habits form that allow your daily diet adherence to just be plain easier. Because adherence is easier, even your low motivation, low willpower days will be less a struggle than they were earlier in the diet.

In order for habits to form, good adherence must happen in the early phases of the diet. Keeping in mind that strict adherence will eventually usher in some relief from the difficulty of dieting in the form of habit can help motivate adherence early on. The weeks immediately before habits mature are some of the toughest times during a diet. To speed the arrival and maturation of habits, set up diet and lifestyle to be conducive to habit formation. Learn to meal prep and make it a regular practice that happens on the same day each week. Keep a regular schedule: train on the same days weekly and wake, train, and go to sleep at as similar times in the day. Have go-to sources of on-the-go healthy options so that you do not fall off track as easily. Once you have automated dietary practices, habits catch on that much quicker and before you know it, diet adherence something you do almost by default.

Passion

If you are working on body composition changes for long enough, usually years, you might get to quite liking the process of running a diet. Getting to create performance-supporting, healthy meals, reaping the fat-loss and muscle-gain benefits, and the very experience of having that much control over how you look and feel can be addicting. Many people grow to love the process so much, that they develop a true passion for it, which means that adherence stops being a concern almost altogether.

You can engender passion by choosing diet goals that are challenging yet realistic, sticking to your plans, and experiencing repeated successes. Every success will compound your positive associations with the dieting process. You can work on creative ingredient options for fat-loss and muscle-gain meals, focus on enjoying the challenges as well as the results, and connect with other individuals who have similar diet goals and mindsets. Fundamentally, passion is not a choice, and its development or lack thereof will depend on the individual. Making sure the goals you choose are for you and not to please or impress someone else can make its development more likely. The good news is that passion is not mandatory for success; although it does make dieting easier, well-ingrained habits alone can get you to nearly any realistic goal.

PRACTICAL RECOMMENDATIONS FOR ADHERENCE SUCCESS

Long-term thinking goes a long way in tolerating the acute discomforts of dieting for body composition. Focus on the final goal rather than temporary hunger on a fat-loss diet or extra fat on a muscle-gain diet. Another psychological trait that supports successful dieting is an internal locus of control. This means that rather than blaming external elements for any failure of the diet, you determine what you could have done differently to maintain adherence. Ultimately the success of the diet depends on your actions alone, and although roadblocks will inevitably arise, it is your choice to overcome them or not. Having an internal locus of control—feeling responsible for both successes and failures—helps you to avoid repeating lapses in adherence. If you blame work for being too busy for you to leave to get a meal or blame the airport for having no healthy options, every time work is busy or you have to fly, you will have the same problem. If instead you consider what you could have done to avoid these issues (keep a protein bar in your purse at work and pack some healthy meals for flights), likelihood of adherence in the future goes up with each obstacle encountered.

Finally, adherence to a diet depends in large part on your dedication to the proposed goal. Achieving the goal you have set for yourself must be more important than temporary pleasures like eating donuts (if you are trying to lose fat) or having abs (if you are trying to gain muscle). All achievements require trade-offs; the great thing about diet trade-offs is that they are temporary. Donuts can be a part of your life post fat loss in moderation without having to relinquish any of the lost weight. Abs (maybe even bigger ones) can be yours again after your muscle-gain phase is completed and you have moved on to fat loss and then weight maintenance. Learning to be disciplined enough to adhere strictly to a diet and reach your body composition goals makes non-dieting periods all the more enjoyable.

CHAPTER SUMMARY

- The ability to adhere to the diet plan directly influences how successful that diet will be.
- Do your best to plan dieting periods so that they are generally free from travel, competitions, or other obligatory distractions.
- When choosing the length and intensity of a dieting phase, realistically consider your own individual tolerance to the discomforts and unpleasant changes associated with that diet.
- Adherence begins with inspiration, then hinges on motivation, intention, discipline, habit, and passion, in that order. Taking care to cultivate each of these constructs as they become relevant during the course of the diet can greatly boost adherence.
- There will always be obstacles and challenges to adherence during a diet, but focusing on long-term goals and maintaining an internal locus of control can help you stay on track.

CHAPTER 8

Hunger Management

People eat for many reasons: for pleasure, out of boredom, due to social pressure, in order to adhere to a diet plan, and most obviously because of hunger. Hunger is an essential signal for the maintenance of life—busy people might forget to eat occasionally, but they probably never risk starvation, thanks to hunger. During fat-loss diets, hunger increases, so forgetting to eat is even less a problem—in fact, hunger can go from a reminder to a constant nuisance during a hypocaloric phase. On the other hand, on a muscle-gain diet, hunger can all but disappear, making it difficult to get in all the food needed for weight gain. In either case, understanding and managing hunger can improve the success of diets and the comfort of their execution.

FAT-LOSS DIETS—THE HUNGER PROBLEM

Hunger is a universally experienced drive, but some people are more prone to hunger than others. Those who grew up with less focus on nutrition and meal-timing structure or who have eaten poorly for much of their life will struggle more with hunger than the average person, especially on their first attempts at dieting. Hormonal fluctuations can also influence cravings. Habitual emotional eating will allow some people to break from their dietary restrictions more readily when stressors arise.

Bodies also have settling point weights and during weight loss, hunger will be increased to push back to those settling points. Settling points can be shifted, but only after months at a new weight. This means that it will take months after a fat-loss phase for the body to "recognize" the new, lower weight as normal and for hunger (even at an isocaloric intake) to diminish. Anyone who is running multiple fat-loss phases over time will have to face the pressure of shifting these multiple settling points. When someone starts from a very overweight point, each subsequent shift downward to a new settling point will be increasingly difficult.

Those with very low daily calorie expenditure (those with desk jobs, long commutes, and so on) will not need to eat as much and may face more hunger as a result. Many people struggle with low output, low intake days more than days when they workout and get to eat more. The very act of chewing more food can decrease perceptions of hunger even if the daily caloric deficit is equivalent.

Under hypocaloric conditions, both overall hunger (the body's signal that calories are needed) and hunger cravings (the desire to eat for the sake of pleasure) increase. Regardless, hunger will be greater under these conditions than during isocaloric dieting. Some of the most reliable ways to promote weight loss include bariatric surgery (which reduces stomach size and results in feelings of fullness from lower volumes of food) and appetite-suppressant drug therapy, both of which act by reducing hunger.

A secondary effect of constant hunger is stress. Warding off intrusive thoughts about eating food and sticking to your plan are difficult. Social events that might normally be relaxing can become a source of stress when you have to fight temptation throughout the experience. Stress can in turn initiate *additional* cravings. Adding cravings on top of fat-loss diet hunger makes adherence to a diet even less likely. Stress also causes the release of hormones such as cortisol which, when chronically elevated, can have negative effects on body composition. It is commonly believed that stress prevents fat loss, but the truth is that elevated cortisol levels increase catabolism of both fat and muscle. Any fat that is gained or maintained during periods of chronic stress is often the product of consuming extra calories. Assuming that the caloric deficit is maintained, elevated cortisol will more often consume muscle resulting in overall loss of weight and strength. Chronically high cortisol also interferes with the recovery and adaptive processes (as does lack of sleep which hunger can also contribute to). This means that the chronically stressed will see poorer performances in their sport and fitness pursuits. So not only does stress directly degrade body composition, it also reduces the training performance that would usually help maintain body composition.

Limiting the lengths and intensity of fat-loss diets (see chapter 9) can help prevent hunger from being as salient a source of stress. Hunger will always be present to some extent during even the best-designed fat-loss diet, however, so it must be managed as well as possible.

HUNGER MANAGEMENT STRATEGIES

Choose Higher Volume Food Options

After eating a meal, satiety can be signaled to your nervous system by calorie amount as well as by the degree of tissue stretching in the stomach. While planning meals with greater calorie intake can help you feel satisfied, this will negatively impact weekly weight-loss rate. Eating less calorie-dense foods that occupy more stomach volume can exploit the latter signal, allowing more weight loss while still feeling sated between meals (figure 8.1).

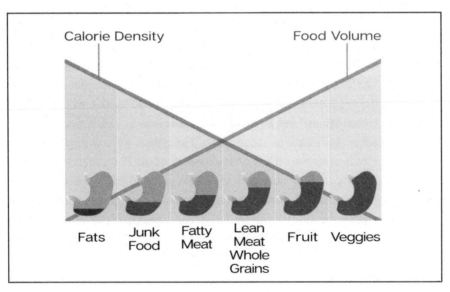

Figure 8.1. *Categories of food listed from left to right as lower to higher volume (food volume) and higher to lower calorie (calorie density). Note that the lower volume and more calorically dense a food, the less filling it is (represented by fullness of stomach images).*

Use the Food Palatability Reward Hypothesis

The Food Palatability Reward Hypothesis (FPRH) explains a very simple phenomenon: When food is tasty, we tend to want to eat more of it. Conversely, when food is bland or boring, we tend to have less desire for it. Though this may seem like common sense, FPRH's implications for dieting are underrecognized. Tasty foods are often calorie dense; assuming you do not eat more than your diet's daily limit of calories, these foods will often leave you feeling unsatisfied. This makes us crave more of that particular food. These cravings can be very powerful, making sticking to the diet plan much more difficult. There is something to be said for the famous advertising slogans of popular snack foods: "you can't eat just one" or "once you pop you can't stop." Similarly, appetizers get their name from the fact that they whet the appetite for more food. The tastiness of high palatability foods along with the lack of fullness from the portions allowed on a diet mean you are often worse-off for having eaten them. Limiting or avoiding highly palatable foods (consuming lower palatability ones) can make fat-loss diet adherence easier and more likely. It is much harder to overeat broccoli and chicken than it is pizza or cheesecake. Even a very tasty sauce on your diet lunch might leave you wanting more, whereas finishing the unseasoned version could leave you feeling full. Table 8.1 is a list of carbohydrate food sources ranked by palatability. Similar indices could be made for protein sources or whole meals, but carbs are an easy example.

Table 8.1. *Examples of foods that fall into general levels of palatability*

Palatability Index Examples
Low
Vegetables, Plain Oatmeal, Plain Potatoes
Moderate
Whole Grain Breads, Pasta, Rice, Beans
High
French Fries, Ice Cream
Very High
Chips, Cookies, Cakes, Candy Bars

If you compare table 8.1 to figure 8.1, you might notice that foods that are highly palatable overlap with foods that have high calorie density and low volume—so you can eat less of them for equivalent calorie amounts. Conversely, less palatable foods like veggies are also high volume and low-calorie density, making them filling, low-calorie options that can be especially useful on a fat-loss diet.

Increase Protein Intake

Research shows that of the macronutrients, protein is the most satiating. Some recent studies have even shown that carbohydrate-based foods prepared to look and taste like high-protein foods have higher anti-hunger effects than in their conventional form. This means that some of the anti-hunger properties of protein are perceptual or texture mediated. It is still likely that the molecular structure of certain proteins has an impact on satiety as protein shakes have been shown to have substantial anti-hunger effects even though they are liquids. Consuming more than the minimum recommended protein might therefore help with diet adherence. In order to increase protein intake while staying within CCH constraints, some other macronutrient benefits will have to be traded away, but if the result is better adherence, it is likely worthwhile. For example, raising the protein intake on a calorie-restricted diet for an active person might require carb reductions, reducing training energy and impeding recovery to some extent. If this means that this individual sticks to their diet rather than giving in to hunger, they are more likely to reach their fat-loss goals. Fats should be cut before carbs for satiety purposes, as well as for energy maintenance and recovery. Carbohydrates are not as satiating as protein on average but are more satiating than fats. Fats are highly calorie dense and highly palatable—they take up less space in the stomach and their tastiness can initiate cravings.

Bias Nutrient Timing

Even in the depths of a very calorie-reduced diet, hunger levels can vary across a given day. Many people are much less hungry in the morning compared to when they return home after the stress of a long day. These people are more likely to cheat on their diet in the evening. Such hunger can be managed by altering mealtimes and sizes. Eating smaller, mostly-protein meals with longer meal intervals earlier in the day and larger, multi-macro meals with shorter intervals in the evening can make adherence easier. If your hunger predictably sways in certain ways throughout the day, you can construct your nutrient timing around it to some extent. You might be trading off best meal-timing choices for comfort, but if this substantially increases adherence, the trade-off is again worthwhile. For example, hard workouts can reduce appetite for an hour or more by activating the fight-or-flight response—if hunger is really bothering you at other times, you might skip the small anabolic benefit of eating soon after your workout so that you can save more food for hungrier times. This is a good strategy when deep into a fat-loss diet or when hunger is strongest. At this point you might be eating lower carbs and be insulin sensitive at all times of the day, so moving your post-workout meal will have a lower magnitude of effect anyway. Remember that at best nutrient timing contributes 10% toward your results, so this effect is small, but still significant in either case.

Eat Higher Fiber Foods

Fiber is not a significant calorie source by itself, but rather acts as a hunger suppressant. Higher fiber foods include veggies, fruits, and whole grains, which already rank high for anti-hunger due to their high volume and lower palatability. The higher the fiber content in a food item, the more it suppresses hunger. Digestion of any other food consumed along with fiber will be slowed as well, increasing the duration of fullness experienced after any meal containing fiber. For example, chicken breast with white rice on the side might keep you full for a couple hours whereas chicken breast with fruits and veggies in place of rice is likely to keep your hunger low for even longer. This increase in satiety time may help save your willpower for other diet and life-related challenges.

Reduce Liquid Calories

Liquid calories are easy to consume in large amounts without getting very full and should be avoided when on a fat-loss diet. In some cases, even intra-workout shakes should be dropped, and those calories added to whole foods post workout to decrease hunger and improve adherence.

Drink Calorie-Free Fluids Before Meals and Eat Slowly

Studies have shown that people feel fuller when they drink fluid right before eating a meal. This can reduce the amount of food you eat when not on a formal meal plan and can make you feel more satisfied after a small meal during a structured fat-loss diet. Drinking fluids before eating stretches your stomach and increases fullness signals even before you have started eating. If you are struggling with hunger, drinking 8 to 24 oz of any calorie-free beverage before each meal can help. Eating slowly can also increase end-of-meal satisfaction. Signals for fullness are not instantaneous, and more time spent eating can mean more satiety by the time your plate is cleared. Additionally, the act of chewing might have some fullness-signaling effect, so making sure to chew food thoroughly might also increase satiety. Chatting with friends, watching a show, or otherwise engaging in something other than eating can help prolong meal consumption. If you can make habit of eating slowing and drinking calorie-free liquids beforehand, you will have a built-in anti-hunger strategy that takes hardly any preparation or effort.

Increase Caffeine Consumption

Caffeine benefits a fat-loss diet threefold. When consumed in a drink, like any other liquid, the caffeine source will take up some stomach space, making you feel a bit fuller. More importantly, caffeine is an appetite suppressant and so can actively reduce your hunger throughout the day. Finally, caffeine makes you feel more energetic, which can promote more movement (higher non-exercise activity thermogenesis: NEAT) and better training. These benefits as well as generally feeling more energetic while on a fat-loss diet can make adherence much easier. It is important to note that caffeine sources with extra calories (coffee with milk or sugar, full sugar soda, or energy drinks) will nullify these benefits for fat loss. On a hypocaloric diet, stick with diet sodas, energy drinks, and plain coffee with sugar-free sweetener or very low-calorie creamer options in small amounts.

MUSCLE-GAIN DIETS—THE FOOD AVERSION PROBLEM

In the quest for fat loss, hunger is your enemy, but when trying to maintain a hypercaloric state during a muscle-gain phase, it can be very helpful. Muscle-gain dieting requires us to eat more food than is required to maintain our bodyweight, which usually means more food than we might want to eat. Hunger becomes a precious resource deeper into such a diet phase. The human body is good at regulating drives (like hunger) to maintain homeostasis, so the longer hypercaloric intake is sustained, the less hunger will be experienced. Similar to the fat-loss diet temptation to eat more, those deep in a muscle-gain phase are tempted to avoid eating–this is falling off of the wagon in the context of muscle-gain diets. For those who have never dieted to gain, it can be hard to imagine a state in which you avoid eating, but this feeling during muscle gain is as real as hunger on a fat-loss diet.

While lack of hunger will inevitably come up for almost everyone at some point during a muscle-gain phase, there are factors that contribute to its likelihood. Some people just have baseline lower appetites for genetic, personality based, or even medication mediated reasons. These are the people who "forget to eat" when busy, and while this may sound blasphemous to some, individuals with this tendency do exist and for obvious reasons have a harder time keeping up a caloric surplus.

Another impediment to success on a hypercaloric diet is a high baseline energy expenditure. If you have any very physical career or high daily NEAT, achieving a caloric surplus will require that much more food. As discussed earlier, your body will push your hunger to match the calories needed for your current settling point. While you can move this point upwards, the further you get from your genetic settling point (your natural weight had you not been taking active steps to put on muscle mass), the more difficult achieving new, higher settling points becomes. At some point, (perhaps around 50 lb. beyond your genetically natural weight), you might have to eat more than you want to *just to maintain*. Consuming mainly junk food might be a strategy that allows easier consumption of requisite calories for gain, but in the long term this comes at the cost of health and to some extent acute muscle gain. Junk food tends to be very high in fat (usually the least healthy types), and exceeding fat intake recommendations means you might not get the small but notable benefits of higher carb intakes. Some occasional junk food can be helpful on a muscle-gain phase, but getting most of your calories from healthy whole food options is still best practice.

HUNGER PROMOTION STRATEGIES

Like excessive hunger, excessive fullness warrants some food choice strategies to minimize stress and maximize adherence. Following are descriptions of some of these strategies, which not surprisingly consist of the inverse of anti-hunger recommendations.

Choose Lower Volume Food Options

If extra calories are coming primarily from more carbs to maximize anabolic effects, you are already limiting the most calorically dense food you can eat (fats). Even in this case, carbs can come primarily from grains and less from fruits and veggies to reduce fullness. Within your grain choices, white rice and pasta are less filling and therefore more recommended than oatmeal and other lower density grains. As the muscle-gain diet progresses, making the trade-off of some anabolic effects in order to decrease carbs and increase fat might make getting your requisite calories a bit more tolerable.

Use the Food Palatability Reward Hypothesis

Highly palatable foods are less filling and tend to make you want to eat more of them—perfect for a muscle-gain diet. Altering cooking methods and seasoning can help make foods tastier and easier to eat. Some occasional junk food items in an otherwise healthy muscle gain phase can also be a good idea, particularly toward the end when eating is especially difficult.

Decrease Protein Intake

As mentioned in chapter 3, protein requirements for muscle maintenance are slightly lower on a hypercaloric diet due to the energy surplus. Protein is very filling, so dropping protein intake to as low as 0.8 g of protein per pound of bodyweight per day (the hypercaloric minimum) on a muscle-gain diet can get you the same muscle growth benefits with a bit less struggle. This strategy allows you to allocate more of your caloric budget to less filling options, easing the burden of overeating.

Bias Nutrient Timing

Just as during a fat-loss phase, eating more food when you tend to be hungrier can be beneficial for muscle-gain diets. Muscle-gain phases will inevitably require you to eat when you are not hungry, but moving more food to times when you are more hungry, or at least less food averse, can reduce this stress.

Eat Lower Fiber Foods

Due to the large amounts of food required for a hypercaloric diet, the risk of eating insufficient fiber for health are minimal even if you are avoiding high-fiber foods. Thus, when in a muscle-gain phase and struggling with appetite, swap out up to half of your higher fiber foods for lower fiber options—exchanging brown rice for white rice for example. You will still get plenty of fiber for your health but will save yourself some of the discomfort.

Increase Liquid Calories

Using protein powder, a carb powder like Waximaize, and perhaps some whole milk or canola oil is a great way to get in needed calories without chewing or taking up much stomach space. During and after workouts, combinations of whey protein and highly glycemic liquid carbs can easily increase your calorie total with the added benefit of fast digestion—ideal for meals around workouts. As long as most of your meals are whole food, you will get your needed micronutrients. Having some meals as shakes around your workout or at low hunger times is an excellent means of keeping you less overfull throughout the day.

Avoid Calorie-Free Liquids and Eat Sooner and Faster

The anti-hunger section recommended drinking extra fluids before your meal to stretch your stomach and reduce hunger levels. To generate more hunger, we take the opposite road. Avoid drinking large amounts of liquids before eating a meal. Fullness signals start being sent as soon as you begin eating, so your best bet for getting more food in before you feel full is to eat your food more quickly. This does not mean eating excessively fast and risking choking. Chew at a normal pace, but instead of taking a break here and there to chat, watch TV, or scroll through your phone, keep eating without long pauses until you finish. This way, by the time your stomach's stretch and calorie detection mechanisms have alleviated hunger, you might already be done with your meal.

Decrease Caffeine Consumption

As an appetite suppressant, caffeine should be minimized whenever you are struggling to eat enough. Even if you are so desensitized that caffeine does not suppress hunger, it can still be helpful to avoid or reduce caffeine anytime you are not in a fat-loss phase so that it can have a potent effect again when it is needed.

PRACTICAL APPLICATION

All these recommendations can be synthesized into a basic recommended protocol for dieting. The techniques for reducing or promoting hunger can be used in increasing amounts across a given diet phase. For example, at the start of a fat-loss diet, you might not be very hungry or tired quite yet. No need to drop to high volume, low palatable food and ramp up caffeine to a maximum just yet. Start adding these manipulations as the side effects of a hypocaloric dieting ramp up in order to increase your comfort and likelihood of adherence. For hypercaloric dieting, decrease food volume and increase food tastiness and liquid meals as you get fuller and struggle more to get all your calories across the diet. There is no need to incorporate the strategies from this chapter any more than is needed for your best comfort and adherence; these tools should be used to the extent that they are helpful, not fully implemented at the start of any diet just on principle.

CHAPTER SUMMARY

- Hunger management strategies can be very useful for both weight-loss and weight-gain periods.
- During weight-loss periods, strategies such as increasing protein, consuming liquids before meals, eating high-fiber foods, eating foods low in palatability, and supplementing with caffeine can be effective tools for decreasing cravings and hunger.
- During weight-gain periods, strategies such as decreasing protein to minimum values, increasing liquid calories, reducing fiber, and eating tastier foods can be effective tools for getting in all the necessary calories when fullness or lack of desire to eat can become impediments.
- A slow increase in the usage of these strategies across a given diet phase is wise— there is no need to use all of them at once or at all, they can be implemented as needed.

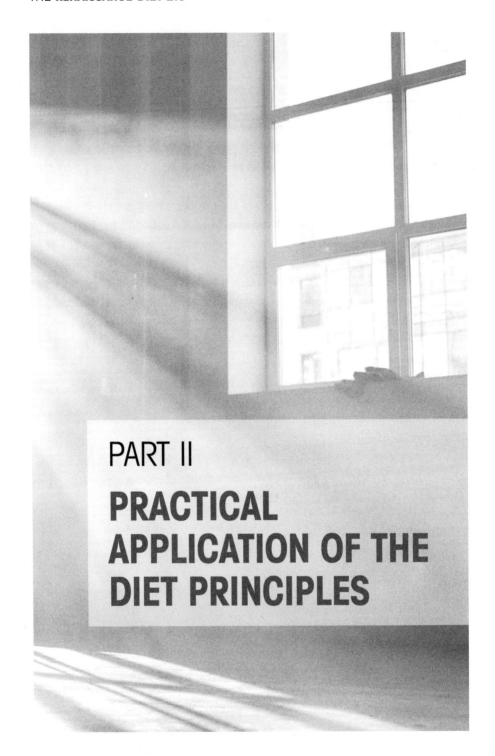

PART II

PRACTICAL APPLICATION OF THE DIET PRINCIPLES

CHAPTER 9

Nutritional Periodization

A periodized plan progresses in a logical, organized fashion with a specific goal in mind. Within the context of nutrition, periodization means that diet phases are not random, but rather they are strategic and purposeful. Periodized nutrition (as well as periodized training) is absolutely necessary in order to maximize the chances of achieving any long-term fitness goals. Before we can design a systematic, goal-oriented nutrition plan, we need to set upper and lower bounds for the rate, duration, and magnitude of weight change during the individual diet phases within that plan.

WEIGHT-LOSS RECOMMENDATIONS

Weight-Loss Rates

Weight-loss rates of between 0.5 and 1% bodyweight per week is likely best under most circumstances. The temptation in fat-loss diets is often to lose more quickly, which can be detrimental to sustained losses, muscle retention, long-term fitness, and even health. The recommended rates of loss increase likelihood of sustained success and maintained health, while still being fast enough to observe and quantify changes.

Weight-Loss Duration

Fat-loss phases are likely most effective with the least downsides when run for between 6 to 12 weeks. There are very few negative side effects of running a very short fat-loss diet (aside from not losing much fat), but since it is difficult to differentiate fat loss from water-weight changes until at least two weeks of data are collected, a low end minimum for weight-loss duration should be three weeks. On the upper end, between 12 and 16 weeks of dieting, chances of declining adherence and rebound gain increase steeply. By 16 weeks most individuals are at chronic dieting risk, and their chances of rebound weight gain is high. It is much better to lose 15 lb. during a successful 12-week fat-loss phase than it is to shoot for 20 lb. across 16 weeks, burn out, regain 10 lb., and have worked longer and harder for a what will feel like a disappointing failure. For this reason, although 16 weeks is within the range of safe fat-loss diet durations, we recommend 12 weeks of fat-loss dieting for most people. Setting fairly extreme upper and lower bounds, fat-loss duration should likely be done for no less than 3 weeks and no more than 16 weeks at a time, with 6 to 12 weeks being a more conservative ideal.

Single Phase Weight-Loss Limits

No more than 10% of total bodyweight should be lost across any single dieting phase. It is important to note that hitting maximum losses is not mandatory; the negative side effects of hypocaloric dieting might overwhelm some individuals by the time they have lost 6% of their total bodyweight. A slower pace and shorter diets can greatly increase the chances of sustained weight loss for many people. For those looking to lose weight across multiple phases, we recommend no less than 3% of bodyweight lost per phase (aside from perhaps the final phase if you have very little left to lose). The reason for this is mainly psychological. Losses smaller than 3% are not very noticeable and tend to demotivate people.

It should be intuitive that longer diets should be less aggressive to mitigate all the negative side effects of weight loss which develop in a rate-dependent manner. Recommended loss rates are between 0.5 and 1.0% bodyweight per week. Shorter end diets of around six weeks are better done with loss rates of around 1% bodyweight per week, whereas longer diets can be executed at slower paces. To attain our maximum total loss of 10% bodyweight, a diet of at least 10 weeks must be run in order to avoid exceeding rate limits. If you prefer to stay on the slower end of the weight-loss pace, around 0.5% bodyweight per week, the most you can lose within the upper end of the recommended duration of 12 weeks is 6% bodyweight— still an impressive change.

Reasons for Upper Limits on Weight-Loss Phases

Training Volume Limitations

Unfortunately, lowering training volumes on a fat-loss diet are not viable if your intention is to actually lose fat. High-volume hypertrophy training is needed to counter the catabolic effect of the hypocaloric condition and prevent muscle loss. In simpler terms, your fat-loss diet is telling your body to lose muscle, so your weight-training workouts must provide a stimulus to tell it to keep that muscle instead. As discussed earlier, the signal produced by high-volume training diminishes over time and will eventually be unable to prevent muscle loss. A low-volume, resensitizing training phase is needed when this happens, and fat-loss diets should not be attempted during low-volume phases or muscle will be lost. Thus a well-constructed lifting plan dictates the need for the limited duration of fat-loss phases.

Muscle Loss Risk

While limiting diet duration, doing proper training, and paying good attention to nutrition can prevent muscle loss during a hypocaloric diet to a great extent, these

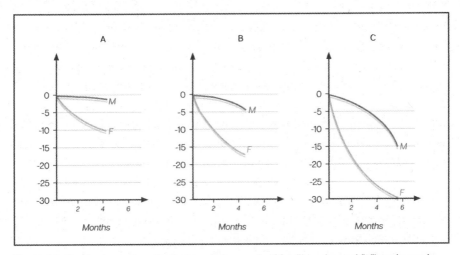

Figure 9.1 *Graphs show a hypothetical example pounds of fat (lines denoted "F") and pounds of muscle (lines denoted "M") lost across different diet paces and durations. A. When losing weight across recommended durations and magnitudes (up to about 16 weeks at a time, 10% bodyweight total), muscle loss tends to be minimal. B. Losing much more than 10% bodyweight in 16 weeks' time will result in much more fat loss, but much more notable muscle loss risk. C. As diet duration is extended beyond the maximum recommendation (appx. 3-4 months) and pace of loss is increased, muscle wasting becomes an increasingly larger concern.*

measures are not infinite in power (figure 9.1). Loss rates faster than 1% bodyweight per week or losing more than 10% of your bodyweight in one go increase the likelihood of muscle loss. This is especially true for those with more weight-training experience. More advanced lifters need to be even more careful about muscle loss in fat-loss phases.

Performance Decrement

If you normally perform at a high level in your chosen sport on 3,000 calories per day, a 1,500 calorie per day deficit is not sufficient for even minimal performance. Further, a cut of this magnitude will almost certainly result in muscle loss. Muscle loss will diminish performance even more and will result in long-term effects on performance well past the diet. This is a scenario in which your body is breaking down muscle tissue to support vital functions, leaving you weaker than you were before and at greater risk for severe fatigue. The longer you remain in a hypocaloric state, the more your body reduces energy output during planned exercise. Further, being hypocaloric for extended periods leads to accumulating fatigue which diminishes performance even further over time.

Health

On the extreme end of excessively long or harsh weight-loss periods, serious health risks, vitamin and mineral deficiencies, and the chance of incurring serious injury increase. These risks probably initiate at around 2.0% bodyweight loss per week or past 16 weeks of consistent deficit, depending on the size of the deficit, and increase from there. Also, at very low body fat percentages (under 15% for females and 5% for males), hormonal axes are thrown off and normal health is unlikely. For females, excessively low body fat results in a drop in estrogen production which degrades bone density in the long term. Health can begin to decline from excessive dieting even before these body fat minimums are reached. The high stress hormone environment of a hypocaloric state weakens the immune system considerably and the loss of muscle caused by other factors in long-term dieting also correlates with a decline in many other parameters of health.

Slower Metabolism and Lower NEAT

Body metabolic speed decreases by a small fraction during fat-loss dieting. The longer you diet, the lower metabolism falls. It is unlikely that metabolism drops caloric expenditure more than 10%, but that is still 10% less calories needed for weight loss, increasing the difficulty of maintaining a deficit. In the case of rebound eating, this adds to the amount of weight that will be gained as a result of extra calories. The human body is also very good at reducing its baseline energy expenditure when it perceives that you are starving, which is how long periods of fat-loss dieting are "seen" by your physiology. On an excessively long diet, your body can decrease total energy expenditure by up to one-third from normal conditions. This means that maintaining the same deficit will require a calorie decrease of up to another 33% compared to the start of the diet (on top of metabolic changes). This leads to even more hunger and fatigue, both of which reduce chances of adherence. As with metabolism decreases, substantially reduced calorie expenditure increases the amount of weight gained from lapses in adherence.

Poorer Sleep

The longer a hypocaloric phase persists or the more intense it is, the worse the quantity and quality of sleep will become. Hunger often plays an additional role, its presence making it more difficult to fall asleep. Sleep is important for health, recovery from training, and fitness improvements. Further, the growth hormone (a very powerful fat burner) is secreted primarily during deep sleep, making sleep critical in the fat-burning process. A lack of recovery due to poor sleep also increases chances of muscle loss. Running fat-loss diets to the point where sleep is impacted, therefore, begins to defeat the very purpose of those diets, increasing chances of negative body composition changes.

Increasing Stress Hormones

Stress hormones can cause increases in muscle loss when elevated for too long. Another unfortunate effect of chronically elevated stress hormones is that they tend to cause water retention. This can mean static readings on the bathroom scale for weeks at a time even if fat is actually being lost. Because water weight often deposits subcutaneously (under the skin), it is difficult to differentiate from fat tissue, which can make your appearance seem unchanged even when you are losing fat. If neither the scale nor the mirror seem to indicate progress, it adds even more psychological fatigue and stress.

Increased Hunger

As we have already seen, hunger is one of the most predictive influencers of adherence. If a diet is pushed too long or too hard, this basic drive will overcome the willpower of most sane individuals. Across a fat-loss diet, hunger, food reward (food tasting better), and preoccupation with food (cravings and intrusive thoughts) all increase. These factors powerfully multiply the chance for a lapse into uncontrolled eating. Even if a diet of excessive length or harshness is completed without a cheating episode, the radically increased hunger and food-seeking tendencies created by it will make the following maintenance phase exceptionally difficult.

Fatigue

As you lose weight, your body's ancestral anti-famine mechanisms kick into gear along with all of the already mentioned side effects of long-term dieting. High levels of fatigue also impact motor learning abilities. This means that if you are trying to learn new sports skills or sharpen existing ones during a long or harsh fat-loss diet, your ability to do so will be hampered. As people adopt a hypocaloric diet for weight loss, they often add extra cardio or additional training to help maintain a caloric deficit. The additional fatigue from the added cardio compounds the already high fatigue levels from the diet and regular training, ushering in the negative effects even sooner. While adding cardio on a fat-loss phase is not necessarily contraindicated, this is yet another reason to take the limitations to fat-loss phases seriously.

Accumulated Psychological Issues

Those who have dieted for fat loss themselves or have coached others through the process know that one predictable effect of dieting is dwindling motivation. All other factors aside, the monotony of constant restriction is taxing. Can you have pizza with your friends Friday night? Nope, it does not fit your diet. Sunday morning brunch? You have to order egg whites while everyone else has mimosas and tasty treats. Drinks with a friend going through a crisis? Alcohol does not fit in your plan. The lack of freedom to indulge at all wears on a person, and the effect is real and significant, even if they are still managing hunger, sleep, and fatigue well. Why does the diet-caged bird sing? Because it can smell bacon cooking as it looks down at its egg whites and dry oats. If you are that caged bird, it is best to end the diet before you succumb to lapses in adherence. Further, extended diets tend to be less and less productive as time wears on. If someone is eating less and training more, but seeing little results, they will often give up. This results in poorly executed maintenance phases and rebound weight gain. End-of-diet low energy expenditure and high hunger levels make rapid weight regain easier, so some diet motivation is still required to slowly ease into the post-diet maintenance phase.

Reasons for Lower Limits in Weight-Loss Phases

Inefficient Fat Loss and Psychological Fatigue

The main issue with losing weight more slowly than is necessary or in excessively small amounts per phase is simply lost time. Most people are motivated by progress. If they see weekly changes on the scale, in the mirror, or with how clothes fit, their chance of continuing adherence is higher. Related to the above point, the excessive time it may take to lose the desired amount of weight very slowly can wear on individuals. Hypocaloric diets are inherently psychologically and physiologically stressful and will always affect performance on some level. There is a lot to be said for getting in, dieting at an efficient but safe pace, and finishing up so that you can get back to living a balanced life.

Measurement Error

Excessively small losses are difficult to track as is achieving tiny caloric deficits day to day. Keeping bodyweight losses large enough to be measured week to week and calorie deficits large enough to be measured accurately day to day is important for any significant progress to be made and tracked.

WEIGHT-GAIN RECOMMENDATIONS

Starting points for weight-gain phases can also affect the proportion of muscle to fat gained. To some extent, the leaner you are when starting a muscle-gain phase, the more favorable your P-Ratio will be, with optimal starting points lying somewhere between 10-20% for males and 15-27% for females (figure 9.2).

Weight-Gain Rates

The best muscle gain rates can be generalized to between 0.25% and 0.5% bodyweight per week. This range allows calorie surpluses and weight changes to be detectable, but still keeps muscle to fat gain ratios in a favorable zone.

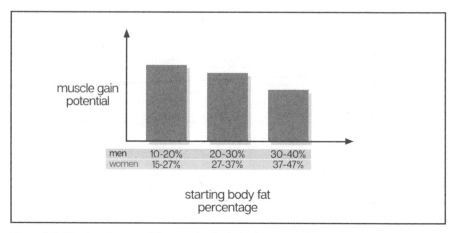

Figure 9.2. *Muscle gain potential at starting body fat for men and women.*

Weight-Gain Duration

Muscle gain durations likely to be most effective, but have the fewest potential downsides, are between 6 and 16 weeks. Gain phases can be run outside of this ideal range but might not be optimal. Our top end recommendation for muscle gain duration for beginners is a maximum of 24 weeks and a maximum of 16 weeks for more advanced lifters (who gain muscle less efficiently and are less sensitive to training stimuli). The absolute shortest duration during which a reliable measurement of changes in tissue weight can be made is three weeks, but this short a muscle-gain phase runs the risk of being pointless. Six weeks is a more ideal minimum recommendation as it allows for meaningful progress while avoiding many of the pitfalls of having too short a gain period.

Single-Phase Weight Gain Limits

Total weight gain during a single hypercaloric phase is also a factor to consider in your diet design. We recommend maximum total of 10% bodyweight gain for beginner to intermediate and 5% for advanced lifters across any single gaining period (figure 9.3). A minimum of 3% bodyweight gain is recommended as it is unlikely that anything less than this will alter the muscle settling point. Recall that best outcomes come from weight gain rates of 0.25 to 0.5% body weight per week, so take this into consideration along with total weight gain limits and diet duration recommendations when constructing your diet. Some simple math clarifies why a 3-week muscle-gain phase, while not entirely unproductive, is not ideal. Gaining the minimum 3% of bodyweight across 3 weeks means a 1% bodyweight gain rate per

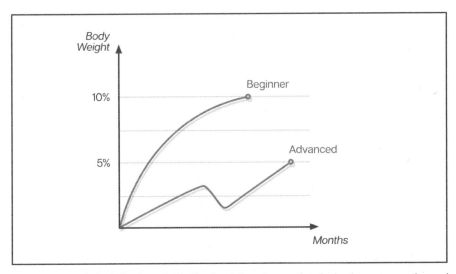

Figure 9.3 *Graph depicting hypothetical bodyweight gain over time for beginner versus advanced lifters.*

week–double the recommended maximum rate of gain. This means a poorer P-ratio (more fat and less muscle gained) than if the same 3% bodyweight gain had been achieved across a longer period. Finding a diet with a rate, duration, and total weight change that fit within the recommended ranges will yield the best outcomes and have fewer downsides.

Reasons for Upper Limits in Weight-Gain Phases

Training Volume Limitations

High-volume training is essential for efficient muscle growth, but over time the body becomes desensitized to its effect (figure 9.4). If one continues to gain weight after the body has become insensitive to high volumes of training, fat will become the primary tissue gained. An intelligent plan, therefore, typically incorporates an isocaloric, low-volume training period (at least one mesocycle; approximately one month) in order to resensitize muscles every three to six months (erring on the side of more often for more advanced lifters).

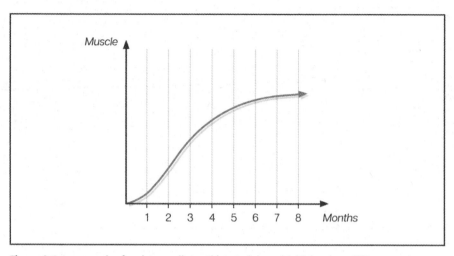

Figure 9.4 *An example of an intermediate athlete training with high volume lifting over time. This curve is prolonged in beginners and reaches a plateau sooner in advanced lifters.*

Decline in P-Ratio

The faster your rate of weight gain and the longer the duration of your weight-gain phase, the worse your P-Ratio. As calories increase to cause gains approaching 0.5% bodyweight per week, the ratio of muscle to fat gained becomes less and less favorable. Past about 0.5% bodyweight gain per week, almost all additional weight will be gained in fat. Likewise, once someone has gained 5% of their bodyweight or more in a single stretch, a growing proportion of gains will be fat. Beginner and intermediate may be able to gain at desirable P-Ratios a bit longer but will most likely benefit from staying at or under 10% total bodyweight gain per phase. Those with more experience or poorer muscle-gain genetics should err on the more conservative end.

Fat Cell Hyperplasia

If you gain large amounts of fat in one interval, either by gaining too fast, too much, or for too long, your fat cells can actually multiply (fat cell hyperplasia; figure 9.5). Once a fat cell exists, it is yours for life; you can empty it of its contents on a fat-loss diet, but it will not disappear.

Having more fat cells has been shown to make people hungrier on average and that much more likely to gain more fat at any time in the future. There is no appreciated metric for the amount of fat gain needed to cause marked fat cell hyperplasia, but the less fat you accrue in a single period, the more you will minimize this possibility. As fat cells multiply, so do skin cells; these new skin cells are generated to encompass growing fat volume. Excess skin can remain for years or, short of surgery, for life after weight loss. Limiting the magnitude and duration of gain phases avoids making future fat gain easier, future fat-loss diets harder, and prevents the formation of excess skin.

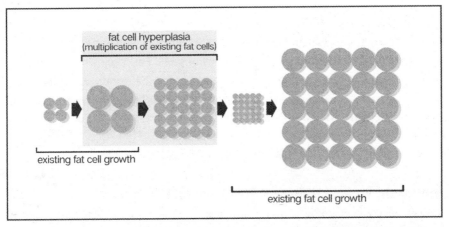

Figure 9.5 *Gaining weight leads to the growth of existing fat cells (depicted as enlarged circles of the same number). Gaining an excessive amount of weight can lead to fat cell hyperplasia–fat cell multiplication after maximum per-cell size is reached (depicted by increases in the number of circles).*

Performance Decrement

Depending on your sport, excessive weight changes, particularly excessive fat gain, can negatively impact your range of motion and ability to perform. In some sports, such as powerlifting, some extra weight might improve leverages for performance on some lifts, while decreasing performance in others. Too much extra fat can also push you into the next weight class and require larger totals to be competitive. For most sports, carrying around extra weight makes you less economical in your movement, can impede range of motion, decrease movement speed, negatively influence sport skills and techniques, and decrease your power to weight ratio.

Health Decline

A heavier bodyweight or higher body fat percentage can become a risk factor to general health and can lead to higher blood pressure, dyslipidemia, and cardiac and kidney stress. You might feel relatively unconcerned about these risk factors if you are exercising regularly and feel physically well, but they can cause problems in the long term. Minor health issues such as these can eventually prevent you from engaging in your normal training program and over time can precipitate more serious and debilitating conditions. In this sense, we want to stay healthy both for its own sake and for the sake of maintaining a fit lifestyle.

Psychological Effects

Very few people look lean and defined at the tail end of a muscle-gain phase thanks to the extra fat that comes with these types of diets. For many who care enough about physique to be engaging in muscle gain, this can be emotionally challenging. This is not true for everyone, but for a majority, putting a cap on weight gain can help with morale.

Reasons for Lower Limits in Weight-Gain Phases

Inefficient Muscle Gain and Psychological Fatigue

This drawback is mainly a matter of less time-efficient progress. Muscle is hard to gain, and the gains come very slowly, but keeping muscle while losing excess fat is much less difficult. So if you gain more muscle by being a little more aggressive in your weight gain, it is often worth it. Similar to fat-loss diets, a lack of tangible progress can also be demotivating on muscle-gain diets. Structured diet and training for muscle gain is psychologically fatiguing—slow progress compounds this.

Measurement Error

Some weight changes are too small to accurately measure or track. For example, if your goal is to gain 0.1% bodyweight per week, and you weigh 150 lb., after four weeks you should gain 0.4% of your weight or 0.6 lb. This is a very minor change that could just as well be attributed to water weight increase from hormones, stress, scale error, salt consumption, and even humidity. In a scientific setting, the difference in your weight would be deemed insignificant because you could not rule out these other factors, and even though your digital bathroom scale might show your weight to one decimal place, many of these instruments are not truly precise with weights this small. Similarly, gaining across less than three weeks or gaining less than 3% bodyweight results in changes that are small enough to be difficult or impossible to measure. Even if these small changes could be confirmed to be tissue changes, the percentage of the increase that consisted of muscle tissue would be close to insignificant and not at all measurable.

Following a diet for extremely small goal changes is equally difficult. Using the previous example, in order to gain 0.15 lb. per week, a surplus of 75 calories per day is needed. Consider this: The difference between an overfilled tablespoon and a normally filled tablespoon of peanut butter can be 100 calories. The error from this one serving is larger than the daily surplus needed in this example. Unless you weigh literally every gram food that goes into your mouth, taking the ripeness of apples and the exact cooking temperature of rice into account, it is simply not practical to have daily caloric intake precision to the nearest 100 calories.

No Settling Point Change

We mentioned earlier that muscle tissue can have its own settling point, such that once you have gained muscle, it is relatively easy to maintain. The two factors in settling point change are the magnitude of the weight change and the duration for which the change was maintained. If we put on a half-pound of muscle over the course of two weeks, it is more likely to be lost when we switch to a fat-loss phase. If we put on a half-pound of muscle over the course of eight weeks, the total change or duration, respectively, are more likely to shift our settling point and increase chances of maintaining those gains over a fat-loss phase.

Lack of Training Momentum and Muscle Growth Mechanism Limitations

Some of the biochemical processes underlying muscle growth take weeks to be completed. Many of the initial responses to training are neural alterations and realignment of tissues to accommodate new lines of pulling force and so on–non-muscle growth adaptations. During those initial weeks, resources that could contribute to more muscle growth are used instead for these prerequisite processes. Only after weeks of hypertrophy training will responses shift to being mainly muscle-growth related, so you are best served extending gain phases into this period. In addition to this, muscles take time to assemble new functional sarcomeres (contractile units of muscle tissue) and to allow satellite cells (muscle cell precursors) to donate their nuclei for more muscle growth. Termed "preparatory hypertrophy," this process is still being studied, but likely takes several weeks or more. Further, slowly building up to greater and greater training volumes and intensities over multiple consecutive weeks results in training that could not otherwise have been achieved. Such training stimulates levels of muscle growth that could not be reached across shorter periods of build-up. You must train for several weeks in order to work up to the most growth-stimulating training. If your muscle-gain phase ends before you can reach this more stimulating volume and intensity, you miss out on a large portion of your muscle-gain potential.

WEIGHT MAINTENANCE RECOMMENDATIONS

Maintenance Between Consecutive Weight-Loss Phases

The goal of maintenance after a fat-loss phase is to keep bodyweight stable and slowly recover from the accumulated diet fatigue. Increasing calories slowly as metabolism and NEAT return to normal allows us to maintain an isocaloric condition across the post-diet recovery period (figure 9.6). Once the negative changes resulting from the fat-loss diet have been resolved, another fat-loss diet phase can be started. Starting another fat-loss diet before a full recovery has been made can mean all the risks from hypocaloric dieting come up sooner and stronger, decreasing your chances of success and increasing your chances of rebound gain. The transition period after a fat-loss diet is as important to sustainable weight loss as the diet itself.

This transition from end of diet to full physiological and psychological recovery usually takes between two-thirds and one times the length of the fat-loss phase that preceded it. This period may be extended after more intense diets or after multiple diet and maintenance phases have been run consecutively. Individual variation also exists for maintenance duration needs. If you are more prone to cravings, have a history of weight gain or yo-yo dieting (dieting weight off only to quickly regain it), we highly recommend you make your maintenance phases at least as long as their preceding fat-loss phases. This means weight loss goals take longer to complete, but if the alternative is gaining the weight back and never getting to your goal, this is a price worth paying.

Recovering from one fat-loss phase before starting another is critical. Individual recovery needs to vary, so we can use some cues to assess how well we have recovered and guide the duration of maintenance. The pleasure of our eating experiences can be a very good indicator of how recovered we are from a fat-loss phase. If your bland diet food still tastes amazing and cheat meals or treats take you to a paradise beyond this earth, no matter how long you have been maintaining, it has not been long enough. If thoughts of food still dominate your day and you do detailed planning for your next indulgence a week in advance, you are not ready for another fat-loss phase. Once you are eating normally (mostly healthy options with some indulgent meals and treats sprinkled in) and not fixated on food or having addict-like tendencies in relation to it, you might be ready for another fat-loss phase.

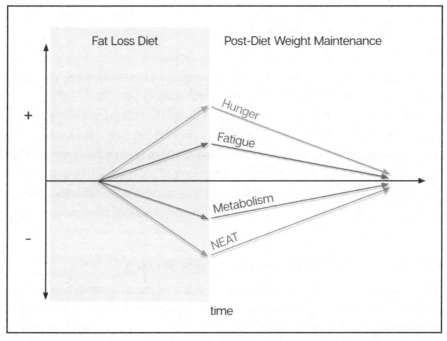

Figure 9.6 *A theoretical graph shows NEAT and metabolism decreasing across months of dieting, while hunger and fatigue increase. Recovery from these processes occurs across the following period of post-diet maintenance.*

Your weight stability is another measure you can use to gauge your readiness for another fat-loss diet. If your daily calories have been around the predicted amount for weight maintenance for four weeks or more and weight is stable, this is a good sign that you are fairly recovered.

Another telling sign is if after an indulgent weekend (once the bloat wears off) your weight bounces right back to the range it was in the week before. If you still have to restrict calories to stay within your maintenance weight range or gain and maintain a pound or two heavier from an indulgent weekend, your energy expenditure is likely not yet recovered enough to diet again.

Even if you are not exhibiting any eating behaviors indicative of diet fatigue and are maintaining weight at predicted calorie levels, we recommend waiting at least two-thirds the length of your preceding fat-loss phase before beginning another. The upside of saving yourself a few weeks in the long run is not worth the potential setbacks of insufficient maintenance.

If you find yourself struggling with maintenance phases, gaining back more than you should and requiring extremely long periods to recover from diets, you might consider taking a long break from dieting and making your fat-loss phases less aggressive. Many people believe that they must set the maximum goals allowable on their fat-loss journey. Popular diets, reality show fat-loss rates, and social media transformations show such rapid and extreme changes in such short periods that even the maximum realistic rates of loss seem slow. What is less often publicized is the abysmal rate of weight rebound gain in these instances. We cannot emphasize enough how important it is to be patient in order make weight loss sustainable in the long term.

Maintenance Between Gain and Loss Phases

After a muscle-gain phase, at least one month should be spent on maintenance before starting a hypocaloric diet. This amount of time allows for settling points to adjust and is enough time to run at least one low-volume mesocycle for resensitization to high-volume lifting. Strength athletes should spend more time in maintenance after a muscle-gain phase than those interested in only general fitness and physique. This is because expressing the strength gained by adding muscle takes more time and progression through low-volume strength mesocycles.

Strength athletes should wait a minimum of two months before beginning a fat-loss diet. Those who have a more difficult time gaining and maintaining muscle should also consider longer maintenance periods between muscle-gain and fat-loss diets as a longer maintenance period decreases chances of muscle loss.

Maintenance Between Gain Phases

Programming a maintenance period in lieu of a fat-loss phase between muscle-gain phases is a technique that can only be used by beginners who make it through a long hypercaloric phase without gaining a substantial amount of fat. Under these circumstances, dieters can program an isocaloric phase with low-volume training (for resensitization) and then begin another muscle-gain phase without needing to cut fat. The low-volume isocaloric phase should last at least one mesocycle (around 4-6 weeks). There is little detriment to a longer low-volume period aside from lost time that could be spent gaining muscle in the next hypercaloric, high-volume phase.

NUTRITIONAL PERIODIZATION

Periodization for Long-Term Muscle Gain

It is unrealistic to achieve most desired strength or physique goals in a single muscle-gain phase. For most people, this is a years- to decades-long project that requires periodization of diet phases to complete in a healthy, efficient manner. For muscle gain, 3% bodyweight in *muscle tissue* gain per phase is about the limit for anyone who is not a complete beginner. Recall that this is not total bodyweight gained, just the portion of total bodyweight gained that is muscle tissue and not fat or water. Overall goals to gain more than 3% bodyweight in muscle tissue should be planned over multiple gain phases broken up with maintenance and fat-loss phases.

As discussed, two of the main factors limiting duration of muscle-gain phases are fat accumulation and the need for low-volume training phases. A smaller but real concern is loss of new muscle in a prolonged fat-loss phase before the settling point has shifted. To account for this, there are two main periodization strategies for muscle gain. The more conventional of these is to program a gaining phase followed by a period of maintenance to establish new settling points and resensitize with low-volume lifting before beginning a fat-loss phase.

For example, with this conventional strategy, a 150-lb. athlete might gain 6% in bodyweight over 12 weeks, taking her to 159 lb. After a four-week weight maintenance phase, this athlete can run a fat-loss diet for 8 weeks and lose 4% bodyweight in fat, dropping her to 153 lb., ideally landing her at a similar body fat percentage to her starting point. That is around 3 lb. (or 2% of bodyweight) in muscle tissue gained across 24 weeks, an excellent result that an early intermediate might be able to obtain.

The second approach to long-term muscle gain takes shorter, more aggressive phases of fat loss called "minicuts" between multiple muscle-gain phases. The same example athlete gaining from 150 lb. to 159 lb. across 12 weeks would, rather than beginning a maintenance phase, immediately start a four-week minicut and lose around 1% of bodyweight per week before beginning another muscle-gain diet. The aggressiveness of the minicut will facilitate rebound gain, making it easier for her to gain muscle on this next round of hypercaloric dieting. In this strategy the athlete will gain a similar amount of muscle and lose a similar amount of fat, but across 16 weeks rather than 24. The minicut option does risk muscle loss a bit more than the conventional strategy due to the aggressive cut, but the eight-week time savings makes up for this and then some in a long-term muscle-gain plan.

For those running only a few muscle-gain phases or athletes whose training limits the number of high-volume lifting phases they can do in a given year, conventional periodization is likely best. For physique athletes or anyone who wants to gain as much muscle as possible over a long period, the minicut strategy might be beneficial. Long-term, traditional fat-loss phases and maintenance phases are needed occasionally even with the minicut periodization strategy. For more information on the structures and recommendations for minicuts, please see our *Minicut Manual* (available at renaissanceperiodization.com).

Periodization for Long-Term Fat Loss

For those looking to lose more than 10% bodyweight or who want to run multiple, conservative diets to get to a 10% loss, a series of diets with weight-maintenance phases in between is needed. One of the main factors that differentiates short- and long-term fat-loss goals is the presence of transitional maintenance phases between fat-loss bouts. If you run just one fat-loss phase, maintenance will consist of easing slowly back into eating more and then remaining in a comfortable, flexible state of isocaloric balance for life. When multiple phases are run, each diet becomes a bit more difficult and each maintenance phase requires more care and sometimes more time. Even when the maintenance between diets is done very well, some phase-to-phase diet fatigue accumulation will occur. This means the longer you have been running fat-loss and maintenance phases consecutively, the longer your maintenance phases will need to be and the more care they will require.

Imagine you are a 250-lb. person whose goal for good health and fitness is 175 lb. Your first fat-loss diet might take you to 225 lb. (the maximum 10% bodyweight decrease) over 12 weeks. You might be eager to continue your weight-loss progress and spend only the minimum of two-thirds the length of your fat-loss phase (8 weeks) recovering, increasing calories and maintaining.

Because a little weight increase is normal across this phase, you start your next 12-week fat-loss diet at 230 lb. Thanks to your leaner starting point and some residual diet fatigue, you lose only 20 lb. this phase. To make sure your third fat-loss phase is successful and sustainable, you might take a full 12 weeks to maintain and then start a shorter, 8-week fat-loss phase next. This time you drop another 15 lb. (down 7% bodyweight) and end at 195 lb. You have now been on your journey for a full year. One year and 55 lb. down and so close to your goal of 175. At this point, a prolonged period of maintenance (6 months or more) is likely a good idea before the final push to your end goal.

Over years of experience with hundreds of thousands of clients at Renaissance Periodization, we have found that individuals who try to diet, even with maintenance phases, for longer than a year usually end up losing steam and rebounding. For recovery to be more complete, increasingly longer periods of maintenance should be taken after each fat-loss diet in a series. Complete recovery results in a subsequent ability to efficiently lose weight and sustain that weight loss. Many find it frustrating to take this slow approach, but lifelong sustainability is worth a few months of waiting.

In our example, you might take six whole months of maintenance at 195 before pushing on to 175. Think of the months at 195 in this case as the highest camp prior to summiting Mount Everest. If we get to the high camp, rest for five minutes, and just rush for the summit, we are likely to fail, and often disastrously so. Our bodies and minds have not yet recovered from the climb or adjusted to the new conditions at this altitude. Life circumstances and responsibilities can be as unpredictable as mountain weather and such setbacks and delays should be expected—prefect progress is rarely made. You can see the summit from the highest camp, just as you feel close to 175 lb. while maintaining at 195, but please take our word for it, the rush is not worth the consequences of never getting to the goal.

CHAPTER SUMMARY

- The processes of gaining muscle and losing fat should be periodized—strategically planned and implemented.
- Weight loss rates of 0.5 to 1.0% bodyweight lost per week for durations of 6 to 12 weeks are recommended in most cases.
- Weight gain rates of 0.25 to 0.5% bodyweight gained per week for durations of 6 to 16 weeks are recommended in most cases.
- Maintenance phases between multiple fat-loss diets should generally last two-thirds to one times the length of the fat-loss phases that preceded them and may need to be extended incrementally when multiple fat-loss and maintenance phases are run consecutively.
- Long-term muscle gain strategies generally involve a cycle of weight gain, followed by maintenance, and then fat loss before repeating.
- Long-term fat-loss strategies generally involve periods of weight loss interspersed with maintenance phases until the desired body composition is achieved.

CHAPTER 10

Designing Your Diet

Now that we have covered the basic principles of diet for body composition and performance outcomes, we will go step by step through the process of building and adjusting your own diet.

CALCULATING CALORIES

As we have learned, calorie balance is the most important aspect of diet for weight change and performance. When designing a diet, the first step is to calculate approximate calorie intake needs. We recommend you design an isocaloric diet first, and then adjust for muscle gain or fat loss, if needed. Of all the elements that determine caloric needs, bodyweight and activity level are the most informative. Together, these two variables give us a sufficient estimate of daily caloric needs. After weighing ourselves to obtain bodyweight, we can categorize our daily activity across four general levels, which are

1. non-training
2. light
3. moderate, and
4. hard.

Non-Training Day

A day on which you do not do any formal exercise.

Light Day

Light day training describes most workouts of up to an hour long. If these workouts are done at room temperature, you will finish with a bit of sweat on your shirt. A light day workout is psychologically fairly easy, even if the lifts are heavy, because the workload is so small. Calories burned during a light day workout should be around 300 or less for most body sizes.

Light day workouts include mobility or technique sessions, individual metcons, small body part workouts (like arms or delts) for bodybuilding, or peaking sessions for powerlifting with most reps in the 1 to 3 range. Light day lifting workouts should include no more than 10 total working sets (non-warm-up sets). Recreational activities such as light hikes or long walks can also fall into this category.

Moderate Day

A moderate day training session should typically last one to two hours with minimal down time. At room temperature, your clothes will be roughly half wet from sweating. This kind of training is psychologically more difficult than a light day and average calorie burn is around 500 calories for most body sizes. These workouts might include a metcon followed by lifting, a lifting session with 10 to 25 working sets, and large body part training such as training back, chest, legs, or push or pull workouts.

Hard Day

A hard training day session will typically take more than two hours. In room temperature, this workout will leave your clothes soaked in sweat. Calories burned will be around 1,000 for most body sizes. Such workouts are psychologically challenging and can include workouts with more than 25 working sets, highly voluminous workouts for lower body or whole body, and workouts that combine strength, weightlifting, metcons, and volume work in the same session.

Table 10.1 contains maintenance calorie estimates for bodyweight ranges and categories of activity. These initial estimates need not be perfect as once you start tracking your weight you can use that data to adjust the diet and determine more precise maintenance calories amounts.

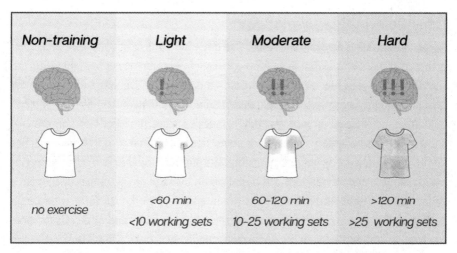

Figure 10.1 *Quick guide to classifying your day as non-training, light, moderate, or hard. Going from no training to hard training; psychological difficulty, sweat production, amount of time spent training, and working sets for lifting sessions increase.*

Table 10.1 *This table shows estimated daily isocaloric calorie needs for by bodyweight for non-training, light training, moderate training, and hard training days. These estimates are averages based on data collected from subjects of different sizes engaged in various levels of activity. The calorie recommendations here are good starting points for designing a weight maintenance diet but should be adjusted based on the dieter's weight change results.*

Bodyweight (lb.)	Approximate Weight-Maintenance Calorie Needs			
	Non-training Day	Light Day	Moderate Day	Hard Day
100-115	1300	1500	1700	1900
116-130	1500	1700	1900	2100
131-145	1700	1900	2100	2300
146-160	1800	2000	2250	2450
161-175	1900	2100	2400	2600
176-190	1950	2200	2500	2750
191-210	2000	2300	2600	2900
211-230	2150	2500	2800	3100
231-250	2300	2700	3000	3300
251-275	2500	2900	3250	3600
276-300	2700	3100	3500	3900

Daily Calorie Need Variability

Not all non-training days are the same. One day you might sit at your work desk, then go home at night and watch movies on your couch. Another day you might visit a job site and be on your feet all day, then go on a date in the evening and walk on the beach for hours. These two example non-training days require very different calorie amounts, and increasing your rest day calories to meet the needs of non-exercise activity can be necessary. Similarly, training does not come in only three volumes (light, moderate, hard); in reality, caloric output for training is a spectrum. Our listed calorie recommendations are based on an average of the ranges within each classification. These recommendations are intended to work well for a wide range of dieters. If you know you tend to err on the higher or lower end of a classification, tracking weight and adjusting calories accordingly—which we will cover shortly—can dial your diet in.

It is well established that most people overestimate the number of calories they burn, so when assessing your workouts, read the listed criteria and examples for light, moderate, and hard days and make sure that your workout fits all of the points for the classification. When preparing for a fat-loss diet, err on the side of the lighter classification if you are unsure. If you end up losing a little too fast, adding more food is an easy solution. If you need to gain weight, erring on the side of the harder workout category is a good way to prevent any wasted time maintaining weight. Again, misjudgments can be fixed quickly with food reductions if you find yourself gaining too fast.

Example Calorie Assignment

As we walk through the steps of creating your own diet, we will use the following example for a 155-lb. female starting a fat-loss diet and doing physique-based weight training. We will begin by calculating her calorie needs for maintenance based on her weight and workout schedule:

Mon, Wed, Fri: 2.5 hours of training consisting of a cardio warm-up and 30 working sets.
Tues, Thurs: 1.5 hours of training consisting of a cardio warm-up and 15 working sets.
Sat, Sun: Rest/no training.

Using figure 10.1 to classify training days and table 10.1 to determine caloric needs according to her weight and activity, our example's daily caloric intake should look like this for weight maintenance:

Mon, Wed, Fri: 2,450 calories (hard training day).
Tues, Thurs: 2,250 calories (moderate training day).
Sat, Sun: 1,800 calories (non-training day).

Once calories have been determined, the next most important diet principle can be applied within those caloric constraints: macronutrients.

CALCULATING MACROS

Now that we have determined daily calories for maintenance, we can allocate macronutrients based on these values. To do this we must first determine ideal ratios of each macronutrient and calculate trade-offs between them to assign appropriate amounts within the calorie constraint.

Protein Calculations

Because protein is generally the most important macronutrient for body composition and performance, you should calculate protein needs first when assigning macronutrients for your diet. The recommendations on protein from chapter 3 indicate that 1 g of protein per pound of bodyweight per day is a good recommendation for those engaging in general resistance training. Thus, we will set protein intake for our 155-lb. female example at 155 g per day.

Carbohydrate Calculations

As discussed in chapter 3, there are ranges of recommended carbohydrate intake depending on sport. Differing training phases and differing days will require different daily carbohydrate amounts. For any type of athlete or fitness enthusiast, daily recommendations should fall within the recommended average ranges but be tuned up or down according to daily activity levels.

Table 10.2 lists minimum and recommended starting carb intake for weight maintenance.

Table 10.2 *Recommended starting carbs for each daily training classification.*

Training	Carb Intake Minima (per lb. per day)	Recommended Starting Carbs (per lb. per day)
Non-training day	0.3 g	0.5 g
Light day	0.5 g	1.0 g
Moderate day	1.0 g	1.5 g
Hard day	1.5 g	2.0 g

We recommend you not go any lower than the minimum values when putting together your maintenance diet. On the other hand, programming more carbs is fine as long as your protein and minimum fat needs are being met. The recommended carbohydrate amounts in the far-right column are a good place to start.

Fat Calculations

Once you have calculated your protein and carbs, your fat calculations are already done—you can simply allot the remaining calories to fat. For example, a non-training day for our 155-lb. female using the recommended starting carb intakes is as follows:

Her protein intake is 155 g and because protein has 4 calories per gram, this means she gets 620 calories from protein. Her carb intake is 155 lb. x 0.5 g carbs = 77.5 g. At 4 calories per gram this gives her 310 calories from carbs. Total calories so far without fats added are 620 calories from protein + 310 calories from carbs = 930 calories. Since our 155-lb. example gets 1,800 calories on a non-training day, 1800 - 930 = 870 calories remaining for approximately 97 g of fat (recall that fat contains 9 calories per gram).

Always double-check that your final fat calculations amount to at least 0.3 g of fat per pound of bodyweight per day so that health is supported. If your diet calculations have left you with less than your minimum fat needs, reassess and move some calories from carbs to fats.

Calculating Trade-Offs Between Macros

Fitness enthusiasts who do not compete have a bit more leeway for preference when choosing how to distribute calories between fats and carbs. Leaning toward the lower end of recommended carb intake and increasing fats is an option if they prefer. Some athletes need to continue to perform at a high level even during non-competition training and cannot sacrifice as much performance for weight-loss progress as those interested in fitness for fitness sake. If your training demands higher performance even on a fat-loss diet, biasing more calories toward carbs on training days at the cost of fats can be a good strategy. Imagine that the latter is the case for our example athlete. To figure out the maximum carb amount for her on a hard day, we would start with her calorie and protein needs and the minimum fat allowance (from chapter 3). This way we can maximize the amount of carbohydrate she consumes without going below recommended protein or minimum fat.

Total calorie allotment: 2,450

Total protein needed: 155 g
155 g of protein x 4 calories/gram of protein = 620 calories from protein

Minimum fat intake: 0.3 g per pound of bodyweight per day
155 lb. x 0.3 = 46.5 g of fat per day
46.5 g of fat x 9 calories/gram of fat = approx. 420 calories from fat

Fat + protein calories: 420 + 620 = 1,040 calories

Total calories minus those used for fat and protein: 2,450 − 1,040 = 1,410 **calories remaining**
1,410 calories ÷ 4 calories/gram of carbs = approx. 350 g of carbs per day (or roughly 2.3 g of carbs per pound of bodyweight per day)

Thus approximately 350 g of carbs per hard training day is the maximum carb intake for our example that will still allow her get enough protein and fats to support vital function, composition, and performance. If you have no pressing needs for performance during a fat-loss diet, start at the recommended carbohydrate values from table 10.2. From there, you can adjust carbs within the minimum to maximum range according to preference as long as you keep daily calories constant by adjusting fats as well. Taking the recommended carb amounts for our 155-lb. example, we can come up with macros for every day of the week, as shown in table 10.3.

Table 10.3 *Daily calorie and macros assigned based on the weight and activity level of our example athlete*

Day	Category	Calories	Protein (g)	Carb Need	Carbs (g)	Fats (g)
M, W, F	Hard	2,450	155	2x155	~310	~65
Tu, Th	Moderate	2,250	155	1.5x155	~230	~80
Sa, Su	Non-Training	1,800	155	0.5x155	~80	~100

Note: If you are a serious endurance athlete, please see chapter 14 for more detailed information on assigning carbohydrates for competition. If you are an advanced dieter, you can adjust protein intake based on the guidelines in chapter 3 for hypocaloric versus hypercaloric diets and training type. If you train more than once per day, err on the side of more carbs within CCH for best recovery and see chapter 13 for more details on multiple daily training sessions.

DETERMINING MEAL CONTENT AND TIMING

The following step-by-step process will help you stay within meal and macronutrient timing recommendations based on your schedule (while suiting your preferences when possible):

- Choose meal number.
- Assign morning and bedtime meals.
- Schedule pre- and post-workout meals.
- Adjust protein content to meal intervals.
- Adjust carbs to training times.
- Adjust fats away from training times.
- Consider an intra-workout shake.

Walking through these steps with our 155-lb. example:

1. Choose meal number.

As discussed in chapter 4, four to six meals per day is the best intersection of physiological ease and real-world feasibility for adherence. If you train more than once per day, we recommend erring on the side of more meals since you need pre- and post-workout fuel for each training session. For our example athlete, we will use a five meal per day schedule.

2. Assign morning and bedtime meals.

When you wake, you are in a fasted state which is highly catabolic to muscle tissue and does not support recovery. Eating as soon as possible after getting up in the morning is recommended, so we can schedule the first meal within an hour of waking. Likewise, to limit the amount of time that our bodies are in a fasted state while sleeping, eating right before bed is helpful. We will schedule the last meal of the day within an hour before bed. Table 10.4 shows our example athlete's schedule as well as her morning and bedtime meals assigned according to her wake and sleep times. We will use her hard days as our first example.

Table 10.4 *Setting up meal timing. The first step is to assign first and bedtime meals to soon after waking and right before sleep, respectively. The shaded cells highlight new additions to the diet program as we make them.*

Example Schedule:

	MON	TUES	WED	THURS	FRI	SAT	SUN
Wake time	7:00am	7:00am	7:00am	7:00am	7:00am	9:00am	9:00am
Training time	5:00pm	5:00pm	5:00pm	5:00pm	5:00pm	N/A	N/A
Bedtime	11:00pm	11:00pm	11:00pm	11:00pm	11:00pm	11:00pm	11:00pm

(continued)

(continued)

Meal Number	Hard Day Mealtimes	Non-Training Day Mealtimes
1	7:30am	9:30am
2		
3		
4		
5	10:00pm	10:00pm

3. Schedule pre- and post-workout nutrition.

Pre- and post-workout meals must be placed strategically around training to support best results. A pre-workout meal should be consumed at least 30 minutes before training to prevent gastrointestinal distress, but no more than 4 hours before for energy supply and anti-catabolism. To prevent workout-induced muscle loss and support recovery, the post-workout meal should be eaten within an hour after training. Table 10.5 shows this timing based on the athlete's 5 pm training time.

Table 10.5 *Setting up meal timing. After assigning waking and bedtime meals, pre- and post-training meals should be assigned. The shaded cells highlight new additions to the diet program as we make them.*

Meal Number	Hard Day Mealtimes	Non-Training Day Mealtimes
1	7:30am	9:30am
2		
3	3:00pm (pre-training meal)	
4	7:30pm (post-training meal)	
5	10:00pm	10:00pm

Now that we only have one meal left to fill in for training days, the timing is simple. We need to spread our protein as evenly as we can, so placing meal 2 evenly between 7:30am and 3:00pm (around 11:00-11:30 am) is a great option. A real world job might mean that our athlete has lunch break at 12 pm. Fortunately, placing her second meal at 12 pm does not mean an extended (over 5 hour) meal interval. Since 12 pm will be more convenient, it will likely be better for adherence and has no downsides.

For her non-training weekend days, meal timing is just a matter of evenly distributing meals, with perhaps a small bias towards more meals and smaller intervals at times when our athlete is hungrier. For example, if she tends to get hungrier at night, we can space meals 1 and 2 four hours apart, meals 2 and 3 three and a half hours apart and the remaining meals three hours apart. This will make evening hunger less difficult to deal with, improving adherence. This is shown in Table 10.6.

Table 10.6 *Setting up meal timing. After assigning waking, bedtime, pre-, and post-training meals; remaining meals can be programmed keeping intermeal intervals in mind. On rest days these remaining meals will include all meals aside from waking and bedtime meals since there is no training. The shaded cells highlight new additions to the diet program as we make them.*

Meal Number	Hard Day Meal Times		Non-Training Day Mealtimes
1	7:30am		9:30am
2	12:00pm		1:30pm
3	3:00pm (pre-training meal)		5:00pm
4	7:30pm (post-training meal)		8:00pm
5	10:00pm		10:00pm

4. Adjust protein content to meal intervals.

Spreading your total protein intake evenly across meals makes food preparation much easier, so in most cases this is the best option. We can take the approximately 155 g of protein that our athlete needs and divide across five meals, giving us 31 g. To keep things simple and give a few more grams of protein at bedtime, when the meal interval will be longer, we can assign 30 g to meals 1 through 4 and 35 g to the evening meal. This is shown in table 10.7.

Another option, though one that makes cooking and planning a little more complicated, is to add some protein to meals before longer meal intervals, taking it from meals before shorter intervals. It is also possible to find the per-hour protein needs and assign exact grams of protein per meal according to exact meal interval. Again, this is unnecessarily complicated in most cases. It might come in handy for those who are awake for 24 hours at a time or have otherwise odd schedules or more extreme meal spacing.

Table 10.7 *Assigning protein to individual meals. Protein can be distributed evenly in most cases (unless intermeal intervals are less than 3 hours or more than 6 hours, which warrants smaller or larger amounts of protein per meal, respectively). In the case of extreme meal timing (not shown here) hourly protein needs can be calculated to support shorter or longer intermeal intervals. The shaded cells highlight new additions to the diet program as we make them.*

Meal Number	Hard Day Mealtime	Protein/Meal (155 g total)	Non-Training Day Mealtime	Protein/Meal (155 g total)
1	7:30am	30 g	9:30am	30 g
2	12:00pm	30 g	1:30pm	30 g
3	3:00pm (pre-training)	30 g	5:00pm	30 g
4	7:30pm (post-training)	30 g	8:00pm	30 g
5	10:00pm	35 g	10:00pm	35 g

5. Adjust carbs to training times.

Carbohydrate distribution should be biased toward meals in the workout window. Table 10.8 gives some basic estimates to start with.

Table 10.8 *Assigning carbohydrate to individual meals should take training into consideration, with more carbs assigned around training. Suggested percentages of daily carbs are listed for different daily meal number options.*

4 meals per day	
Pre-workout meal	25% daily carbs
Post-workout meal	35% daily carbs
Bedtime meal	25% daily carbs
Remainder	15% carbs to remaining one meal
5 meals per day	
Pre-workout meal	20% daily carbs
Post-workout meal	30% daily carbs
Bedtime meal	20% daily carbs
Remainder	30% spread across remaining two meals

6 meals per day (1x daily workout)	
Pre-workout meal	18% daily carbs
Post-workout meal	25% daily carbs
Bedtime meal	18% daily carbs
Remainder	39% spread across remaining three meals

The exact distribution can be amended if you train earlier or later in the day, but these are good, rough estimates to start with. There is also room here to make modifications for convenience. For example, measuring carb amounts such as 50 g, 50 g, 25 g, 25 g, will be easier than something like 61 g, 48 g, 22 g, 19 g when preparing meals and the difference in effect is insignificant. If we take the information from Table 10.8 and use it to distribute "hard day" carbs (310 g carb allotment), we can fill in carb amounts for training day meals in our example. This is shown in table 10.9.

Table 10.9 *Assigning carbohydrates to meals for hard training days. Using table 10.8, we calculate grams of carbs per meal for our example athlete. The shaded cells highlight new additions to the diet program as we make them.*

Meal Number	Hard Day Mealtime	Protein/Meal (155 g total)	Carbs/Meal (310 g total)
1	7:30am	30 g	~15%: 45 g
2	12:00pm	30 g	~15%: 45 g
3	3:00pm (pre-training)	30 g	~20%: 65 g
4	7:30pm (post-training)	30 g	~30%: 95 g
5	10:00pm	35 g	~20%: 60g

For non-training days, carbs are distributed evenly across all meals or across a few meals at times when hunger is worse. We know from her macro calculations that our athlete gets approximately 80 g of carbs on non-training days. We also know that she tends to be a bit hungrier later in the day. Taking the latter into consideration, we can assign her non-training day carbs as shown in table 10.10.

Table 10.10 *Assigning carbohydrates to meals for non-training days. Using table 10.8, we calculate grams of carbs per meal for our example athlete. Because there is no training, carbs can be organized roughly evenly across meals to make meal preparation easier. The shaded cells highlight new additions to the diet program as we make them.*

Meal Number	Non-training Day Mealtime	Protein/Meal (155 g total)	Carbs/Meal (80 g total)
1	9:30am	30 g	0 g
2	1:30pm	30 g	~25%: 20 g
3	5:00pm	30 g	~25%: 20 g
4	8:00pm	30 g	~25%: 20g
5	10:00pm	35 g	~25%: 20g

6. Adjust fats away from training times.

Fats follow an inverse pattern to carbohydrates with respect to timing around workouts; we want less fats in meals near training. The closer to the workout, the fewer fats. The process for determining fat distribution per meal can look something like as shown in table 10.11.

Table 10.11 *Assigning fats to individual meals should take training into consideration, with less fat assigned around training. Suggested percentages of daily fats are listed for different meal types.*

Calculating Per-Meal Fat on Training Days
1. Pre-workout meal: • if within 2 hours of workout, 10% daily fat • if within 4 hours of workout, 20% daily fat
2. Workout shake: 0% fat
3. Post-workout meal: 10% daily fats
4. Distribute remainder of fats evenly over other meals

Applying those criteria to our example (with 65 g of fat on hard training days) and rounding fat grams for ease, we get the distribution shown in table 10.12. Note that once the pre- and post-workout meals are assigned 10% daily fat each, a disproportionate remainder of the fats are allotted to the nighttime meal. This will help with bedtime satiety but is not a mandatory distribution.

Table 10.12 *Assigning fats to meals for hard training days. Using table 10.11, we calculate grams of fats per meal for our example athlete. The shaded cells highlight new additions to the diet program as we make them.*

Meal Number	Hard Day Mealtime	Protein/Meal (155 g total)	Carbs/Meal (310 g total)	Fats/Meal (65 g total)
1	7:30am	30 g	45 g	~20%: 15 g
2	12:00pm	30 g	45 g	~20%: 15 g
3	3:00pm (pre-training)	30 g	65 g	~10%: 5 g
4	7:30pm (post-training)	30 g	95 g	~10%: 5 g
5	10:00pm	35 g	60 g	~40%: 25 g

For non-training days, we again just distribute fats evenly or by preference across meals. We determined earlier that our example athlete gets 100 g of fats on rest days. We will allot a bit more fat at later meals for her evening hunger, but other than that, distribute them fairly evenly. This is shown in table 10.13.

Table 10.13 *Assigning fats to meals for non-training days. Using table 10.11, we calculate grams of fats per meal for our example athlete. Because there is no training, fats can be organized roughly evenly across meals to make meal preparation easier. The shaded cells highlight new additions to the diet program as we make them.*

Meal Number	Non-training Day Mealtime	Protein/Meal (155 g total)	Carbs/Meal (80 g total)	Fats/Meal (100 g total)
1	9:30am	30 g	0 g	10 g
2	1:30pm	30 g	20 g	15 g
3	5:00pm	30 g	20 g	25 g
4	8:00pm	30 g	20 g	25 g
5	10:00pm	35 g	20 g	25 g

7. Consider an intra-workout shake.

For harder workouts, a shake can provide some small but meaningful benefits. To program a shake, subtract about one-half of your pre-workout meal's protein and carbs, and allot these to your shake. Unless you are training for over an hour within the moderate category at least, a workout shake is not necessary. See table 10.14 for a meal schedule including an intra-workout shake.

Table 10.14 *Adding an intra-workout shake to hard training days. Carbs and protein are subtracted from the pre-training meal and added as whey protein and liquid carbohydrate to be consumed during training. The shaded cells highlight new additions to the diet program as we make them.*

Meal Number	Hard Day Mealtime	Protein/Meal (155 g total)	Carbs/Meal (310 g total)	Fats/Meal (65 g total)
1	7:30am	30 g	45 g	15 g
2	12:00pm	30 g	45 g	15 g
3	3:00pm (pre-training)	15 g	35 g	5 g
Shake	5-7pm	15 g	30 g	0 g
4	7:30pm (post-training)	35 g	95 g	5 g
5	10:00pm	30 g	60 g	25 g

FOOD COMPOSITION CHOICES

For health reasons, we highly recommend getting most of your calories from minimally processed, whole food sources, with exceptions being vegan protein sources and some higher glycemic carb options around the training window. The "processing" of plant protein often improves digestibility and can increase the health benefits in that sense. Higher glycemic carb sources that digest faster thanks to processing can be advantageous after training when quick delivery of glucose to muscles offers more benefit. Here is a brief sample of some foods you can use for each macro category:

Example Lean Protein Sources:
- Chicken or turkey breast fish and shellfish
- Tofu and other low-fat soy products
- Mycoprotein
- Lean beef and any other lean meat
- Egg whites
- Fat-free or low-fat dairy

Example Veggie Options:
- Broccoli
- Spinach
- Lettuce
- Onions
- Tomatoes
- Peppers
- Asparagus
- Zucchini
- Squash
- Cauliflower
- Celery
- Carrots
- Cucumbers

Example Healthy Carbohydrate Sources:
- Fruit
- Whole-grain bread
- Whole-grain rice
- Oatmeal
- Sweet potatoes
- Pasta
- Corn
- Whole-grain crackers and wraps

Example Higher Glycemic Index Carbohydrate Sources for Post Training:

- Fruit bars
- Toaster pastries
- Kid's cereal
- Low-fat baked goods
- Fat-free candy
- White rice
- White bread

Example Healthy Fat Sources:

- Nuts
- Nut butters
- Canola oil
- Olive oil
- Flaxseed oil
- Avocado

We recommend having veggies with most non-shake meals as fiber, vitamins, minerals, and phytochemicals support health. Consuming high-fiber, high-volume veggies will help with satiety on fat-loss diets as well. Lower fiber, lower volume foods cause less gastrointestinal distress when eaten pre-workout and can be easier to eat right after training as well, so decreasing or eliminating veggies from the workout window meals can be helpful.

Using lean protein sources is also recommended. For best health, fats should come mainly from mono- and polyunsaturated sources. Animal fat is generally saturated, and although eating fatty meat occasionally will likely cause no harm, getting a large portion of your fats from saturated sources is not recommended. Eating fattier meats also makes macro calculations more complicated. When choosing foods to meet our macros, we have to remember that there are very few pure-macro foods. While lean steak is mostly protein, it does have some fat; while pasta is mostly carbs, it does have some protein; and so on. You can go about adjusting for these "ancillary macros" in a few different ways. Macro tracker apps and websites will count all macros from each food you log in for each meal, main and ancillary alike. The only problem with this is that you will have a hard time discerning how much protein came from higher quality, complete sources and what came from grains and nuts. If you use a tracker, as you prepare your meals, be sure to confirm that you are getting most of your protein from high-quality sources.

Another option that is a bit less tedious than logging every food you put in your mouth is the following algorithm: For every approximately 150 lb. of bodyweight, subtract 5 g of each macro from your per meal macro needs. For example, if you weigh 150 lb. and need 30 g protein, 45 g carbs, and 10 g fat per meal, choose a protein source with 25 g of protein, a carb source with 40 g of carbs, and a fat source with only 5 g of fat. Double this (subtract 10 g from each macro) if you weigh 300 lb., and so on. On average, you will get very close to covering the ancillary macros this way, and your portions will be close enough to actual macro needs to make your diet effective, especially in the longer term of weeks of dieting.

Taking food composition into account, some sample meals for our athlete might look like table 10.15.

Table 10.15 *Example food composition choices to fill the meal-to-meal macronutrient assignments we have developed thus far for our example 155-lb. athlete on hard training days.*

Meal Number	Hard Day Mealtime	Protein/Meal (155 g total)	Carbs/Meal (310 g total)	Fats/Meal (65 g total)
1	7:30am	30 g from egg (whites)	45 g from toast	15 g from egg (yolks)
2	12:00pm	30 g from turkey + cheese	45 g from bread/fruit	15 g from cheese
3	3:00pm (pre-training)	15 g from steak	35 g from rice	5 g from steak
Shake	5-7pm	15 g from whey protein	30 g from Gatorade	0 g
4	7:30pm (post-training)	30 g from skim milk and whey protein	95 g from cereal	5 g from cereal
5	10:00pm	35 g from ground turkey	60 g from pasta	25 g from olive oil

ADDING SUPPLEMENTS

Because supplements contribute only minor differences in outcome, adding them to your nutrition program is a matter of personal choice. If the stress of more things to consider and schedule will make you less adherent, you are better off not adding supplements. In the long term, the small differences that supplements make can add up, so more experienced dieters who are comfortable with other aspects of diet design might be well served to add them. We will go through how and when to use the most recommended supplements later.

Caffeine

If you are taking caffeine for anti-hunger and focus enhancement on a fat-loss diet, a good plan is to take some in the morning and some midday, so long as the second dose does not affect your sleep. If you are taking caffeine for workout energy enhancement, taking it 15 to 30 minutes before your workout begins is a good strategy. For workouts later in the day, experiment with very low doses or taking the caffeine even earlier than 30 minutes before your workout and find a regimen that will not keep you from falling asleep at night. If you are new to caffeine consumption or have not had any in a while, it is best to start slow, adding 25 to 50 mg of caffeine per day. You will become desensitized to the effects of caffeine over time, so gradual increases across a fat-loss diet can be helpful. Our advice is to increase caffeine intake by 25 to 50 mg per day when you feel like you need more, and not by greater amounts at any one time. Normal ranges of caffeine consumption can offer many benefits at little or no risk to your health, but anything over 300 mg of caffeine at a time or 1,000 mg per day is best avoided. Those who approach these high levels might do well to consult with a medical professional. Even when tolerated well, higher doses of caffeine (especially consumed closer to bedtime) can interfere with sleep, which interferes with recovery.

It is also a good idea to take caffeine breaks occasionally. The best time to take a break is during maintenance or muscle-gain periods when you have more energy from food and are not struggling with hunger. Coffee, tea, soda, and energy drinks are all fine caffeine sources pre-workout. Carbonated beverages may be more difficult for some to tolerate before a workout, so individual experimentation with different sources is wise.

An example caffeine usage protocol follows. Note that increases and decreases are gradual–suddenly dropping from high consumption to zero can cause headaches and fatigue, and ramping up too quickly can leave you jittery and sleepless. Also note that caffeine is used most during times of lower energy or more difficult training. Caffeine dosing times are listed as AM (morning consumption), pre-workout (consumption before training), and PM (afternoon consumption).

> **Muscle-Gain Phase** *(ramping up across 2 months):*
> No caffeine → 25-50 mg pre-workout

> **Maintenance Phase:**
> Break from caffeine

> **Fat-Loss Phase** *(ramping up across 3 months):*
> 25 mg AM → 50 mg AM + 25 mg PM → 75 mg AM + 25 mg pre-workout + 50 mg PM

> **Post-Fat-Loss Maintenance Phase** *(ramping down across 2 months):*
> 50 mg AM + 25 mg PM → 25 mg AM

Whey Protein

Because whey protein is a very high-quality, fast-digesting protein, it is ideal for an intra-workout shake or as a part of a post-workout meal. For workout shakes, combine with fast-digesting carbs (see Carbohydrate Formulas). Start sipping the shake before you train, drink two-thirds during, and finish the remainder right after the workout. This gives you enough nutrients for all the beneficial intra-workout functions without risking gastrointestinal distress. Whey is not a good option for any other meal replacement on its own, but it can be combined with slower digesting carbs and fats or in a mix with casein protein to slow its absorption for this purpose.

Casein Protein

Casein protein is very high quality but very slow digesting and due to the latter unique property, it is best used before long meal intervals or at bedtime. Its slow-release effect can be extended even further with the addition of fats, fiber, or other slowly digested food. It is best not to use casein as a protein source during the workout window.

Carbohydrate Formulas

There are two kinds of supplemental carbs that can be effective: very quickly digesting carbs and very slowly digesting carbs. Fast-digesting carbs follow recommendations described for whey protein; they are best used within the workout window. Some examples of quickly digesting carbs include Gatorade, Powerade, and Dextrose-based carb powders. You can use juices and coconut water as well, but the digestion speeds will be significantly lower than for specially formulated carbohydrate drinks and these are therefore not as ideal.

If you need a carb supplement that acts as a meal replacement, Waximaize or similar slow-digesting carb powders can be mixed with casein protein powder to provide a meal replacement shake. This can be a good option toward the end of a hypercaloric diet when drinking some of your meals might be appealing. This option is also convenient when traveling or without access to refrigeration–bringing a powdered mix of whey, casein, and Waximaize and simply adding water might be a very workable meal solution in these cases.

Creatine

The only currently confirmed safe and effective type of creatine is creatine monohydrate. Luckily, this type is the most commonly sold and by far the cheapest. We recommend using creatine for up to three months at a time and taking one-month breaks between stretches of use. Although it is likely that it can be taken indefinitely and be effective and safe, there is a chance that taking breaks will revamp endogenous creatine production. This supplement must be taken consistently every day to support fitness outcomes–taking creatine two or three times per week will have almost no effect. It takes about a week of consistent use (around 3 g per 100 lb. of bodyweight per day is recommended) for creatine to fully load in the muscles and have an effect. Dose timing is minimally important, although some data suggest that creatine is best absorbed when taken with carbs and might be better absorbed when ingested post workout.

This supplement is most useful during muscle-gain or fat-loss phases. Maintenance phases are therefore ideal for a break in creatine use if you choose to take one.

When taking creatine, weight gain of 1 to 3% of bodyweight is not uncommon. Be aware of this potential weight gain when starting to track your weight for a hypo- or hypercaloric diet phase. It can be helpful to begin supplementation two to three weeks before you start your diet so that you can get a stable baseline bodyweight before you begin tracking changes.

Multivitamins

While multivitamins and minerals cannot replace all of the nutrients from a whole-food diet, they can be helpful when consuming less total food on a fat-loss diet or when skipping veggies at the end of a muscle-gain diet. Taking the recommended dosage listed on your multivitamin is best practice.

Omega-3 Fat Supplements

EPA (Eicosapentaenoic acid) and DHA (Docosahexaenoic acid) supplements are good options for Omega-3 supplementation. Fish oil is another option, but capsules can go rancid, losing their effectiveness over time. The American Heart Association recommends 1 g of combined EPA and DHA per day, but more or less might be prudent depending on the amount of Omega-3-rich food sources you consume. Following the recommended dosage on the bottle is a good place to start.

Table 10.16 shows an example of how all the above supplements might be integrated into our sample diet plan.

Table 10.16 *Example supplement choices and timing for our 155-lb. athlete*

Meal Number	Hard Day Mealtime	Supplements
1	7:30am	Meal + coffee, multivitamin, creatine
2	12:00pm	Waximaize and whey + casein shake with nuts if too busy to eat a meal
3	3:00pm (pre-training)	Meal + tea
Shake	5-7pm	Whey protein and dextrose powder
4	7:30pm (post-training)	Meal with half needed protein from whey
5	10:00pm	Meal with casein as protein source, Omega-3 supplement

CHAPTER SUMMARY

- The first step in designing a diet is to estimate daily calorie needs based on bodyweight and activity level.
- Breaking down calories into daily macronutrients starts with protein, as it is the more important and least variable of the three macros.
- Daily carbohydrate intake is determined by the amount of training done each day and can vary from day to day.
- Daily fat intake is determined by using the remaining calories for fat after protein and carbohydrate demands are met (so long as the health minimum of 0.3 g of fat per pound of bodyweight per day is achieved).
- For most people, daily macronutrient intake should be broken down into 4 to 6 meals per day.
- Map out morning, bedtime, pre-, and post-workout meals first, then any remaining meals can be spaced out evenly throughout the day.
- In most cases, protein can be distributed evenly across all meals.
- Carbohydrates should be higher, and fats should be lower in meals around training.
- Once the numerical content of each meal is determined, food composition, and supplement choices can finalize the meal plan.

If you like to understand the science behind your nutritional choices but would prefer for seasoned PhDs and Registered Dietitians to design your diet, RP is at your service.

From our premium, fully personalized one-on-one coaching plans to our tried and true but more DIY best-selling diet templates, we have you covered!

Check out www.renaissanceperiodization.com for more information.

CHAPTER 11

Tracking Your Weight and Adjusting Your Diet

TRACKING BODYWEIGHT

Changes in metabolism and other compensatory mechanisms will adjust your body's calorie needs across a dieting period. Weight loss will naturally slow during a fat-loss phase and calorie intake will need to be decreased to maintain a constant rate of loss. Likewise, weight gain will typically decrease across a hypercaloric phase and calorie increases will be needed to continue progressing. In order to determine when and how much to adjust your diet, you will need to monitor your progress. Progress can be assessed on a large scale using metrics such as body fat percentage tests, how your clothes fit, and how you look in the mirror, but making adjustments to your diet in real-time requires a more quantifiable metric. Bodyweight averages are specific enough for this purpose and are very easy to implement.

When you are hypo- or hypercaloric, your tissue weight will be changing, but due to water weight noise, this can only be reliably measured by tracking average changes across multiple weeks. For example, if you were on a fat-loss diet and the scale suggested you had gained a pound across one week, the reality might be that you were retaining two pounds of water weight, but had lost one pound of tissue. In this situation, the scale would not be a good reflection of fat loss because the water weight was able to mask the tissue changes.

Fortunately, body water changes rarely accumulate consistently over time like tissue weight gain or loss, so across the weeks and months of a diet, scale weight will reliably measure progress. In this example, if you continued to lose one pound per week, this would eventually be larger than any amount water weight could mask on the scale.

Average weight should be compared week to week using two to three weigh-in data points. Weighing daily is an option, but it is unnecessary and adds additional variability that can lead to stress. Day to day changes will not be clear on the scale, and seeing the daily number can overwhelm and demotivate some people. Weigh-ins should be done under the same circumstances each time to avoid additional variability. Taking your weight first thing in the morning before eating and after using the restroom is a good choice.

Tracking Weight for Maintenance

Imagine that our 155-lb. female athlete was running a six-week maintenance diet; she would want her average weekly weight to be approximately 155 lb. To keep from adjusting the diet because of water weight changes, she should set a range of plus or minus 1.25% bodyweight as her "acceptable" range. For a 155-lb. person, 1.25% is approximately 2 lb. This means that changes of plus or minus 2 lb. from 155 lb. are not cause for alarm during maintenance. So a range of 153 to 157 lb. is acceptable, as long as the weekly averages are not trending reliably up or down. It is also important to note that a single weight outside of this "safe range" should not be cause for alarm; more than one in a row may indicate a trend, but any one weigh-in can be an outlier for a number of reasons. Taking a weekly average gives a clearer picture of weight movement than any one weight can.

To get a good weekly average, our athlete chooses two weigh-in days per week, Tuesday and Friday. She knows Tuesday comes after a hard training day and Friday comes after a moderate training day (per her schedule in the last chapter), so she can expect that her Tuesday weight might be a bit higher than her Friday weight thanks to extra carbs and inflammation (fluid retention) from a harder workout the night before.

In addition to looking at her weekly weight averages, our athlete assesses week to week changes in average weight. Imagine a scenario where she starts at 153 lb. and slowly moves up to 157 lb. across weeks and is indeed gaining, despite the fact that all weigh-ins were within the acceptable range. Average weekly weight would be moving up in this case, but be close to 155 lb. If this were the only data we assessed, we might miss the trend toward increasing weight.

We look at the difference between each week's average weights; the average of the *change* in weight should be close to zero. In the example weight log in table 11.1 and graph of this log in figure 11.1, we see that weight dropped by 2.5 lb. from week 1 to 2, but then went up 0.6 and 2.6 lb. between weeks 2 and 3 and weeks 3 and 4, respectively. On average this change is close to zero, nothing to worry about. The overall average weekly weight change across the full six weeks is +0.06 lb.–a weight of less than one-tenth of a pound–an amount not even measurable on any standard scale. This means that our athlete successfully maintained her weight.

Table 11.1 *A table of tracking bodyweight fluctuation on an isocaloric diet. Goal weight and actual weigh-ins for two days per week are listed. Average weight for the week is calculated as the average of the week's two weigh-ins. Week-to-week weight changes are calculated by subtracting the current week's average weight from the previous week's. Average weight change across the full six weeks is calculated as the average of the weekly weight changes.*

Week	Goal Weight	Tuesday	Friday	Average Weight for the Week	Change From Last Week
1	155	155.4	156	155.7	N/A
2	155	153	Forgot to weigh	153	-2.5
3	155	154.4	152	153.2	+0.2
4	155	156.6	155	155.8	+2.6
5	155	156.2	153.5	154.9	-0.9
6	155	156	155.4	155.7	+0.9
					Average change: +0.06 lb.

If our athlete had gone based on the change from her week 1 average (155.7) to her week 2 weigh-in (based on only one weight since she forgot to weigh-in Friday), she might think she had lost 2.5 lb. Based on this she might have increased her calorie intake to maintain weight. After assessing the third week, however, where there is no change, we can see that she was better off not adjusting her diet; there is no need for adjustment based on a single anomaly.

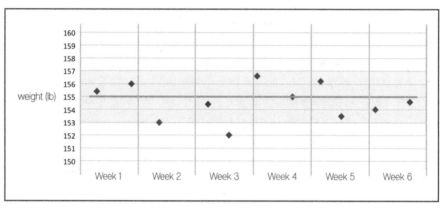

Figure 11.1 *A graph of the weigh-in data from table 11.1 (on an isocaloric diet). A solid line indicates the target average weight of 155 lb. across six weeks. The shaded region indicates the expected range of normal weight fluctuation on an isocaloric diet. Black diamonds indicate specific bi-weekly weigh-in data points. This graph is a visual representation of normal weight fluctuation across weeks during weight maintenance.*

Tracking Weight for Muscle Gain

For muscle gain we can identify target weights for each week that fit our goal gain pace. We will use our 155-lb. example female, trying to gain at the rate of 0.5% bodyweight, or 0.8 lb. per week for six weeks. As long as weight is trending up and week-to-week increases are averaging around 0.8 lb., we know that she is on the right track despite weekly fluctuation. An example weight log and graph for this are shown in table 11.2 and figure 11.2, respectively.

In the example weight log shown in table 11.2, you can see that from week 1 to week 2 she gains more than the target 0.8 lb., but from week 2 to week 3 her weight drops slightly. Since the previous change was a bit above the desired rate, the average of the two is closer to target gain. In the following week change we see a 2.4-lb. increase and now can definitely rest assured that weight is being gained. Gains seem to slow toward the end of this six-week phase, but when we average weekly changes, our athlete has actually hit her target weekly rate exactly—gaining 0.8 lb. per week on average across six weeks.

Table 11.2 *A table of tracking bodyweight fluctuation on a hypercaloric diet. Goal weight and actual weigh-ins for two days per week are listed. Average weight for the week is calculated as the average of the week's two weigh-ins. Week-to-week weight changes are calculated by subtracting the current week's average weight from the previous week's. Average weight change across the full six weeks is calculated as the average of the weekly weight changes.*

Week	Goal Weight	Tuesday	Friday	Average Weight for the Week	Change From Last Week
1	155.8	155.4	156	155.7	N/A
2	156.6	158	156	157	+1.3
3	157.4	157.2	156	156.6	-0.4
4	158.2	158	160	159	+2.4
5	159	159	159.4	159.2	+0.2
6	159.8	159.4	160	159.7	+0.5
					Average change: +0.8 lb.

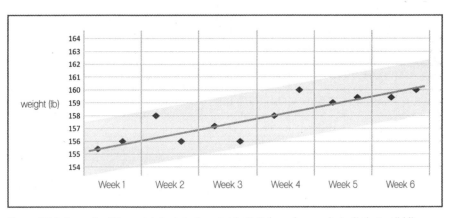

Figure 11.2 *A graph of the weigh-in data from table 11.2 (on a hypercaloric diet). A solid line indicates the target average weight gain from approximately 155 to 160 lb. across six weeks. The shaded region indicates the expected range of normal weight fluctuation on this hypercaloric diet. Black diamonds indicate specific bi-weekly weigh-in data points. This graph is a visual representation of normal weight fluctuation across weeks during weight gain.*

Tracking Weight for Fat Loss

Imagine our 155-lb. example athlete chooses a 1.0% bodyweight or 1.5-lb. loss per week for a six-week fat loss diet. An example weight log and graph for this are shown in table 11.3 and figure 11.3, respectively. You may notice that in week 4, both weigh-ins are outside of the approximate goal weight range. This is what we refer to as an outlier in statistics—a data point that falls outside of an expected range, but which does not represent the trend. These week 4 weigh-ins are outliers. Given that our example athlete is a female, one explanation is that she was experiencing some hormonal bloat during week 4 that faded during week 5. Week-long weight bumps can also happen due to higher salt intake, particularly tough workouts, and many other reasons. This is a concrete example of two or more weeks' worth of weigh-in data being needed to drive appropriate diet change decisions.

Table 11.3 *Tracking bodyweight fluctuation on a hypocaloric diet. Goal weight and actual weigh-ins for two days per week are listed. Average weight for the week is calculated as the average of the week's two weigh-ins. Week-to-week weight changes are calculated by subtracting the current week's average weight from the previous week's. Average weight change across the full six weeks is calculated as the average of the weekly weight changes.*

Week	Goal Weight	Tuesday	Friday	Average Weight for the Week	Change From Last Week
1	155	155	153.8	154.4	N/A
2	153.5	154	152.2	153.1	-1.3
3	152	152	151	151.5	-1.6
4	150.5	153.6	152	152.8	+1.3
5	149	150	148	149	-3.8
6	147.5	148	146.5	147.3	-1.8
					Average change: -1.4 lb.

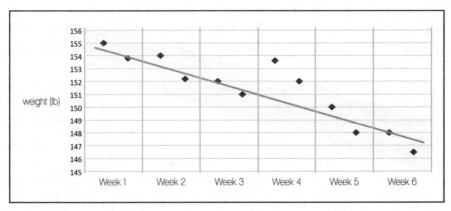

Figure 11.3 *A graph of the weigh-in data from table 11.3 (on a hypocaloric diet). A solid line indicates the target average weight loss from approximately 155 to 148 lb. across six weeks. The shaded region indicates the expected range of normal weight fluctuation on this hypocaloric diet. Black diamonds indicate specific bi-weekly weigh-in data points. This graph is a visual representation of normal weight fluctuation across weeks during weight loss.*

ADJUSTING THE DIET

When after two to three weeks of assessment, weight is not moving as expected, it is time to make adjustments to your diet. When and how much to adjust your diet under various circumstances will be outlined in this section. Following is a reminder of some critical information for making such diet adjustment calculations:

1 lb. of tissue = approx. 3,500 calories
1 g of fat = 9 calories
1 g of carbohydrate = 4 calories
1 g of protein = 4 calories

This means that every extra 3,500 calories ingested results in roughly 1 lb. of bodyweight gained, and every 3,500 calorie deficit results in approximately 1 lb. of bodyweight lost. This information can be used to appropriately adjust your diet based on targeted losses, targeted gains, or the need to alter your diet to maintain weight. If you need to lose 1 lb. per week, you simply drop 3,500 calories from your diet per week. For other weekly weight change amounts, simply multiply the weekly weight in pounds by 3,500. For example, if you are looking to lose approximately

173

0.8 lb. per week, you need a weekly calorie deficit of 0.8 x 3,500 = 2,800 calories. Across the seven days of the week, this translates to a 2,800 ÷ 7 = 400 calorie deficit per day.

When altering your diet, the calories per gram of macro value can be used to determine how much of any given macro must be cut to achieve the desired calorie change. If you needed to cut 400 calories per day and were doing so by reducing fats, 400 calories is approximately 400 ÷ 9 = approx. 44 g fat. Fat has 9 calories per gram, so dividing the calorie amount you need to change by the calories per gram of the macronutrient you will alter gives you the grams of macronutrient you must change. This can be done by modifying a single macro or a combination of macronutrients to achieve the desired calorie change.

Adjusting a Long-Term Weight Maintenance Diet
(These instructions are *not* for a maintenance diet immediately following fat loss or muscle gain.)

1. Construct an isocaloric diet.
2. Run this diet for three weeks, tracking weekly weight averages.
   a. If weight is within the acceptable +/- 1.25% range from your maintenance weight and weekly changes are close to zero on average, you are maintaining. Continue to track to confirm that weight stays steady.
   b. If weekly weight changes across three weeks are showing an average increase, calculate the number of calories that would yield that average increase. For example, take the increases observed in table 11.2 (muscle-gain weight log: +1.3 lb. from weeks 1 to 2 and -0.4 lb. from weeks 2 to 3), and imagine these weigh-ins were collected on a maintenance diet. The average weekly weight gain here comes out to approximately 0.8 lb. In calories, 0.8 lb. is roughly 3,500 x 0.8 = 2,800 calories—so in this example the maintenance calories were over by 2,800 per week or 2,800 ÷ 7 = 400 per day. In this case, 400 calories should be subtracted per day to achieve weight maintenance. Weight should then be monitored for another two to three weeks and adjusted again if needed.

c. If weekly changes across three weeks show an average decrease, calculate the number of calories that would yield that average decrease. For example, if someone trying to maintain weight observed the decreases in table 11.3 (fat-loss weight log: -1.3 lb. from weeks 1 to 2 and -1.6 lb. from weeks 2 to 3), the average weekly weight loss here is approximately 1.5 lb. In calories, 1.5 lb. is roughly 3,500 x 1.5 = 5,250 calories–so in this example the maintenance calories were off by 5,250 per week or 5,250 ÷ 7 = 750 per day. In this case, 750 calories should be added per day to achieve weight maintenance. Again, weight should then be monitored for another two to three weeks and further adjustments made if needed.

Adjusting a Fat-Loss or Muscle-Gain Diet

Construct an isocaloric diet.

1. Add or subtract the daily calories needed to create your surplus or deficit. To do this, take your desired weekly percentage bodyweight change and convert to pounds. So if you weigh 155 lb. and are looking to gain 0.5% bodyweight per week, this translates to approximately 0.8 lb. per week. In calories this means you need 0.8 x 3,500 = 2,800 extra calories per week, or 400 extra calories per day. If, on the other hand, you are looking to lose at a rate of 1% per week, this translates to approximately 1.5 lb. per week. In calories this means you need a weekly deficit of 1.5 x 3,500 = 5,250 calories per week–a 750 calorie daily deficit.
2. Adjust your daily maintenance intake according to the needed surplus or deficit.
3. Run this diet for three weeks.
   a. Similar to your maintenance adjustment, if you find your target losses or gains are off, take the average observed weekly change and compare it to your desired weekly change. Make adjustments in daily calories accordingly. If your target weight loss per week is 1.5 lb. and you find that after three weeks of tracking that you are losing only 1 lb. per week on average, you need to decrease calories in your diet enough to lose an extra 0.5 lb. per week. In calories this is 3,500 x 0.5 = 1,750 calories. To subtract 1,750 more calories per week, 1,750 ÷ 7 = 250 calories per day need to be dropped.
4. Continue to assess weight changes across weeks and adjust when your desired pace of loss or gain slows on average across two or more weeks.

Tips for Adjusting Calories via Macronutrients

Calorie changes are created by increasing or decreasing the amount(s) of one or more macronutrients. Merely adjusting calories up or down without regard for macronutrient amounts would still result in weight changes, but body composition would not necessarily change as desired. For example, if calories were cut evenly from all macros to create a calorie deficit, the deficit would certainly result in tissue loss, but might cut protein below minimum levels resulting in muscle loss. Considering which macros to adjust when making adjustments to your diet is important business. We have discussed optimal and minimum macro amounts for various circumstances, training, and goals. These largely dictate the choice of which macros to cut or add when adjusting a diet, but preference and practicality should also be considered.

Macro Adjustments During Fat-Loss Phases

Fats offer no unique physiological advantage when consumed over their minima on a fat-loss diet, so cut fats first on hypocaloric diets. If further cuts are needed once fats are at minimum levels, another macro must be considered. Protein is the most important macronutrient, so as long as this was not programmed above physiologically required levels from the start, it should be left alone. Carbohydrates are therefore the next to be cut. Once carbs are at their minimum for anti-catabolic effect and fats are at their minimum for health, individuals are generally at the tail end of their weight-loss phase—going lower than this is seldom necessary. In some extreme cases (dieting in the last few weeks before a bodybuilding competition, for example), taking carbs all the way down to their sensible minimum (0.3 g per pound of bodyweight per day, as recommended in chapter 3) might be a necessary trade-off to complete the fat-loss phase. If you are not a competitive bodybuilder and get to this point, it is probably time to end your diet and lose any remaining fat in a subsequent fat-loss phase as pushing a diet this hard can lead to rebound weight gain.

Macro Adjustments During Muscle-Gain Phases

Practicality can play a bigger role in food choice during muscle-gain phases. As long as protein and carbohydrates are at the recommended anabolic levels and fat is at least at minimum levels for health, the difference between adding calories via more fat, more carbs, or more protein is very small. Protein is the most expensive and most satiating of all the macros, so eating more of it is pricier and will make it harder to finish your meals, so we can probably rule protein out as a best choice. Choosing between adding carbs versus fats is a matter of trade-offs. The primary trade-off is optimal effect versus ease of adherence. Fats take up less space in the stomach and contain more calories per gram than carbs, but carbs are more anabolic. Table 11.4 lists the pros and cons of increasing calories via fats or carbs. Due to their anabolic potential, carbs should probably be added first, up until this becomes cumbersome enough to put adherence at risk, at which point further additions can come from fats.

Table 11.4 *The benefit of adding calories via carbs versus fat on a muscle gain diet.*

Adding Calories via Carbs	
Outcome Pros	**Adherence Cons**
Allows for more anabolism.***	Higher volume makes it harder to consume as much.
	Low-fat/high-carb food is less common.
***Anabolism is weighted heavier than other pros as it has a larger influence on outcome.	
Adding Calories via Fats	
Adherence Pros	**Outcome Cons**
Fats are easy to add to food.	Leads to slightly higher adiposity than excess carbs.
Low volume makes it easier to consume more.	
	Less anabolism than with added carbs.
High-fat/high-carb food is more common.	

TRANSITIONING FROM ONE DIET PHASE TO ANOTHER

There are several diet transitions that require different adjustments, and we will go through instructions for each:

• Transitioning from fat loss to maintenance
• Transitioning from muscle gain to maintenance
• Transitioning from fat loss to muscle gain
• Transitioning from muscle gain to fat loss (to mini-cut)
• Transitioning from fat loss (mini-cut) to muscle gain

Transitioning From Fat Loss to Maintenance

1. Determine your current calorie intake as well as estimated average calorie maintenance requirements for your weight and training level from table 10.1 in chapter 10.
2. Find the calorie amount exactly between the current calorie intake and estimated average maintenance requirements you determined in step 1 and increase your calorie intake accordingly. If your intake at the end of a fat-loss diet was 1,500 calories on a light day and estimated light day calories from table 10.1 for your new weight were 2,500, you would begin eating 2,000 calories on a light day to start maintenance.
3. Assess your weight for two weeks.
    a. If weight is maintained, wait another week and then increase calories by around 20% per day. Continue to do this every three to four weeks as long as weight is maintained and until calorie amounts are close to estimates in table 10.1 for your new weight and level of daily training.
    b. If weight is still decreasing, assess the average decrease in pounds, convert to calories, and add this weekly amount. If your weight is still dropping by an average of 0.5 lb. per week, add 3,500 x 0.5 = 1,750 calories per week. Once weight is stable for two to three weeks, follow instructions in subpoint a.
    c. If weight is increasing, continue the current diet until weight is steady for three weeks and then follow the instructions in subpoint a.

Transitioning From Muscle Gain to Maintenance

When transitioning from a muscle-gain phase to maintenance, your strategy will depend on whether you are still gaining at the end of your diet or not. In the latter, you can continue eating exactly as you are and maintain. Follow the instructions here in the former case:

1. If you are still gaining at the end of a muscle-gain phase, you will need to reduce your calorie intake to get to an isocaloric state. We recommend calculating your weekly calorie surplus based on average weight gain over the final two weeks of mass and decreasing your intake by that amount. If you were gaining approximately 0.8 lb. per week on average at the end of your muscle-gain phase, you will need to subtract 0.8 x 3,500 = 2,800 calories per week to be isocaloric.
2. Run this diet for three weeks.

3. Reassess average weight changes. If your weight is stable, you can continue this diet for the remainder of your maintenance. If weight is decreasing or still increasing, alter calories accordingly, reassessing average changes every two to three weeks until your weight is stable.

Transitioning From Fat Loss to Muscle Gain

1. Eat at your estimated maintenance calories for your current body weight. Because you have been on a fat loss diet, your daily caloric needs for your current weight will be lower than expected and the estimated maintenance calories will therefore provide a surplus.
2. Run this diet for three weeks.
   a. If weight is increasing, carry on with this diet until pace slows for two to three weeks.
   b. If pace slows or is under target, calculate the needed calories to increase gains to the desired pace. If your target gain pace is 0.5% bodyweight (approx. 0.8 lb.) per week and you are gaining at an average pace of 0.4 lb. per week over the last two weeks, you need to add enough calories to increase weight gain by another 0.4 lb. per week. Additional calorie needs are therefore 3,500 x 0.4 = 1,400 calories per week, or 1,400 ÷ 7 = 200 calories per day.

Transitioning From Muscle Gain to Mini-Cut

1. Start with your current calorie intake (as if this were your maintenance) and follow instructions for adjusting a fat-loss diet. The only difference between a mini-cut and a conventional cut is that target weight loss pace will be slightly faster as mini-cuts are meant to initiate rebound gain in a subsequent muscle-gain phase.

Transitioning From Mini-Cut to Muscle Gain

1. Calculate your estimated maintenance calories based on bodyweight and activity levels and then add a surplus as you would when starting any muscle-gain phase. Because of the short duration of the mini-cut, diet fatigue is less severe and your predicted maintenance calories should be fairly accurate.
2. Follow adjustment steps from the muscle-gain diet section.
3. Weight gain and loss is a lot like launching a guided rocket to a target. The initial launch points the rocket in the right general direction, and then small

adjustments keep the rocket on track from there. Nutrition is a bit like rocket science after all!

CHAPTER SUMMARY

- Tracking bodyweight is your best means of assessing and adjusting any diet.
- Bodyweight measurements should generally be taken two to three times per week under the same conditions to allow for average weekly comparisons.
- During a weight maintenance phase, bodyweight should remain stable within ± 1.25% of bodyweight over time on average.
- Changes should never be made to a diet based on a single weigh-in.
- Two weeks of weight tracking are needed at minimum to establish weight change trends or lack thereof.
- During fat-loss and muscle-gain phases, trend analysis is used to determine if the average change per week is congruent with the goals of the diet phase over time.
- Adjusting any diet will be based on the needed changes in bodyweight, which can be converted into calorie and then into macronutrient adjustments.

CHAPTER 12

Monitoring Body Composition Changes

While a bathroom scale is the perfect tool for assessing changes across the timescale of individual diets, bodyweight does not indicate muscle-to-fat tissue ratios. Measuring our body composition occasionally is helpful in order to monitor long-term progress. Before we go into the available metrics for this assessment, we will outline typical target body fat percentages for health and for performance in various sports.

NORMATIVE STANDARDS IN BODY COMPOSITION

A socialite was once quoted as saying, "You can never be too rich or too thin." We can debate the accuracy of the "too rich" part, but science is quite clear that there is such a thing as "too thin" in terms of health and fitness. For some sports, such as bodybuilding and physique, "too lean" for best health is a state that can be safely reached only *temporarily* in order to step on stage and compete. For other sports such as powerlifting, higher body fats can support better leverages and recovery for good performance. When choosing a body composition goal, you should first consider health and then sport performance and aesthetics according to your preferences. Please note that the following values and discussion is meant only for healthy adults. There are very different standards for children and other special populations such as pregnant women, nursing mothers, or those with medical issues.

Body Composition and Health

Males

Body fat recommendations differ for males versus females due primarily to differences in sex hormones and essential body fat. Males who want to prioritize health are best served keeping body fat between 10 and 20%. Some males who are genetically leaner may be able to safely maintain between 5 to10% body fat, but for most, staying above 10% is best. Dropping below 5% very temporarily for physique competitions, photoshoots, or the like should pose no threat to health, so long as this leanness is not maintained longer than a few weeks. For males, body fat above 20% begins to correlate with negative long-term cardiometabolic health outcomes, and by 30% body fat these risks start to increase more rapidly. Even at a healthy body fat percentage there is some risk of negative health outcomes with higher body weight, but gaining enough muscle to be at this risk is rare without anabolic steroids, which carry their own set of health risks (and legal risks in most countries).

Females

To prioritize health, females should maintain their body fat between 15 and 30%. Females have higher recommended body fat levels for best health because they have essential body fat required by their reproductive systems that males do not. When the body fat percentage gets too low, it can result in amenorrhea (loss of menstruation) for females of childbearing age and decreased estrogen levels that affect other hormones. Chronically low estrogen levels from excessively low body fat in females can negatively impact bone health, leading to increased risk of osteopenia and osteoporosis. On the other end, body fat levels over 30% for females start to correlate with negative health outcomes, and these risks increase with body fat percentages from that point.

Body Composition and Wellness

Health and wellness are two aspects of overall well-being. In the context of body fat, health is how well your body systems are operating at a particular body fat percentage, whereas wellness is the quality of life you experience while maintaining at that point. For most, staying at the leanest end of the healthy body fat ranges requires the kind of meticulous dieting that saps a lot of joy and energy from the rest of life. On the other hand, body fat levels toward the upper end of the healthy ranges start to affect mobility and daily energy levels. Individual preference, sport needs, and genetics will help determine where within the healthy range you are most comfortable. In some cases, one might put wellness aside for sport goals or put aesthetic ideals aside for a more enjoyable life.

Body Composition and Performance

Leanness levels optimal for sport are not always those best for health and wellness. Table 12.1 lists approximate body fat percentage ranges for best performance by sport and sex.

Table 12.1 *Body fat percentage ranges for best performance*

Sport Category	Male Body Fat	Female Body Fat
Physique competition (temporary, on stage %)	Sub 5%*	6%-10%*
Distance running	5%-10%*	10%-15%*
Fitness sport	5%-15%*	10%-20%*
Weightlifting/Powerlifting	10%-15%	15%-25%
Court, mat, and field sports	10%-15%	15%-25%
Strongman/Strongwoman	15%-25%	20%-30%

*Keep in mind that these lower end body fat percentages are not generally maintained by athletes year round and are not ideal for health if maintained for more than a few weeks at a time. Physique competitors especially should not maintain the body fat percentages they reach for competition day any longer than necessary.

Some people are genetically predisposed to maintaining higher body fat percentages and may need to diet very hard to get to the optima for their sport. If maintaining the recommended leanness for your sport is an endeavor that ends up degrading your performance, choose a body fat percentage somewhere between your natural default and the sport's optimal range.

PRIMARY BODY COMPOSITION ASSESSMENT METHODS

When muscle-gain and fat-loss phases are repeated across years, we may weigh more than when we started our fitness journey but have a lower body fat percentage. This is where body composition tracking can be helpful for quantifying progress. There are quite a few tools available for assessing body composition. These tools have varying costs and accessibility as well as varying levels of accuracy, precision, and reliability. Some methods are more informative and worthwhile than others; you should choose the most accurate and reliable option(s) available to you.

Body Mass Index (BMI)

Description

BMI is a value obtained by dividing a person's bodyweight in kilograms by the square of their height in meters. These values are used to determine how likely it is that an individual of a certain height and weight is overfat. For example, someone who is 250 lb. and 6'8" is less likely to be overfat than someone who is the same weight at 4'8". BMI classifications are as follows: Values under 18.5 kg/m2 are considered underweight, values from 18.5 to 25 kg/m2 are considered normal weight, values from 25 to 30 kg/m2 are considered overweight, and values over 30 kg/m2 are considered obese.

Accessibility/Cost

If you have a scale, a calculator, and know your height, you can easily calculate your own BMI in just a few minutes without any additional cost.

Precision/Reliability/Accuracy

The BMI value itself is very precise and reliable, but its meaning is not. A very lean muscular person often falls under the classification for overweight or obese using this scale, despite a low body fat percentage. There is no reliable formula for translating BMI values into body fat percentages. When estimating any one individual's body fat, especially if they train with weights or play sports, BMI is very inaccurate. For estimating approximate body fat percentages in samples of thousands of people, BMI is a bit more accurate, but still mis-classifies subsets of the group.

When to Use

Although cost free and easy to calculate, because of its inaccuracy for individual body fat calculations, BMI is one of the less helpful means of assessing body composition. Your doctor or insurance agent might use it to assess the likelihood that you are overweight to the point of health risk, but BMI has little relevance for tracking physique and fitness changes.

Body Circumference Methods

Description

You can measure your waist, hip, and other body part circumferences, and track these over time. Lost fat will result in decreasing numbers, though this can be confounded if muscle is also gained.

Accessibility/Cost

If you have a tape measure, you can obtain body part circumferences in several minutes. These measurements can be more difficult to do accurately on yourself, so you might need some help from a friend or family member.

Precision/Reliability/Accuracy

Because exact placement and how tightly you squeeze the tape can alter the measurement, precision and reliability for this method is low. Some tape measures have a pressure moderator which obviates the tightness problem, but placement on the body is still an issue. Differences in water weight can also confound body part measurements. Waist circumference is more accurate than other body parts due to less muscle change confounds in that region—if you lose fat and gain arm muscle your numbers might not change, but abdominal muscles tend to grow less and will influence waist measurement much less than fat loss. This method does not translate well to body fat percentage but can help you qualitatively determine whether you are growing or shrinking.

When to Use

You can use circumference measures at the beginning and end of each diet phase. For example, you can measure your waist a week into fat loss (when body water has settled) and a week before the phase ends (before body water bounces back up from additional food).

Tips on How to Use

Be as consistent as you can with pressure and placement. Standardized protocols for each measurement site have been developed and can easily be found online. Having someone experienced administrate the measurement is even better. It is also helpful to standardize the time of day and level fullness and hydration you have when measuring. Using circumference measures too often does not provide meaningful data. Even once-weekly measures tell you more about how much body water you are carrying or how swollen your muscles are than they do how much fat you are losing. If you use this method, measuring every two to four months is best.

Rep Strength

Description

The amount of weight you can lift for a certain number of consecutive repetitions (6-15 reps in particular) on familiar exercises can be a proxy for how muscular you are. Rep strength does not provide any information about body fat percentage, but loss of strength can be an indicator of muscle loss, particularly if this information is used in concert with another measure of body composition that supports the same conclusion.

Accessibility/Cost

If you train regularly, you already have this information available.

Precision/Reliability/Accuracy

Because your strength can vary from workout to workout and day to day, this is not a very precise method, and, as mentioned, cannot tell you anything about fat levels. Due to workout energy variance and the changing levels of fatigue, reliability of this method is low on a weekly scale, but over months and years you can draw some conclusions about muscle mass. This method is qualitatively accurate in that steady long-term increases or decreases in rep strength usually indicate muscle gain or loss respectively. It is important to note, however, that strength gains and losses are not always due to muscle mass changes. Quantitatively it gives us little information regarding the amount of muscle lost or gained and gives no information about body fat levels.

When to Use

This method can be used as an indicator of muscle retention. It is best to compare rep strength month to month. Using it any more frequently is going to tell you a lot more about your fatigue states than about your muscle mass levels. It is also best to use in combination with other measures since strength changes without muscle mass change do occur. A good time to use this method is during a fat-loss diet; you can use rep strength maintenance as decent assurance that muscle is being maintained. Although a loss in rep strength from month to month does not definitively mean loss of muscle, it can at least prompt further investigation. Likewise, rep strength increases on a weight-gain phase are a good sign (though not definitive evidence) that muscle growth is happening.

Tips on How to Use

Keep a journal of your training numbers and current bodyweight, especially on the basic movements like squats, pull-ups, benches, shoulder presses, upright rows, curls, and so on. If your bodyweight is going down month to month but your strength for reps is stable or increasing slowly, you are almost certainly maintaining your muscle. If you are losing rep strength within 5% of your best efforts, you might just be fatigued temporarily from a hypocaloric diet, and not actually losing any muscle. If you have lost 10% or more of your strength, then you are more likely to be losing muscle and need to reassess your diet strategy. Conversely, if you are not gaining rep strength month to month on a muscle-gain phase, you are not likely gaining muscle. Do not use rep strength with novel moves, because most of the monthly improvement will be technique based (you will get better at the movement and be able to lift more because of this efficiency) and may not reflect muscle mass changes.

Progress Photos

Description

Comparing photos of your body over time can give you a rough idea of body composition changes.

Accessibility/Cost

A camera and the same clothes and lighting are all that are needed for this assessment.

Precision/Reliability/Accuracy

Even with before and after pictures in the same clothes and same light, this method is entirely subjective. The angle of the camera and hydration levels can alter your appearance in photos. Photos can be more useful for those who have had their body fat measured with other devices and know what they look like at certain levels of leanness. For example, a bodybuilder might know from previous measurements that when his top abs show up, he is at around 15% body fat. Many people, regardless of experience, can have trouble making self-assessments. Finding a coach or honest friend to help judge comparisons can be helpful.

When to Use

Using progress photos can be a supplemental way to validate scale changes across a diet. They can also be a qualitative means of visualizing aesthetic changes across months and years. Photographs cannot be used to precisely determine body fat percentages or to quantify muscle gain, but they can be reassuring when scale results are confusing.

Tips on How to Use

Taking photos in the same bathing suit or underwear, in the same place, with the same lighting, and at the same angle will help standardize your pictures for better analysis. Visual changes may be best observed every four weeks or so, since changes on a shorter scale might be difficult to discern. That being said, subjective measures like photo assessment cannot compete with objective tests.

Skinfold Analysis

Description

A special caliper device is used to pinch and measure the thickness of folds of skin at standardized locations on the body. More fat under the skin makes these folds thicker, and equations are used to estimate body fat based on these measurements. Individual distribution of fat can alter these results in some cases as can variations in caliper use technique and exact placement of calipers. There are two main approaches to using calipers. The first is having a professional do a conventional full three- or seven-site test. The second is to perform a single site test on yourself. The latter, while even less accurate than a three- or seven-site test, can be used to track relative changes. In this case, ignore the percentage calculated and just assess how it changes over time.

Accessibility/Cost

Calipers can be purchased online from anywhere between $30 to $100. Skinfold analysis is best done by a highly experienced practitioner. Unfortunately, most people—and even personal trainers who are not trained in skinfold analysis—cannot perform this test reliably. A proper three- or seven-site skinfold test amounts to about 15 minutes of you standing in your underwear with a trained expert.

Precision/Reliability/Accuracy

When used correctly, calipers can be fairly precise and reliable. Reliability depends on the person applying the calipers; having the same person apply the test the same way each time is best. Skinfold analysis cannot determine extremely accurate body fat percentage values but can be used to reliably track trends.

When to Use

Caliper assessment will give you a general idea of trends when done every six months to a year. Self-tests can be done weekly to track relative changes as well.

Tips on How to Use

All the skinfold sites have standardized measurement protocols that can be easily found online. When doing your own caliper measurements, make sure to measure in the same location each time using the same protocols. The spot an inch directly to the left or right of your belly button is an easy-to-use and easy-to-replicate measurement site. Again, this measurement will not accurately tell you how lean you are, but the changes over time can give you an idea of which direction you are trending. Another option is to measure your skinfold values and correlate them occasionally with a more reliable measure of body fat such as a DEXA scan (to be covered later). Once you have a general idea of what skinfold measurements correlate with what body fat percentages according to the DEXA scan, you can begin to use skinfold values to more reliably estimate your leanness. If skinfold measurement will be your primary means of assessing body composition, get measured by the same trained professional every time and avoid getting measured more than twice per year as the variability in the measurement calculations is too large to accurately reveal changes on a smaller scale.

Bioelectric Impedance Analysis (BIA)

Description

BIA works by sending a harmless electrical current through your body and measuring it as it comes back out. Because fat impedes current more than lean tissue, the more current the machine detects, the less fat it estimates you have. BIA machines range from handheld options to tools imbedded in bathroom scales, to standing four-point measurement systems. InBody scans, Tanita scales, and Omron handheld devices are common options.

Accessibility/Cost

You can find BIA devices at many gyms and supplement stores, purchase handheld options, or get a bathroom scale that includes one. It takes just a few minutes to take the BIA test and get a reading. Costs range from around $35 to $50 to own a device or pay for a scan.

Precision/Reliability/Accuracy

BIA is not very precise; its estimate can be off by up to 10% from your actual body fat percentage. It is decently reliable. If you standardize your body water content for every measurement, you can get a reasonable idea of trends in body fat changes using BIA. This is because each measurement should be off by a similar amount, allowing relative changes to be tracked despite inaccurate body fat percentage values.

When to Use

You can use a BIA at the beginning and end of any major diet phase if you do not have access to any more precise measurement devices; just take the exact numbers with a grain of salt and look only at relative changes.

Tips on How to Use

As mentioned earlier, keeping a similar hydration level at each measurement will help reduce variability. If you need accurate body fat measures, the BIA is not a good choice, but it can be useful for trend analysis across a dieting phase.

Air Displacement Plethysmography Device (Bod Pod)

Description
This method measures air displaced by your body inside a chamber to determine body volume. The device then uses this information in conjunction with your bodyweight to estimate your body density. Because body fat is less dense than bones, organs, and muscle, equations can be used to predict how much of you is fat and how much is lean tissue. This results in a body fat percentage estimate.

Accessibility/Cost
Bod Pods can often be found in bigger cities and on college campuses. Most facilities will charge $30 to $100 for a test. The whole test takes about 15 minutes and requires you to be in minimal, tightly fitted clothing with a swim cap to make sure that hair and clothing do not contribute much to your volume measurement.

Precision/Reliability/Accuracy
If the Bod Pod is maintained and calibrated properly and if tests are run under consistent conditions, measurements are fairly precise and reliable. As usual, for body fat measurements, accuracy is not perfect–though this method is more accurate than any we have discussed so far.

When to Use
Similar to caliper tests, Bod Pod assessments are best done twice a year so that body changes are large enough to be assessed over the measurement error of this test. Those who are uncomfortable in enclosed spaces might struggle with this test as it requires they be locked in a small, enclosed space for several minutes.

Tips on How to Use
The test administrator will give you all needed instructions. Bring form-fitting clothes and be prepared to sit very still for a few minutes during the test.

Underwater Weighing/Hydrostatic Testing

Description

In this test you are dunked underwater and weighed while submerged. Because we know the density of water, how much you weigh underwater tells us how dense you are, estimating your lean tissue to fat ratio.

Accessibility/Cost

There are only a small handful of these setups left. They were more common in the past, especially in exercise science laboratories, and you could pay for a test, but this is much less common today. The reason for this is that the more recently developed Bod Pod gives very similar results but is simpler to use and maintain. For hydrostatic testing the participant must remain completely still, holding their breath underwater for 5 to 10 seconds after exhaling fully. Where hydrostatic testing still exists, costs are around $100 per test.

Precision/Reliability/Accuracy

Precision and reliability for hydrostatic testing is similar to Bod Pod when done under consistent conditions. Accuracy is also similarly low, but trending changes across a year can be accurately assessed.

When to Use

Underwater weighing is best used twice per year to assess larger changes in body composition. If you cannot swim or are uncomfortable exhaling and holding your breath underwater, this is probably not the best test for you.

Tips on How to Use

The test administrator will give you all needed instructions. Bring a bathing suit and a towel.

Dual Emission X-Ray Absorptiometry (DEXA)

Description

A DEXA machine scans your body with two x-rays of different energy levels and assesses how much these are absorbed by your tissue. Bones, other lean tissue, and fat each have different rates of absorption. The energy remaining after the rays have passed through your body can be used in conjunction with your bodyweight to estimate the amount of each type of tissue. Because the DEXA scan can separate bone from other lean tissue and fat, your bone mineral density can also be assessed—an important measure for health.

Accessibility/Cost

Most hospitals and many universities have DEXA scanners. Various companies also offer DEXA scans from their facilities or out of mobile trucks. Scans are generally under $100 per scan. Most DEXA scans require you to lie still for about 10 minutes while a scanner passes over your body.

Precision/Reliability/Accuracy

The DEXA scan is currently the most accurate method of body fat testing available to consumers. Estimated variability is around plus or minus 4%. If you get scans done under similar conditions, results are fairly precise and reliable. Results will vary somewhat even at the same body fat percentage between fully loaded and depleted glycogen conditions or between fully hydrated and dehydrated conditions.

When to Use

Though the DEXA does expose you to x-rays, you get more radiation from a day at the beach and much more on an intercontinental flight than you do from a DEXA scan, so safety is not an issue. DEXA can track fat levels more accurately than muscle levels since glycogen and water changes affect fat less than muscle tissue. DEXA scans for fat totals in pounds can be done every few months for a reliable picture of fat changes. To assess muscle changes, which are slower and more easily affected by other variables, twice per year is probably best practice.

Tips on How to Use

The test administrator will give you all needed instructions. If you are over 230 lb., you might need to find a larger than standard DEXA so that you fit into the scanning area. As with any x-ray technology, consult a medical professional prior to scheduling a scan.

Visual Densitometry

Light absorption imaging technologies are not new, but using optical properties of body tissue for body composition analysis is still developing at the time this book was published. Tissues of different densities absorb, scatter, and reflect light to different degrees. The visual densitometry method takes advantage of this to measure tissue densities and, in conjunction with your weight, calculate relative amounts of lean and fat tissue. Some visual densitometry devices are becoming commercially available, but until this technology is further vetted by exercise scientists, it is not yet recommended. Within the next 5 to 10 years, due to its easy use and potential precision, visual densitometry may become one of the prevalent forms of body composition assessment.

USING BODY COMPOSITION ASSESSMENT IN PRACTICE

Weighing yourself two to three times a week to obtain averages is an important part of tracking short-term progress over individual diet phases. Monitoring long-term body composition requires one or more of the methods discussed in the previous section. Table 12.2 breaks down the timescales and usefulness of some of these methods.

Table 12.2 *Recommended assessment timescales and some notes on each of the methods for assessing body composition. DEXA is the most accurate, accessible, and reliable method for tracking body composition changes, but if you have access to a Bod Pod or hydrostatic testing, these are good options as well. Other methods, such as BIA, skinfold analysis, rep strength assessments, progress photos, and body circumference measures can also be useful, but should be taken with a grain of salt and used in conjunction with each other to determine relative progress.*

Assessment Method	Assessment Timescale	Notes
Progress photos/Body circumference	Every 4 weeks	Progress photos and body circumference measures can help you qualitatively monitor fat loss. Muscle gain is harder to track with these methods.
Rep strength	Every mesocycle	Track every workout and note best efforts at training peaks and see how they compare to previous peaks.
Skinfold	Weekly	Can give you a relative idea of body fat trends in conjunction with other measures
BIA	Every diet phase	Can give an idea of relative changes from the start to end of a diet phase. Exact number cannot be trusted, but direction of change is usually reliable.
DEXA/ Bod Pod/ Hydrostatic	Every 3 to 6 months	When done under similar conditions each time, these are the best methods for tracking long-term body composition changes accurately.

When Progress Is Lacking

If you are gaining too much fat or not gaining muscle on a hypercaloric phase or not losing fat or losing too much muscle on a hypocaloric phase, changes to your diet and training need to be made. You should not conclude that any of these problems are occurring based on one measurement point or one type of measurement alone. Conclusions should be based on several measures over time using more than one measurement tool.

We can feel more confident that diet adjustments are needed when multiple measurements suggest the same conclusion. For example, if your rep strength has decreased across three mesocycles in a row, it is likely that something needs to change. Even if you are using the most precise and accurate measure, more than one data point should be considered before drawing conclusions. Even a DEXA scan can be off for a single reading, but if two scans in a row show the opposite trend from your goals, you might need to reevaluate your approach.

Even if several measures in a row using one measurement method suggest something is wrong, it is wise to confirm using other measurement techniques as well. For example, if your rep strength is not improving, you do not look any bigger in photo comparisons, and your scale-based BIA shows no lean tissue changes, you probably are not gaining much muscle. If only one of your measurements suggests movement in the right direction, waiting longer to draw conclusions is a good idea.

If your goals are not being met, your first move should be to review your diet and training programs to ensure that they are being executed correctly and that there are no extenuating circumstances at play. For example, if you are not gaining much muscle on a series of weight-gain phases, make sure you are adhering to your diet plan, your stress levels are in check, you are getting good sleep, and your training structure is appropriate for hypertrophy, and so on. If all your highest priority diet principles are on point, your training is well designed, and you are very consistent in your adherence, your next move might be to recalibrate your goals. After the first five years of diet and training, progress will begin to slow substantially, and your goals should reflect this.

CHAPTER SUMMARY

- A periodic body composition analysis is the only way to quantify changes in muscle mass and body fat over time.
- Sport specificity aside, men and women who strive to be healthy and fit should maintain a body fat percentage between 10 to 20% or 15 to 30%, respectively.
- There are numerous body composition assessments, all of which can vary in their accuracy, reliability, cost, and practicality.
- The DEXA scan is currently the most accurate and accessible means of assessing body composition.
- Definitive conclusions about body composition cannot be gleaned from any single measurement alone and often need corroboration from multiple assessments using different methods over time to become clear.

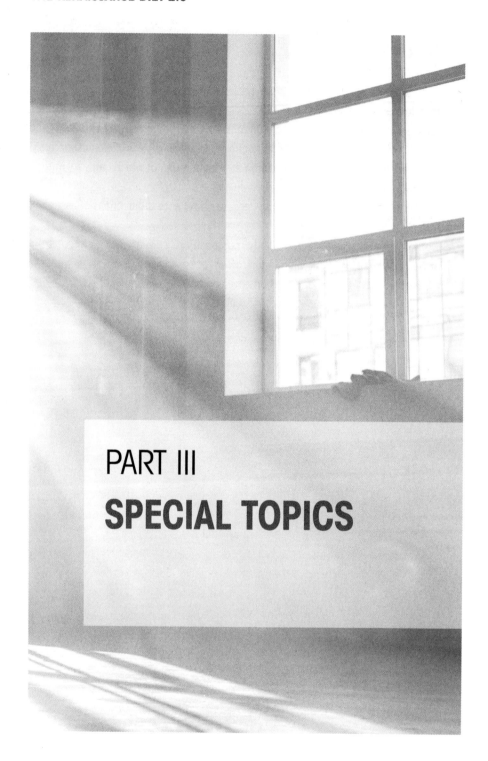

PART III
SPECIAL TOPICS

CHAPTER 13

Special Diet Considerations

The preceding chapters have provided a thorough roadmap to building a basic diet that can be altered for fat loss or muscle gain and encompass many levels of physical activity and different scheduling. However, there are circumstances, schedules, and medical conditions that require additional diet adjustments for best results.

TRAINING TWICE A DAY

Training twice a day will not make you bigger, faster, stronger, or leaner—unless you recover enough from one training session to have a productive second training session, and recover enough from both sessions and across the week to make best rates of progress over the long term. Without good recovery, training twice per day can be worse for your progress than not training at all. Training two times per day can be very productive for muscle growth when timed and fueled well. Minimizing this interference between sessions and maximizing recovery from both sessions can accommodate productive twice-daily training.

Training and Meal Timing Strategies

Ideally you will be well fueled before your first training session (have had at least one meal), have a meal or two between training sessions to recover, and have at least two meals after your last training session to replenish nutrients and help with recovery.

This assumes five to six meals per day, which is recommended when training more than once per day.

The more intense workout should be programmed in the first session. If you have some heavy lifts to do and then a lighter cardio session or higher volume technique work, program your heavy session first. It is more difficult to do workouts of high intensity when fatigued compared to voluminous or cardio based workouts. The consequences of failing a heavy lift are also worse than failing at push-ups, so this recommendation improves both training quality and safety.

Scheduling in the real world is not always flexible enough for perfection. We recommend that you prioritize keeping your sessions as far from each other as you can if you cannot keep the ideal schedule described above. There are other strategies that can further support the effectiveness of training two times per day.

Intra- and Post-Workout Shakes

Your first training session will use up your muscle glycogen, and these stores must be refilled for recovery and fueling your next training session. Drinking a workout shake containing quick-digesting carbohydrates (Gatorade, etc.) during and right after training helps with this. Fast-digesting carbohydrates spare some of your muscle glycogen by making glucose readily available in the bloodstream to be taken up and stored in your muscles—replacing what is being lost. Further, the most efficient time for glycogen resynthesis occurs during and immediately after training, so there is no more effective time to consume carbs.

High-Glycemic-Index Carb Intakes Between Sessions

The time window for efficient glycogen reloading is limited, and the need to restore fuel sources is particularly high when training twice per day. High-glycemic-index carbs have been shown to reload muscle glycogen more efficiently than low-glycemic-index carbs. Avoiding fat and fiber in meals between training also increases digestion speed. This is especially useful when there is limited time between the first and second training session and the need to maximize glycogen reloading is high. Hydration during the inter-workout period is also important for maximal uptake of glucose. About 3 g of water are required per gram of glycogen to be synthesized in muscle or liver cells.

Assigning Carbohydrate Amounts for Twice-a-Day Training

Recall from chapter 10 that we can assign training day carbohydrates based on the general workload classifications of light, moderate, and hard. Generally speaking, when training twice per day, carbs will be assigned at least according to the hardest workout of the day, if not more. In other words, a day with two light sessions or a moderate and a light session would both be treated as moderate. A hard and a light session would be treated as hard. Very hard training days, when a hard and moderate or two hard workouts are performed, require a bit more carbohydrate. In these cases, we multiply hard day carbohydrate recommendations by 1.15. See table 13.1 for a list of these recommendations.

Table 13.1 *This table gives training day classifications for twice a day training according to the two individual workouts performed on that day.*

Workout 1	Workout 2	Classify As
Light	Light	Moderate
Light	Moderate	Moderate
Light	Hard	Hard
Moderate	Moderate	Hard
Moderate	Hard	Hard
Hard	Hard	Hard x 1.15

You may wonder why carbohydrate alteration for a second hard training is only a 15% increase from one hard training session. Recall that the carbohydrates being discussed here are for a full day, and most go toward energy needs across the 20-plus non-training hours. Further, it has been shown that as workout volumes increase to very high levels, NEAT (non-exercise activity thermogenesis, or anything that burns calories but isn't exercise, like daily tasks and errands) typically falls drastically for the rest of the day. This reduces baseline expenditure during non-training hours and makes our additional 15% carbohydrate increase sufficient to fuel the second training session.

OTHER SPECIAL TIMING CONSIDERATIONS

First-Thing Training

If you wake less than an hour before training, there is not enough time to eat a pre-training meal with the recommended percentage of daily carbs, but you can still consume those carbs in liquid form in a workout shake to get a similar effect. Additionally, you can increase the whey protein content of your shake to match pre-training meal amounts. Start sipping your shake when you wake and finish it during your workout. Since this shake will be lacking the small amount of fat you may usually have in your pre-training meal, you can simply move those fats to a later meal.

Late Evening Training

Sometimes life and scheduling leave people with no choice but to train right before bed. While this is not the best option, it is better than not training. The downside is that both the post-workout meal and your bedtime meal need to be squeezed in at essentially the same time. This can leave the earlier meals of the day much more spread out. Not eating, or eating very little, after nighttime training will significantly impede muscle growth, retention, and recovery, so it is likely best to trade the downsides of a hungrier day and fuller evening for progress. There are some steps you can take to minimize discomfort. Increasing the protein and carb content of your workout shake (taking protein and carbs from the post-training meal) can make the amount of food you need to consume between training and bedtime less daunting. Moving all fats to earlier meals can help a bit with hunger across what will likely be longer meal intervals. Skipping veggies in the post-workout meal can also help (you will feel less "stuffed," and one meal without veggies on training days is unlikely to result in any vitamin or other deficiency).

Skipped Meal

If you miss a meal on a maintenance or muscle-gain diet, just spreading the macros of that meal over the next several meals is a fine solution. On a fat-loss diet, you can do the same, or, if you are not overly hungry, you can eat the protein from the missed meal when you remember and skip the fat and carbs. This is not recommended as a regular habit, but if done occasionally it will have limited detrimental effect.

VEGAN DIETS

Although arguably noble and potentially healthy, switching to a diet free of animal products is not–contrary to popular belief–a nutritional cure-all. For every benefit vegans and vegetarians stand to gain, there is a nutritional inadequacy they will need to address with careful dieting and supplementation. This lifestyle is likely beneficial to the environment, is obligatory if your personal morals oppose harming animals, and if done well can support health and fitness. For lacto-ovo vegetarians, eating for best fitness and health outcomes is a bit easier as dairy and eggs can provide much of the vitamins, minerals, and high-quality protein that vegans will need to carefully manage or supplement.

Protein

Most vegan protein is either deficient in some essential amino acids or poorly digested and absorbed by humans. The latter is due to the cellulose content of plant matter. Some exceptions such as mycoprotein, nutritional yeast, and soy exist, but most vegans will want to acquire protein from multiple sources. To ensure enough protein is absorbed and sufficient amounts of all essential amino acids are consumed throughout the day, increasing protein intake by 20% from the recommended range for your sport and personal goals is a good idea. If you are a competitive vegan athlete or want to achieve maximum body composition changes as a vegan, ensuring complete protein intake at each meal can give you an edge. While making sure all essential aminos are in included in every meal is not mandatory for health, the small difference it may make can accumulate over time for better long-term muscle retention or growth.

Carbs

Carb source recommendations for vegans are not any different from general recommendations. What may differ is that many vegan protein sources contain ancillary carbs that will go toward total carbohydrate counts when performing macro calculations.

Fats

Vegan sources of fat are plant based and therefore tend to be mainly monounsaturated and polyunsaturated, making healthy fat intake easier on a vegan diet. There is currently a popular belief that coconut oil is particularly healthy, but coconut-based fats are perhaps the least healthy vegan fat option as they contain saturated fats (which is rare in plants). Coconut oil has even more saturated fat than butter or beef fat. As with non-vegan diets, avocados, vegetable oils, and nuts and nut butters are generally the best options. Even most processed vegan food is free of trans fats and low in saturated fat, making it easier to avoid these less healthy fats.

Mixed Macro Protein Sources

Many vegan protein sources also contain a significant amount of carbs. These must be counted toward daily macros and make diet calculations a bit more complex. Particularly on a hypocaloric diet, fat amounts may need to be set lower from baseline to account for these extra carbs within the CCH (Caloric Constraint Hypothesis). Many vegan protein sources, particularly the processed ones like tempeh and mock meats, have extra fats in addition to extra carbs. On hypocaloric diets, eating leaner protein options and getting fats from other individual sources helps increase food volume and make meals a bit more appealing. If all your macros for a single meal come from a single source, dropping that macro-packed veggie burger on your plate with nothing else can be demoralizing. In contrast, when overly full on a hypercaloric diet, vegan protein options packed with carbs and fats can make the extra eating less oppressive.

Supplementation Differences

For best fitness and health outcomes, the vegan diet requires supplementation. Even when sourced primarily from whole food with a good variety of fruits, vegetables, and vegan protein sources, the vegan diet will lack important components. The following is a list of micronutrients often missing from a vegan diet that may require supplementation.

Zinc

Vegans need about 40% more zinc than omnivores. The approximately 50 mg per day recommended zinc for vegans can be consumed via careful assessment of values in foods or via supplementation.

Iron

Vegans should consume approximately 13 mg of iron per day—twice the dose of iron recommended for people who consume animal products. This is because vegans get less iron in general and because plant-derived iron (non-heme iron) is not as easily absorbed.

Vitamin D

Research on best recommended vitamin D supplementation is ongoing for vegans and athletes. Current data suggest assessing blood levels of vitamin D in individuals and supplementing at higher values (up to 5000 IU per day) when deficiencies are more extreme.

Calcium

Calcium recommendations for vegans are the same as for omnivores (1000 mg per day), but vegans have to work a bit harder to reach this amount. Plant-based sources of calcium include beans, pulses/legumes, and green vegetables. Broccoli, bok choy, and kale are great choices. Spinach and arugula also contain calcium, but along with oxalate, which impedes calcium absorption. Carefully choosing food and tracking calcium intake is recommended.

B12

B12 is found primarily in meat and dairy. One vegan protein source that is usually fortified with B12 is nutritional yeast. (Algae should not be used as a source of B12, as most of it contains factors that hinder B12 absorption). Recommended dosage for adults is 2.4 to 2.8 µg per day.

Creatine

Creatine is found in animal products, but the type sold as a powder supplement is created in the lab without the use of animal products and so is 100% vegan. Although vegans can live without this supplement, it may improve fitness and physique results to a greater extent for them compared to meat eaters. Vegans and vegetarians typically have lower muscle creatine levels, and increasing creatine load in the muscle can facilitate better resistance training performance, resulting in better response and adaptation. Creatine monohydrate should be consumed at the same dosage as recommended for omnivores (3 g per 100 lb. bodyweight per day) as the loading and maintenance process will be the same regardless of starting concentrations. Creatine must be taken consistently as maintaining constant creatine saturation in the muscles provides the best benefit.

FEMALE-SPECIFIC NUTRITION

Dieting During Conception

If the body is changing in weight, especially if it is losing weight, fertility declines. When weight is stable and nutrients are plentiful, the chances for a successful pregnancy increase. Body fat itself is also important for fertility. Body fat levels between 20 and 35% usually best support hormone levels that increase chances of conception.

Nutrition During Pregnancy

A medical professional is always your best source of nutrition information during pregnancy. The information provided here is very general, and your doctor's advice should always take precedence over general guidelines from any book. You should not diet for body composition changes, fitness, and especially not for weight loss during pregnancy. The health and growth of your baby should be your only nutrition goal during pregnancy. Weight gain during pregnancy is expected and necessary. Typical weight gain across the entire first trimester is around 2 to 4 lb., but weight gain increases to about 1 lb. per week in the second and third trimesters. This means that your average daily calorie surplus at this time is around 500 calories. Eating at your maintenance macro intake with whole, healthy foods and adding 500 calories or so from foods you crave can be an easy, healthy, and enjoyable way to fill the surplus need. Pregnancy weight gain should result in roughly 20 to 40 lb. (on the higher end of this range if you tended to stay on the lower end of body fat range before pregnancy and vice versa). Here is a rough estimate of where this weight comes from:

- 8-10 lb. from fat tissue
- 6-8 lb. from the baby itself
- 1-2 lb. from breast volume
- 6-8 lb. from blood and body fluids
- 2-3 lb. from amniotic fluid
- 2-4 lb. from placenta and uterus growth

While pregnant, eat healthy, eat well, and listen to your doctor. Pregnancy is not the time to be concerned with fitness and physique goals.

Dieting Post Delivery

Immediately after delivering, time is needed for healing and recovering before any weight-loss dieting is attempted. First, your body needs calories to heal from giving birth, your hormones need time to return to a normal baseline, and you need to be cleared by your doctor to do the hypertrophy training needed to prevent muscle loss on a hypocaloric diet. Even if you could start a fat-loss diet right after delivery, assessing weight changes would be nearly impossible thanks to larger than normal water-weight shifts in the weeks after childbirth. Your doctor will clear you for full activity at some point after having a baby, at which point you can consider beginning a weight-loss diet. This typically happens around four to six weeks after the delivery.

Dieting While Breastfeeding

Generating breast milk requires about 500 to 650 extra calories per day in addition to your maintenance calories. This decreases as your baby begins to eat other foods in addition to breast milk for their nutritional needs. It is recommended that you get the extra calories mainly from healthy whole foods during this time.

Protein should be increased by around 25 g per day from your recommended daily total to support milk production. Once you are cleared for activity and start a fat-loss diet, it is recommended that you lose no more than 1% bodyweight per week as long as you are breastfeeding in order to maintain an adequate, healthy milk supply. During this time, keep an eye on milk production. Speak with your doctor and reduce weight-loss pace or end the fat-loss phase if milk production is suffering. Your baby's health should be your first priority.

Dieting During and After Menopause

Resting metabolic rate and hormone levels decrease during menopause—the former is mainly mediated by muscle loss throughout life, so weight training can do a great deal to limit this effect in women. In other words, if women lift weights, they tend to preserve more muscle mass, have higher metabolic rates after menopause, and are able to eat more while maintaining weight as they age.

Along with lifting, increases in calcium and vitamin D can support bone health in postmenopausal women. Taking care to get fats from unsaturated sources and to eat plenty of whole grains, fruits, and vegetables is even more important after menopause as declining estrogen production increases cardiovascular disease risk.

Increasing soy intake might also reduce blood pressure and help with hot flashes, as phytoestrogens in soy can simulate the effects of estrogen in the body to a small extent.

The important thing to note is that age has less an impact on fitness-related goals for women compared to men and is largely mediated by muscle loss (which can be prevented to a large extent with weight training). Older women may not gain muscle as quickly or recover as well as they did when they were younger, but making body composition and fitness progress is still very much possible and has added health benefits.

Hormone therapy during and post menopause is also an option. Such therapy is not for everyone, but it can make a big difference for some in terms of potential for body composition change and is something to consider discussing with your doctor.

YOUTH NUTRITION CONSIDERATIONS

Diets for Young Athletes

Nutritional recommendations for young athletes focus primarily on helping kids develop healthy eating habits. When teaching children and young people about nutrition, classifying any food as "good" or "bad" should be avoided. Such extreme ideas can contribute to negative relationships with food where some foods are taboo and guilt-inducing even in moderation. Our best advice is to try to encourage positive, inclusive moderation for less healthy foods rather than negative, exclusive avoidance or elimination.

Calorie intake needs vary drastically for children because of body size differences, activity levels, and growth rates. A pediatrician can tell you how your child's weight and growth rates compare to averages and give advice on how to modulate your child's eating habits when needed. If your child is somewhat overweight, lowering calories is not recommended in most cases. Encouraging or increasing physical activity and adjusting the child's diet toward healthier foods are best recommendations. A growth spurt will often follow weight gain, so it is rare that a child should be put on a calorie-restricted diet. Because children are still growing, hypocaloric diets are almost never a good idea. Too much weight monitoring and diet structuring are not generally necessary or healthy for children as long as they are eating mainly healthy and staying active; over-monitoring and over-structuring a child's diet can encourage unhealthy eating patterns as they develop.

As a child grows, their body weight increases, so their protein needs increase accordingly. Between 0.5 and 1.0 g of protein per pound of bodyweight per day is a healthy range for most children. This recommendation is the same for both males and females. Carbohydrates should contribute to at least half of a child's daily calories, mostly from whole grains, fruits, fruit juices, and vegetables. Carbs should be eaten with nearly every meal and spread evenly throughout the day. Whole fruit should be chosen more often than fruit juices, but excess fiber can cause gastrointestinal distress more readily in children than adults. For this reason, up to half of a child's carb intake can come from white breads, pasta, and white rice to allow the consumption of enough carbs without overloading on fiber. Fats are also critical to proper growth and development. Polyunsaturated fats in particular and especially the essential fats are important for brain and nervous system development. It is likely wise to limit saturated fat intakes to 10% or less of total calories while keeping total fats at around one-third of total calories.

Work with your pediatrician to make sure your kids are not excessively over- or underweight and are meeting their nutritional needs while being positive about food and discouraging avoidance practices. This will set your children up for higher levels of athletic performance, better health, and positive eating habits. For more information on nutrition for young athletes, check out the book, *Fueling the Adolescent*.

DIETING WITH SELECT HEALTH ISSUES

Hypothyroidism

Hypothyroidism is an autoimmune disease in which the body's immune system attacks its own thyroid hormones. The thyroid gland initially compensates by ramping up hormone production but eventually becomes overstressed, resulting in lower overall thyroid hormone levels. Effects of this disease include impaired glucose control and weight gain. Prescription of synthetic thyroid hormones can be an effective treatment for some. Outside of medical treatment, making healthy diet adjustments can help control symptoms and improve longevity. More evenly distributed carb intake and lower daily carb totals can help with better blood glucose control. Increases in healthy fat consumption can be used to make up for the missing carb calories.

Unfortunately, hypothyroidism increases cardiovascular disease risk as does the weight gain which often accompanies it. For these reasons, lower-than-average recommended body fat percentages can help improve health outcomes in those with hypothyroidism. Between 16 and 25% body fat for females and 6 to 15% body fat for males is recommended. Speaking to your doctor about drug treatment as well as the mentioned diet modification recommendations can help maintain lower body fat percentages.

Hyperthyroidism

Hyperthyroidism is a condition in which the thyroid gland oversecretes thyroid hormones. This can greatly increase energy and glucose utilization in the body, leading to constant risk of liver glycogen depletion and hypoglycemia. If the individual is not sufficiently well fed, tissue wasting (rapid fat and muscle loss) may result. The most common recommendation for hyperthyroidism is increased calories. More protein is needed to offset muscle-loss risk, more carbs are needed to provide enough blood glucose and glycogen to maintain activity levels and mental acuity, and more fats can make the calorie increases tolerable. Higher carbs not only spare muscle protein from being used for energy, but they can also be consumed in much higher amounts pre-, intra-, and post-workout to supply enough energy and fuel for recovery and productive training.

Individuals with hyperthyroidism will require more calories compared to peers with similar body size and activity at every stage of the diet process. This is pretty convenient during weight loss, as only a minor calorie restriction (provided protein is kept high) will result in rapid fat loss. On the other hand, simply maintaining weight can be a chore due to the amount of food that must be eaten. Muscle gain can be oppressively difficult with hyperthyroidism as it requires extremely high calories to overcome the body's rapid metabolic rate. Those with overactive thyroids will often need to use every hunger promotion tactic from chapter 8 and a great deal of willpower in order to gain.

Polycystic Ovarian Syndrome (PCOS)

PCOS is an endocrine disorder that causes ovarian cysts. PCOS causes a host of unpleasant symptoms, some of which are relevant to fitness goals, including decreased metabolic rate (up to 20% fewer calories than their non-PCOS counterparts) and insulin resistance. A diet with fewer calories and evenly distributed carbs across meals is recommended. Abstaining from higher glycemic carbs is also a good idea. For weight-loss purposes, carb cuts to reduce calories might precede healthy fat cuts in those with PCOS. Staying active also directly improves insulin sensitivity and promotes weight loss, which indirectly further improves insulin sensitivity. Medical treatment can include birth control to regulate the timing of periods, metformin for insulin and blood sugar control, and appetite suppressing medication. A trained dietician and medical doctor should approve any diet plan for those with PCOS.

Type 1 Diabetes

Type 1 Diabetes is also commonly called "juvenile onset diabetes" because it affects children in late childhood or early teen years. It is an autoimmune disease whereby the body's own immune system attacks and destroys the beta cells of the pancreas. This makes the pancreas unable to produce insulin and therefore unable to transport glucose into most of the body's cells.

The most relevant and common medical treatment for Type 1 Diabetes is insulin injection to introduce the insulin that is not being produced internally. This means that diet must be coordinated with injections because otherwise a potentially fatal imbalance of insulin and blood sugar may occur. If insulin is injected, but no food is eaten (specifically carbohydrate), blood sugar levels can become dangerously low. This is why those who inject insulin are advised against skipping meals and should eat meals rich in slow-digesting, high-fiber carbs. This includes consuming predominantly whole grains, fruits, and vegetables for carbs and avoiding processed sources for the most part. It is critically important to note that any intentional diet manipulations with Type 1 Diabetics should be done exclusively under direct supervision from a medical doctor or a qualified nutritionist.

Type 2 Diabetes

Type 2 Diabetes or "adult onset diabetes" usually develops in individuals in their 30s and older. It is by far the most common form of diabetes, constituting more than 90% of all cases. In Type 2 Diabetes, a chronic, overwhelming amount of nutrients in the bloodstream has caused peripheral insulin resistance. The pancreas produces even more insulin to combat this lack of sensitivity, and after some time, both high circulating levels of insulin and high levels of blood glucose occur at the same time. If the situation gets bad enough, the pancreas eventually becomes overwhelmed and begins to slow and eventually stop insulin production. This leads to hyperglycemia (excessively high blood glucose), which is a very health-taxing condition that can cause limb loss, kidney shutdown, blindness, and death.

Medical treatment for Type 2 Diabetes can include blood sugar medications to improve insulin sensitivity but can eventually require injectable insulin to supplant the defunct pancreas. Diet recommendations include consumption of evenly distributed, slow-digesting carbohydrates in order to avoid dangerous spikes in blood glucose. Weight loss and fat loss are two of the best ways to minimize the risks of Type 2 Diabetes. The leaner you are and the smaller you are, the more your insulin sensitivity improves. Losing weight before you are at risk of developing Type 2 Diabetes is wise. If you already have Type 2 Diabetes, weight loss and an active lifestyle can only slow the progression of pancreatic dysfunction, not cure it. In any case, increased physical activity and reduced bodyweight and body fat are *very powerful* weapons against Type 2 Diabetes.

Gestational Diabetes

When Type 2 Diabetes is first diagnosed in a pregnant female, it is termed "gestational diabetes." Gestational diabetes can result in adverse perinatal outcomes and can be fatal to the fetus. Medical treatment for gestational diabetes usually involves injectable insulin to lower blood sugar levels, but dietary interventions can also be a part of an effective management strategy. Because of the fragile state of the developing fetus, gestational diabetes is a very serious medical condition, and nutritional therapy must be performed under the guidance of a registered dietician. Normalizing blood glucose levels to keep the fetus safe from hyper- and hypoglycemia is the first priority, and this can be done in part by making sure all meals contain a roughly similar amount of carbs throughout the day. Processed sugar intake should be limited, and the focus should be on consuming vegetables, whole grains, and fruits. Smaller, more frequent meals might also help with normalizing blood glucose levels. Lastly, making sure that weight gain during pregnancy is not excessive can help improve outcomes with this condition.

CHAPTER SUMMARY

- When training more than once a day, daily calorie and carbohydrate amounts need to be raised proportionally to the increase in overall activity.
- Higher glycemic carbohydrates can be especially useful to ensure adequate glycogen restoration when training multiple times per day, and should be consumed in the intra-workout and post-workout meals, as well as in other meals between training sessions.
- Vegans may follow the same general intake recommendations as non-vegans; however, they may benefit from increasing daily protein values by about 20% and more closely monitoring or supplementing their intake of zinc, calcium, iron, B12, vitamin D, and creatine.
- Dieting for weight loss is not recommended for women who are pregnant or trying to conceive, and weight-loss rate should be limited during breastfeeding.
- Dieting for young athletes should involve developing fundamental healthy eating habits, rather than the micromanagement of meals or any explicit dieting for body composition.
- Many select health issues can be better managed through diet and exercise; however, some may require more extensive pharmacology or medical supervision for the best outcomes.

CHAPTER 14

Competition Day Nutrition

Nutritional recommendations for the day of competition can vary a great deal both between different sports and within sports compared to recommendations for non-competition day. When the time has come to compete, the top dietary priorities are to make energy available and avoid gastrointestinal distress. Different sports require different degrees of hydration and electrolyte balance for best performance; meal timing and food composition are also sport dependent. For weight-class competition, the process of cutting body water safely is involved and should be carefully planned and executed. Replenishing fluids, electrolytes, and nutrients after a water-weight cut in time to compete is equally involved and critical for performance.

ENDURANCE SPORT COMPETITION

Carbohydrate loading is one important difference between endurance and other sports but is often overemphasized. As long as glycogen stores are full prior to competing, the exact means of filling these stores will make little difference. The more complicated nutritional differences for endurance events lie in intra-workout carbohydrate consumption, hydration, and electrolyte recommendations. Within these recommendations, there is flexibility for personal preference.

Individual reactions during competition can meaningfully impact performance, so it is especially important for endurance athletes to practice intra-workout nutritional strategies during training to assess their reactions and calibrate their strategies for future competitions.

Week Before Competition

Carbohydrate loading in the week before competition is only necessary for events over three hours. The week of competition, ensure adequate calorie consumption for recovery and glycogen replenishment. You should not be hypocaloric at this time. Shifting some caloric focus from fats to carbs is recommended to ensure maximum recovery of glycogen. This is also a good time to practice your intra-competition nutrition strategies. For events over three hours, start consuming 2 to 3 g of carbohydrate per pound of bodyweight more than normal two to three days out. Choose moderate- to high-glycemic index foods and avoid excess fiber. Overshooting these carb recommendations by a small amount for cycling events can be beneficial. Cycling is less weight-dependent than running, so the downside of a few added pounds from glycogen, water, and gut contents will be vastly outweighed by the benefits of full glycogen stores.

Day Before Competition

To continue carb loading for events lasting over three hours (or to begin loading for shorter events lasting around two hours), consume 3 to 5 g per pound of bodyweight above normal the day before the race. Spread the consumption evenly across the entire day, ideally ending by the evening before your race. If your event is under one hour, there is no need for any extensive carbohydrate loading; in this case, you can consume 0.5 g of carbs per pound of bodyweight more than you otherwise would the day before the race.

Pre-Race Meal

For events lasting more than two hours, you should consume as much carbohydrate as you can stomach without gastrointestinal distress at your pre-race meal. For some people that might be close to 1.0 g carb per pound bodyweight, and for others, it might be no more than 0.5 g carbohydrate per pound bodyweight. Again, practicing with your pre-race meal before long training runs will allow you to determine where you lie on this spectrum of pre-race carb recommendations. Experiment early and often. Rebound hypoglycemia, or "blood sugar crashing," results in intense hunger, shakiness, sweating, faintness, nausea, and fatigue—none of which are ideal for performance. It is generally a safe bet to consume your pre-race meal 90 to 120 minutes prior to race start. Getting a final bite or swig of easily digestible carbs within 15 minutes of starting an event or event warm-up is probably a good idea as well.

Race Day

Carbohydrate Recommendations

When determining intra-workout carbohydrate needs, endurance athletes must consider the potential for gastrointestinal distress along with the absorption rates of the carbohydrate sources they choose. The upper limit of carbohydrate absorption during exercise is approximately 90 g per hour. This has been shown to be largely independent of athlete body mass or size but can vary by up to 20% between individuals. Increasing carbohydrate consumption to beyond 90 g per hour is unlikely to improve performance under any circumstances. As exercise duration increases, so too should the rate of carbohydrate consumption. Table 14.1 lists minimum, recommended, and maximum carb intakes for exercise at different durations. Start with the recommended amount and increase carbohydrate consumption to find where you perform best, up to the maximum. If you begin to have gastrointestinal issues, consider reducing carb content toward the minimum listed. Going below the minimum is not recommended and will likely result in performance decrement.

Table 14.1 *Carbohydrate minima, recommended amounts, and maxima for consumption during endurance competitions of varying lengths.*

Intra-Competition Carbohydrate (grams/hour)			
Duration of Workout	Minimum	Recommended	Maximum
Up to 30 min.	0	10	30
30 min. to 1 hr.	0	20	40
1-1.5 hr.	10	30	50
1.5-2 hr.	20	40	60
2-2.5 hr.	40	50	70
2.5-3 hr.	50	60	80
3+ hr.	60	75	90

Some of these recommendations are slightly higher than research data suggest. The reason for this is that there is a chance of enhancement of glycogen replenishment from slightly overshooting carbohydrate needs, which can be especially useful if your competition involves multiple bouts of endurance activity.

It is inevitable that consumption will not keep up with metabolic carbohydrate demand during long endurance events because the absorption rate of carbohydrates in the gastrointestinal tract during continuous exercise is limited. It is important to maximize the amount of carbohydrate absorbed per unit of time. This can be managed by increasing fructose content in your intra-workout carbohydrate drinks. The more absorption per hour needed, the higher the fructose to glucose ratio should be, up to a maximum of 1:2.

Hydration Recommendations

With steady drinking, most athletes can consume one liter of fluid per hour of exertion without gastrointestinal distress. This is provided that the concentration of the sugar and electrolytes in the water is not greater than that of the fluid in their body, as this slows gastric emptying. It is sometimes advantageous to increase the concentration of sugar for available energy, despite the risk this presents for hydration. This is a much more complex topic, but targeting 6 to 8% sugar in solution is a good place to start. The use of more concentrated beverages should be done with care and practiced before race day to ensure adequate hydration is still possible. Ironically, acute dehydration can also slow gastric emptying rates, making it harder to take in water once dehydration has begun. For the ultra-endurance athlete, it is important to stay well ahead of dehydration. The fuller the stomach is (to a point just shy of discomfort), the faster gastric emptying occurs. Athletes can take advantage of this by consuming fluid regularly enough to maintain stomach volume—every 10 minutes is recommended, with 15 minutes being a likely maximum. Waiting longer than 15 minutes between consumption episodes can result in a decreased gastric emptying rate, less-than-optimal hydration maintenance during endurance activity, and potentially hypoglycemia. Some people elect to stop consuming fluids toward the end of an event to maximize performance. This decision should be made only by advanced athletes seeking to squeeze every last second out of their performance, and even then, it is a gamble.

STRENGTH, POWER, AND COMBAT SPORT COMPETITION

Like most sports, strength, power, and combat sports benefit from full glycogen stores. Unless you need to cut in order to make weight for an event, your goal in the three to four days before competition should be to consume adequate calories to maintain your weight and plenty of carbs to maintain full glycogen stores. The stress and excitement of competition day can make your stomach more sensitive, so eating foods you are used to is recommended to avoid any additional gastrointestinal distress.

If you participate in a sport like powerlifting, strongwoman, or any sport that has multiple events separated by hours throughout the day, fueling across the entire competition is relatively straightforward. This type of schedule gives you time to replenish fluid, glycogen, and calories between events. Low-fat, low-fiber food options and eating and drinking as soon as each event is over is recommended. This practice minimizes chances for digestion to interfere with the subsequent event. Protein is also slow digesting in most forms, so getting your protein from a shake and your carbs from some high-glycemic foods is a good option.

For combat sports that run on a tournament-style schedule with matches or fights separated by much shorter breaks, inter-match nutrient sources must be even more quickly digesting and easy on the stomach. Protein shakes and electrolyte carb beverages are probably your best choice under these circumstances.

Peaking for Physique Competition

Eating to peak for physique competition requires a complex dietary strategy because there is so much individual variation in which protocol will yield best performance. There is an entire industry of contest prep coaches that specialize bringing physique athletes to their peak, and many of these prep coaches are in exceptional demand because of their ability to correctly manipulate the dietary variables based on individual needs. A thorough guide to the physique peaking process and various possible strategies would take an entire book to describe. This section will cover the general structure for effective contest peaking; tweaks will likely be needed based on individual responses. Plenty of practice and some expert guidance is recommended in addition to the following instructions.

The physique peaking process should start about one-and-a-half weeks before the show. Once you begin the peaking process, you should be in an isocaloric state. This means that you must be as lean as needed for your contest one-and-a-half weeks before. Starting your fat-loss diet with this earlier deadline in mind is important.

Macronutrients

During the one-and-a-half weeks prior to the contest, protein intake should be between 1 to 1.5 g per pound per day, and fat intakes should be at least 0.3 g per pound per day, preferably more in order to begin normalizing hormonal levels. The goal for a physique show is to have your muscles appear as large and defined as possible, with visible vascularization under the skin. When you manipulate glycogen stores by increasing carbohydrate intake, you will fill your stores, making your muscles look full, but you will also risk water retention under the skin, making you appear less lean. Your goal is to have filled glycogen stores with minimal subcutaneous water. There are three potential ways of going about this:

1 Coasting In

Rapid elevations in carbohydrate intake are most likely the cause for subcutaneous bloating. One strategy to mediate this issue is to adjust carbs moderately based on appearance. If your muscles look flat, increase carbs, and if you are bloated and seem to be holding water under your skin, reduce carbs. This strategy minimizes risk, but it might not maximize glycogen stores. It takes practice or the help of an experienced coach to perfect.

2 Slow Ramp

We know that the process of storing glycogen and the process of cell hydration can take hours to days to normalize. Thus, another strategy for increasing muscle glycogen can be to increase slowly (adding 50-100 g of carbs per day). While the initial increase in carbs can negatively affect appearance due to water retention, a delay of a day or two can result in improved appearance. A ramp approach should have a top-end target of around 5 g per pound per day by 72 hours before the show. If you see signs of subcutaneous water retention in the 72 to 96 hours before the show, cut carbs by 40%, and you should level out by the show. If you see water retention earlier, keep carbs at the current level until 72 to 96 hours before and then make a new assessment.

3 Depletion Supercompensation

This strategy is probably the most complex and risky, but it has the potential to optimize your appearance. In a process called glycogen supercompensation, muscles depleted of glycogen tend to take it up more readily and in slightly larger amounts for a short period of time. Protocols for facilitating this phenomenon begin with high-volume, full-body training in the last week of a mesocycle and limited to no carbs for two to four days early in the week before the show to deplete glycogen. About 72 hours before the show, a high-carb diet begins (around 3-5 g per pound per day), and supercompensation occurs. The risk with this process is added fatigue and little room for in-process tweaking of your appearance. The upside is that, when done well, supercompensation can give you the fullest possible muscles with the least subcutaneous water and therefore an extra competitive edge. This strategy is worthwhile if you have the experience or guidance to choose the right carb values and timing that work for you. Unless you are familiar with the precise physiological mechanisms underlying this strategy, it is probably best to hire a coach with an upper level education in a sport- and exercise-related field and experience coaching physique athletes.

Water

Increased carbohydrate intake will help pull the water you drink into the muscles. This effect can be enhanced by consuming more water than needed in the one-and-a-half weeks before the show. A good starting point for this water increase is around 50% more than usual. This increase initiates diuresis (more urination), but the extra water intake will still be enough to fill out your muscles.

During the last one to two days before the show, you can reduce water intake back to normal levels. Because this reduction is relatively minor, diuresis will continue, helping to eliminate subcutaneous water. The mild reduction in water consumption is also not drastic enough to drain the water from your muscles or initiate an antidiuretic response which could cause you to hold water under your skin.

Salt/Electrolytes

While manipulating electrolytes can allow you to fine-tune your appearance, this also has the potential to go terribly wrong and be detrimental to your on-stage appearance. We recommend avoiding electrolyte protocols unless you are very well practiced or are assisted by an expert physique coach with a formal education in a sport- and exercise-related field—risks to optimal appearance typically outweigh rewards.

Water-Weight Cuts

While we do not recommend running fat-loss diets up to competitions under any circumstance (and in fact recommend getting down to your competition weight four to eight weeks before the competition), there are some situations in which cutting water can land you in a more beneficial weight class for your sport without sacrificing performance. For safety, health, and ability to recover to full performance capacity, we do not recommend losing more than 5% of your bodyweight in water for any reason. The amount of time you have to rehydrate and replenish after weighing in dictates how much water weight can be safely lost (up to 5%).

Table 14.2 lists the amount of bodyweight that can be lost in water and replenished across specific time periods, along with the setup time required for these manipulations.

Table 14.2 *A list of percentages of bodyweight that can be safely lost as water and replenished during the various time periods between weigh-in and competition as well as the days prior to weigh-in that preparation must begin.*

Time Between Weigh-In and Competition	% Bodyweight That Can Be Lost	Prep Time Needed Before Weigh-In
24 hours	5%	Approx. 7 days
12 hours	3%	Approx. 4 days
2 hours	2%	Approx. 1 day
Mat-side	1% or less	Less than 1 day

Dehydration can be dangerous, especially when approaching losses of 5% bodyweight. Pre-existing conditions can increase these risks further. Though you may have heard of MMA fighters undergoing much more drastic water-weight cuts, this practice is extremely dangerous and can result in death or permanent damage to organ systems. These fighters (who often have doctors on hand and IV-based recovery options) are taking a serious risk losing more than 5% bodyweight via a water cut.

Equally important to cutting water is replenishing what was lost. Electrolyte balance must be returned, glycogen stores must be refilled, and the athlete needs be rehydrated following the weigh-in. This can take as much care and consideration as the water-weight cut itself and is critical for performance. It is best to consult your physician before attempting any of the following dehydration techniques. Once you have a doctor's approval, it is still wise to have someone with you and to proceed with caution.

Mat-Side Weigh-In

For strength or combat sports, a 1% bodyweight drop via dehydration is unlikely to negatively affect performance, so even if competition immediately follows the weigh-in, this level of dehydration can be worth the benefits of getting to a lighter weight class. To decrease bodyweight by 1% through dehydration, water consumption should be minimized starting about 12 hours before weigh-ins. During the 12 to 24 hours before the weigh-in, food volumes (fibrous options) should be reduced and salt intake should be decreased by 70% or more for the day prior and day of competition.

For competitions with a higher endurance component such as combat sports like jiu jitsu (which typically has mat-side weigh-ins), any level of dehydration can be detrimental to performance. In this case, prevention of unnecessary bloat (overhydration) is the most you can do without sacrificing performance. To this end, overly salty foods and high-volume foods should be avoided the day before and morning of a mat-side weigh-in.

Using the earlier chapters of this book to lose fat months prior to competing is the best way to make sure you are on weight and ready to perform in a sport with mat-side weigh-ins.

1 Hour Between Weigh-In and Competition

There is little time to replenish nutrients and water within a two-hour period. A 2% loss of bodyweight is the maximum for this type of weigh-in. About a day of preparation time is needed.

Starting the day before the weigh-in:
- Choose low-volume food options.
- Restrict carbohydrate intake to 0.3 g per poundbody weight or less (the less the better).

- Decrease salt by approximately 70% from normal.
- Stop drinking water approximately 12 hours before weigh-in.

Starting immediately after the weigh-in:
- Consume a minimum of 1 L of fluids per 100 lb. bodyweight.
- Consume approximately 1.2 g per poundbody weight in carbs.
- Consume approximately 0.3 g per pound bodyweight in protein.
- Consume approximately 0.1 g per pound bodyweight in fats.

Sandwiches, low-fat sushi options, rice, pasta, or any other sources of carbs and lean protein paired with soft drinks, sports drinks, and options like low-fat chips are good choices for post weigh-in replenishment. Moderate to fast-digesting macros low in fiber will help the nutrients get to where they are needed in time for you to compete.

12 Hours Between Weigh-In and Competition

The approximately 12-hour period between weighing in and competing allows up to 3% bodyweight loss, but a bit more preparation time is required to safely initiate this level of dehydration. The additional time for replenishment allows more extensive water loss via carbohydrate reduction, which decreases the amount of water held in the body by glycogen. This timeframe also allows water loading early on in order to promote subsequent water loss. Following is a time structure for the process of losing 3% bodyweight, starting four days out from your weigh-in, followed by some detailed explanations for these procedures and a strategy for replenishment.

4 days out from weigh-in
- Restrict carbohydrate intake to 0.3 g per pound bodyweight or less.
- Drink approximately 4 L of fluid per 100 lb. bodyweight per day.
- Consume normal amounts of salt.

48 hours out from weigh-in
- Reduce salt intake by approximately 70% or more.

24 hours out from weigh-in
- Begin restricting water (drink sips of water to swallow food at most).
- Limit food volume.
- Limit fiber.

Carbohydrate Reduction

Glycogen can store up to 3 g of water per gram of carbohydrate. An individual weighing 150 lb. can therefore store roughly 500 g of glycogen and thus 1.5 kg of water. This adds up to 2 kg (4.4 lb.) total weight in glycogen and water. Thus depleting 75% of glycogen results in a weight reduction of approximately 1.5 kg (approx. 3.3 lb.). For a 150-lb. person, that is already over 2% bodyweight.

Glycogen is used during all daily tasks and typically will become depleted after around five days of minimal to no carbohydrate intake. Fats can be increased during this time to make up for the calories lost when carbs are eliminated.

Water Loading

Drinking large amounts of water shifts the body's water retention systems toward diuresis. In other words, if you drink more water than you need, your body will upregulate its systems for water removal, which will come in handy when you are subsequently dehydrating for water-weight loss. Remember during this process that all liquids contain water, and you get plenty of water from food, so these foods and any liquids will also contribute to your water loading. As mentioned previously, hyponatremia can also be a concern when consuming high volumes of water. To be safe, drink enough extra fluid so that you are urinating frequently (every few hours) and your urine is pale yellow, but do not drink much more than 4 L per 100 lb. of bodyweight per day. Watch for symptoms like nausea, headache, confusion, and muscle spasms and stop drinking and consult your doctor if you have these or other symptoms or do not feel well. It is also important to spread your water consumption out across the day. Do not drink large amounts in one sitting—never drink more than 1 L at a time as a rule. The more spread out your intake, the safer. During water loading, your weight will rise for the first several days as you hyper-hydrate. As your water regulation pathways adjust to the higher water intakes and induce diuresis, and glycogen depletion from your low carb diet occurs, your weight will fall.

Salt Restriction

Salt pulls even more water into your tissues than glycogen. Thus, restricting salt intake is eventually going to be a strategy to drop lots of body water. However, the hormonal regulators of salt concentration in the human body are incredibly sensitive and will create an antidiuretic (water retention) effect within hours of salt restriction. For this reason, salt intake adjustments come later in the dehydration process for 12-hour weigh-ins. Continue to eat normal amounts of salt all week before this manipulation is initiated and drink some carb-free electrolyte beverages as a part of your fluid intake.

Water Restriction

During this phase, consume only enough water to be able to swallow your food and nothing more. The diuretic drive from water loading and the release of water from glycogen stores and lowered salt intakes will initiate heavy urination and water-weight loss.

Food Restriction

In the final day before the weigh-in, minimize the amount of food in your digestive tract. Eating very low-volume foods with minimal fiber (since fiber holds water) will reduce digesting food and fecal weight. Skip the fruits and veggies during this time. Casein protein pudding is a great low-volume option that will also make you feel fuller despite its low volume.

Once you have weighed in, replenishing lost fluid, carbohydrates, and electrolytes is imperative for good performance. This process should begin as soon as possible after the weigh-in. More fast-digesting options are better here as there is limited time to complete the replenishment process. Most of your post-weigh-in food should be consumed in the approximately first six hours, especially if the weigh-ins were done the night before a competition, and you need to sleep after replenishing. Fluids can be a bit more spread out as you will have quite a bit to drink in order to replenish, and taking in large volumes at a time can be dangerous.

Starting immediately after the weigh-in, 12 hours before competition:
- Consume approximately 4.0 L of fluids per 100 lb. bodyweight.*
- Consume approximately 25 calories per pound of bodyweight.
- Consume approximately 4.5 g carbs per pound bodyweight.

- Consume approximately 0.7 g protein per pound bodyweight.
- Consume approximately 0.5 g fats per pound bodyweight.

*Spread out drinking volume across the hours of replenishment and never drink more than 1 L of plain water in a single sitting (to decrease risk of hyponatremia). If volumes of more than 1 L at a time are needed to complete rehydration across the approximately first six hours, electrolyte beverages for larger single intakes are recommended.

24 Hours Between Weigh-In and Competition

The strategy for this type of weigh-in is very similar to the 12-hour weigh-in except that we start dropping carbs and water loading a bit earlier to promote more water loss. There will be more time to replenish between weighing in and competing, allowing this water cut to be a bit more extensive, up to 5% bodyweight. This timeframe also allows for a final manipulation when needed and hyperthermic induction of water loss through sweat. Following is a timeline for the 24-hour weigh-in depletion and replenishment strategy followed by some details on aspects of this process. Table 14.3 depicts the timeline for 24-hour weigh-in depletion procedures.

Table 14.3 *This table is a quick reference for the timeline of water loading, carb depletion, salt depletion, water depletion, and hyperthermia that must occur across the seven days leading up to a 24-hour weigh-in, in order for the maximum 5% of water weight to be successfully lost.*

Strategy	Begins	Ends
Low-Carb Eating	7 days out	After weigh-in
Water Loading	7 days out	24 hours out
Salt Depletion	48 hours out	After weigh-in
Water Depletion	24 hours out	After weigh-in
Food Volume Reduction	24 hours out	After weigh-in
Hyperthermia	12-4 hours out	After weigh-in

The justifications for low-carb eating, water loading, salt and subsequent water restriction, and low-volume food consumption recommendations are the same for the 24-hour weigh-in as for the 12-hour weigh-in. See the previous 12-hour weigh-in section for these.

Hyperthermia

This final strategy is used in the last 12 hours or so before the weigh-in itself. By increasing our body temperature, we can initiate sweating and lose even more water weight. The substantial trade-off is that hyperthermia is very fatiguing and is not safe for long periods, so we recommend:

- Using all of the other strategies to the maximal extent before employing hyperthermia.
- Overheating (in the sauna, for example) for no longer than 20 minutes without a break.
- Being observant of your physical and mental state and cooling down when needed.
- Limiting water-weight loss from hyperthermia to approximately 1% bodyweight.

If your vision starts to blur, you lose coordination, or muscle weakness presents, cease your weight cut immediately and seek medical attention. Again we recommend getting clearance from a medical doctor before beginning this process. You should also always have someone with you during hyperthermia (someone who is not also cutting water weight).

Some methods for inducing hyperthermia and water loss through sweat are wearing warmer-than-needed clothing or using a sauna, hot shower, hot bath, or hot tub. Exercising in overly warm clothes is not recommended due to the additional fatigue added by exertion.

Hyperthermia is already a stressful and fatiguing strategy, so minimizing its negative impact is best. If you have fully utilized all of the other strategies and are staying within safe weight-loss ranges, active hyperthermia will be unnecessary.

Replenishment Following a 24-Hour Weigh-In

As with any water-weight cut, the timely replacement of the lost nutrients and fluids afterwards is critical for best performances. After weighing in 24 hours before a competition, replenishment should begin immediately and should be mostly complete 12 to 16 hours later, allowing time for sleep—rest is also critical for resolution of accumulated fatigue from the water cut. When all nutrients are replenished and you are fully hydrated again and ready for competition, your weight should reflect this return to baseline. If morning weight on the day of the competition is still lower than usual, aggressive replacement of fluid and nutrients is still needed.

Starting immediately after the weigh-in, 24 hours before competition:
- Consume approximately 6.0 L of fluids per 100 lb. bodyweight.*
- Consume approximately 35 calories per pound of bodyweight.
- Consume approximately 7 g carbs per pound bodyweight.
- Consume approximately 0.7 g protein per pound bodyweight.
- Consume approximately 0.5 g fats per pound bodyweight.

*Spread out drinking volume across the hours of replenishment and never drink more than 1 L of plain water in a single sitting (to decrease risk of hyponatremia). If volumes of more than 1 L at a time are needed to complete rehydration across the first approximately 2 to 16 hours, electrolyte beverages for larger single intakes are recommended.

Carbohydrate Replenishment

Ingesting 7 g of carbs per pound of bodyweight is a relatively large amount of carbs; carb replenishment should be spread out across the first 12 to 16 hours after weigh-in. There is a limit to the rate at which carbs can be absorbed and resynthesized into glycogen; in general, 1 g per pound of bodyweight every two hours is a good working limit. If you weigh 150 lb., you want to limit your carb intake to around 150 g every two hours–this means that if you have a meal every four hours, you would have 300 g of carbs per meal. Carbs should be relatively low in fiber (to enhance absorption and prevent feeling too full to get in all needed food and liquid); moderate-to-high glycemic (to enhance absorption speed, glycogen loading rate, and total amount loaded); and be from a combination of solid and liquid sources. The "fun" carbs have their day today. Recommended options include low-fat cookies, cakes, snack crackers, chips, as well as kids' cereal; non-fat or low-fat flavored milk; white bread, white rice; and sugary sports drinks, fruit juice, or regular soda (without caffeine).

The Role of Calories in Recovery

Large amounts of calories must be consumed during the first 12 hours after weigh-in for two reasons. First, a hypercaloric diet is one of the best ways to alleviate fatigue, a side effect of the water cut. Second, if recommended carb amounts are eaten but calories are inadequate, much of the carb intake will go to fueling normal body activities and not get incorporated into glycogen reserves. Be careful not to overeat fats and keep fiber low so as not to delay digestion.

Salt Replenishment

There is no need to take salt pills or over-salt your food to replenish electrolytes. Because you are eating fairly large amounts of food, you are likely to get most of the salt you need from this and any electrolyte sports drinks you might be drinking to rehydrate.

Following is a sample meal plan across the 24 hours after a weigh-in the day before competition:

Right After Weigh-In:
Gatorade and whey protein

30 Minutes Later:
A deli meat, white bread sandwich with baked low-fat potato chips, and a glass of water

2 Hours Later:
A low-fat burrito with two glasses of regular caffeine-free soda

1.5 Hours Later:
Non-fat frozen yogurt with sugary toppings and a glass of water

2 Hours Later:
A deli meat sandwich with baked low-fat potato chips and a glass of water

1.5 Hours Later:
Low-fat devil's food cake with a glass of non-fat chocolate milk

3 Hours Later:
Sushi with soy sauce and a glass of Gatorade

1.5 Hours Later:
Poptarts with a glass of non-fat strawberry milk

3 Hours Later:
Teriyaki bowl with just rice and protein and a glass of water

For breakfast the following day, have a meal similar to one of your post weigh-in meals and continue to hydrate.

CHAPTER SUMMARY

- Pre-competition carbohydrate loading is an effective tool for saturating glycogen stores before endurance events or any event lasting more than three hours.
- During endurance events, athletes are encouraged to continue consuming water with electrolytes and carbohydrates throughout the competition; however, they should find dosing strategies that do not cause gastrointestinal distress.
- Most strength, power, and combat sports do not require advanced pre- or competition-day-specific nutrition outside of staying hydrated and well fed in the days leading into competition.
- Peaking for a physique competition requires careful manipulations in carbohydrate, water, and electrolytes and should be done under the guidance of a reputable professional, as it can be dangerous when done improperly.
- Cutting water for a weight class is largely dependent on how much time there is for replenishment of water, nutrients, and electrolytes between the weigh-in and competition.
- Water cutting potentially comes with some substantial risks, including death, so medical clearance and supervision are a must.

CHAPTER 15

Gut Health

The study of the digestion and absorption of nutrients has exploded in recent years. There is a lot more going on than you might imagine after you swallow the last bite of your perfectly designed post-training meal. The human intestinal tract is home to over 100 trillion microorganisms comprised of thousands of species expressing millions of genes. There are about 10 times more bacterial cells in the gut than human cells in the body, and together they weigh about 1.5 kg. These bacteria, collectively known as the gut microbiome, play a role in everything from food digestion and vitamin production to appetite regulation and immunity. They have also been implicated in a variety of other processes in metabolic and cognitive function.

Evidence has been mounting that the types and ratios of an individual's gut bacteria–their enterotype–can even be correlated with their propensity for obesity. Dysbiosis, or a gut microbiome lacking diversity with an abundance of non-beneficial bacteria, has been linked to inflammatory bowel diseases, insulin resistance, and even obesity.

While there is promising evidence that a healthy gut microbiome may contribute to positive health and fitness outcomes, this should only be taken into consideration after you have perfected all of your other diet priorities. A probiotic shake will not cancel out the effects of a poor nutrition and poor planning. Interestingly, a healthy diet itself might be the biggest factor in promoting better gut health.

Supplementation cannot recolonize an individual's gut, but it can enrich certain populations. However, recent research has illustrated potential risks and shortcomings to probiotic supplementation, indicating that this practice should not be recommended wholesale.

EFFECTS OF THE MICROBIOME ON APPETITE AND METABOLISM

Appetite

While the mechanisms are not completely understood, emerging evidence shows that the microbiome can affect hunger-regulating hormones in the gut and the brain. Gut bacteria ferment some fibers and the by-products of this fermentation (short-chain fatty acids) stimulate the production of hormones that signal satiety. Some bacteria can produce certain neurotransmitters and neuromodulators which also suppress appetite, and there also appears to be a link between gut bacteria and the signaling system that drives eating for pleasure rather than hunger. Because hunger and appetite are affected by so many factors, this is an area that requires much more research, but the gut microbiome does appear to play a role in eating behaviors and the propensity for obesity or disordered eating habits.

Metabolism

Skeletal muscle is one of the largest metabolically active tissues in the body, and in healthy individuals it responds rapidly to changes in fuel availability. Diabetes, obesity, and high-fat diets are all linked to metabolic inflexibility, or abnormal skeletal muscle metabolism that leads to more fat storage in the muscle and a reduced ability to use fat for energy. Skeletal muscle cells express immune system receptors that can be activated by lipopolysaccharide (LPS), released from certain strains of gut bacteria. Individuals with obesity or type II diabetes exhibit elevated levels of LPS, the bacteria that release it, and the immune receptor to which it binds. High-fat meals also increase the permeability of the intestines, allowing more LPS to enter the bloodstream. When LPS binds the immune receptors on skeletal muscle, the inflammatory response results in metabolic inflexibility.

While studies in humans are correlational, many studies in mice have shown that colonization with bacteria from an obese mouse to a lean mouse will result in obesity and insulin resistance without a change in food intake. Additionally, feeding studies in humans have illustrated that high-fat meals increase concentrations of LPS in the blood. While the link between obesity and the risk of type II diabetes has long been established, the microbiome is emerging as an important player in this relationship. Further research may give us a clearer picture of how the two are linked.

EFFECTS OF DIET ON THE MICROBIOME

Many factors influence the profile of the microbiome, including age, gender, and drug use, but physical activity and dietary habits seem to have the greatest impact. Exercise and diet are each estimated to account for 20% of the microbial profile. Rapid and long-lasting changes to the microbiome have both been documented, but how profound and sustained any exogenously induced change to the microbiome can be has yet to be fully determined.

Current evidence also shows that some bacteria can change without alterations to predominant metabolic pathways present in the microbiome (i.e., favoring the metabolism of carbohydrate versus protein), so not all observed changes will have any meaningful effect for the individual. Likewise, transient changes in the function of the microbiome can occur without changes to the profile of bacteria present, and this effect may be missed in studies that only examine the organisms rather than their functionality. There are clear correlations between dietary habits and the gut microbiome, but the details and implications are still being studied.

Carbohydrates

High-carbohydrate diets are associated with greater numbers of bacteria more common in exercisers compared to sedentary individuals, but the species of bacteria in this group have a wide array of beneficial and pathogenic effects. It is important to note that because fiber plays such an important role in microbial metabolism, whole grains are preferable to refined grains. Replacing refined grains with whole grains has already been shown to improve appetite control and blood glucose regulation, but also appears to increase the population of some varieties of beneficial bacteria. While there is still much to be learned, it is clear that a high-fiber diet confers many health benefits and may improve the gut microbiome as an added bonus.

Some individuals experience severe symptoms of irritable bowel syndrome after ingestion of certain fibers (those that can be fermented by gut bacteria), and in this case, a low FODMAP (fermentable oligosaccharide, disaccharide, monosaccharide, and polyol) diet is recommended. Reducing the intake of fructose, lactose, sorbitol, and mannitol may reduce the numbers of beneficial bacteria, but it also reduces the symptoms of IBS. A low-FODMAP diet is not intended for long-term adherence, but it is a helpful tool to strategically remove and reintroduce foods to determine their effect on one's gastric issues.

Artificial Sweeteners

The effects of non-nutritive sweeteners, such as saccharin, aspartame, and sucralose, on the gut microbiome are just beginning to emerge. Most of the research thus far has been done in rodent models and still needs testing in human subjects. In one small human study, the ingestion of high amounts of saccharin (equal to the FDA's maximum acceptable daily intake) led to reversible changes in the profile of the microbiome of some participants. When their gut bacteria were transplanted into mice, those mice experienced the same effects. These effects were highly individual, and it is likely that one's susceptibility to these changes is based on their enterotype (i.e., their gut bacteria). Both aspartame and sucralose have been shown to reduce the diversity of the microbiome. While the dose of aspartame in these studies was reasonable (equivalent to 2-3 diet sodas per day), the dose of sucralose was equivalent to an individual drinking one diet soda per 4 lb. of bodyweight per day–a physiologically unreasonable volume.

A great deal of additional research needs to be done in order to conclude whether changes in gut microbiome are seen consistently in humans as a result of consumption of normal-level, non-nutritive sweetener and whether these changes meaningfully impact any fitness or health outcomes.

Calories must be accounted for when replacing artificial sweeteners with a nutritive sweetener, as an excess of energy can cause weight gain. Sugar-sweetened beverages are associated with reduced microbial diversity as well as obesity, so the replacement of regular beverages with diet versions is beneficial, irrespective of microbiome effects.

Low-glycemic sweeteners such as agave nectar, isomaltooligosaccharide (IMO) sweetener, or sugar alcohols, are alternatives to table sugar, but they still contain calories and may cause gastric distress if consumed in high amounts. Based on the evidence thus far, regular consumption of sucralose seems to have the most minimal effect on the microbiome, with saccharine following a close second.

Fats

A high-fat diet (generally defined as one in which more than 40% of calories come from fat) has been linked to low-grade inflammation termed metabolic endotoxemia, wherein pieces of bacterial cell walls (endotoxins) escape the gut and activate an immune response. This process has been implicated in insulin resistance and obesity. High-fat diets also appear to reduce microbiome diversity and promote specific strains of bacteria associated with the development of obesity. Even a high-fat but calorie-restricted diet (a ketogenic diet with lowered carbs to produce a caloric deficit) led to a reduction of certain desirable strains of bacteria. High-fat diets have even been shown to prevent the positive gut microbiome effects seen with physical training; the guts of exercising participants consuming a high-fat diet resembled that of the sedentary control group. This is something to consider when using the CCH to determine fat and carb intakes—keeping your total fat at a level that contributes to less than 40% of total calories is likely a good idea. An active person assigning carbohydrates according to recommendations provided in earlier chapters should have no trouble adhering to this as too many calories will be taken up by carbs to allow for a high-fat diet in most cases.

Saturated fat, monounsaturated fat, and Omega-6 polyunsaturated fats all seem to elicit similar effects on various beneficial bacterial strains, likely because these bacteria specialize in metabolizing specific plant-based compounds. Diets high in animal fats appear to preferentially increase numbers of bacteria which degrade the protective mucus layer of the intestines. This could be one mechanism behind the increased permeability of the intestinal wall during a high-fat diet. Omega-3 polyunsaturated fats do not appear to affect the profile of the gut microbiome. Because epidemiological studies can only illustrate associations, and intervention studies do not keep fiber constant between controls, it is unclear whether a diet high in fat and fiber would have the same effects as the high-fat, low-fiber diets studied thus far.

Protein

Animal Protein

Few studies have examined the effects of high-protein diets on the gut microbiome, and they come with confounding variables since increased protein at the same calorie intake requires a decrease in either fats or carbohydrates. High-protein diets have been linked to improved body composition and reduced appetite. However, epidemiological studies have linked regular consumption of red and processed meats to increased risk of colorectal cancer and inflammatory bowel diseases via products of amino acid fermentation by bacteria. Several studies have shown that high protein intake is correlated with bacterial profiles associated with leanness, but these bacteria also produce compounds associated with colorectal cancer and atherosclerosis. The production of these compounds appears to be higher with habitual ingestion of red meat compared to poultry. Other studies have shown that the effects depend on the specific type of protein; for example, animal proteins and whey protein have been shown to have differing effects. More research is needed to elucidate the best recommendations, and these may differ from person to person.

Collagen

Recently, some fitness celebrities have popularized supplementing with collagen or glutamine to support gut health, but there is no evidence that either product "heals" gut permeability. Glutamine is a prime nutrient for intestinal cells, but a dietary deficiency is highly unlikely; likewise, the amino acids found in collagen are readily available in other protein sources with better digestibility, and non-essential amino acids (including glutamine, glycine, and proline found in collagen supplements) can be made by the body. Due to the low bioavailability of collagen and its lack of essential amino acids, it is not a suitable replacement for whole food or post-workout protein shakes.

Gluten

Gluten is a protein found in wheat, barley, and rye. It can cause severe allergic responses in individuals with celiac disease (CD). A gluten-free diet (GFD) reduces the prevalence of these attacks for affected individuals. Recently, a GFD has become one of the most popular diets worldwide, though there is no evidence that it is superior to any other diet for reducing or controlling bodyweight. Because a GFD excludes some sources of carbohydrates and fiber, it can cause changes in the microbiome. Likewise, the microbiome may play a role in the development of CD, as CD patients characteristically demonstrate dysbiosis even after a GFD is adopted. Removal of gluten from the diet has been shown to modestly increase types of bacteria that metabolize resistant starch, which may be due to greater inclusion of gluten-free carbohydrate sources like potatoes. In mice that were colonized with bacteria from CD patients, immune responses to gluten were much more severe compared to mice colonized with anti-inflammatory bacteria. Some people who do not have CD may experience some relief from general gastric distress on a gluten-free diet. Long-term consumption of a GFD has been associated with weight gain in both children and adults, so there is little justification for adopting this diet to lose weight if you do not have CD.

Probiotics

Probiotic supplementation seems like an obvious intervention to improve the profile of the microbiome and promote gut health. Probiotics—not to be confused with prebiotics—are live bacteria ingested with the intention of enriching the gut. Probiotics may come in the form of capsules or ingested as part of a fermented food product such as yogurt, kefir, kimchi, or sauerkraut. Multiple studies have illustrated a protective effect of probiotic supplementation against high-fat-diet-induced changes in insulin sensitivity and obesity, and many studies have shown that specific probiotic strains improve symptoms of inflammatory bowel disease. All effects are strain specific, and given the variability of individual microbiomes, diets, and study design, it is difficult to make conclusive statements about the effectiveness of over-the-counter probiotics. However, studies consistently show that probiotic supplementation does improve general gastrointestinal tract issues, and the consumption of fermented food items is associated with increased microbial diversity. What the latter means for health and fitness outcomes remains to be seen.

Recent studies have shed light on some of the risks and shortcomings of probiotic supplementation. There is no way to control whether, or where in the gastrointestinal tract, the probiotic bacteria will take up residence. Additionally, a recent study illustrated that supplementation with a multi-strain probiotic after a week of broad-spectrum antibiotics actually delayed recovery of the participants' native microbiome and led to reduced diversity over a month later. It was better to either ingest their own fecal transplant or simply return to their normal habits and allow the microbiome to recover on its own. While probiotics are generally recognized as safe, they are not a necessary addition and may not be effective or beneficial.

It is also important to note that the dosages provided in the studies showing a positive effect are very high–in the 10s of billions–and often contain multiple bacterial strains. Consumers should be aware that dietary supplement labels and contents may not be accurate since they are not regulated under the same auspices as food and drugs. Look for labels from third-party purity tests, such as the United States Pharmacopeia (USP), which ensure the potency of the product. Probiotics must contain live bacteria, and the minimum effective dose appears to be between one million and one billion CFU (colony-forming units). Additionally, it may be prudent to select probiotics that are highest in Bifidobacteria with little to no Lactobacilli, as the former may not take up residence in the small intestine where the acidic environment favors the growth of Lactobacilli.

Prebiotics

Prebiotics are fibers that have been shown to "feed" specific beneficial strains of bacteria. Inulin and beta-glucan are such fibers available in wheat, barley, rye, bananas, onions, and asparagus. Resistant starch is another prebiotic and is found in potatoes, rice, and legumes; cooking and cooling these foods repeatedly will increase the content of resistant starches.

Isomaltooligosaccharide (IMO) syrup is a plant-based sweetener with a low glycemic index and prebiotic effects, making it a prudent alternative to non-nutritive artificial sweeteners. Other beneficial compounds include polyphenols found in fruits and berries. In comparison with potential risks or lack of benefit to probiotic supplementation, it is much simpler to include plenty of fiber in one's diet to support the controlled growth of beneficial bacteria.

EFFECTS OF THE MICROBIOME ON PERFORMANCE

It is difficult to determine a causal relationship between the gut microbiome and exercise performance, but there appear to be some correlations between fitness and some strains of bacteria. In mice, the presence of a complete microbiome led to much higher endurance compared to those who had no gut bacteria or a single strain. Specific bacterial types also appear to be either enriched in physically active individuals, associated with cardiovascular fitness, or increased after an exercise intervention. However, most athletes consume a diet higher in carbohydrates and proteins compared to sedentary people, so it is a challenge to determine the effect of the diet or exercise alone.

There are very few intervention studies that have examined the effect of the microbiome on performance, but in one study, a multi-strain probiotic of 45 billion CFUs trended toward an improvement in triathlon performance. Some studies in cyclists and runners have shown a decrease in markers of inflammation and muscle damage as well as reduced GI distress and incidences of respiratory infections. Even if the microbiome or probiotic supplementation does not directly impact exercise performance, the ability to train with greater intensity, duration, and frequency due to good health should lead to improvements.

CHAPTER SUMMARY

- Eat a primarily whole-food diet that includes whole grains, fibrous and starchy vegetables, fruit, fermented products, products containing polyphenols, and foods with Omega-3 fatty acids.
- Limit dietary fat to less than 40% total calories, with less than 10% calories from saturated fats.
- Limit consumption of red meat, processed meat, some artificial sweeteners, and refined sugars.
- Consider including prebiotic foods in your diet, such as inulin and beta-glucan containing foods, resistant starches, and isomaltooligosaccharide.
- Consider a probiotic with a USP label and at least 1 billion colony-forming units.
- There does appear to be a relationship between the microbiome and exercise; however, at the current time the interplay between the two is not well understood.

CHAPTER 16

Alcohol, Body Composition, and Performance

There are often two extreme opinions on the subject of alcohol in fitness: the first being that it should be avoided at all times by anyone serious about their fitness or athletic goals, the second being that alcohol does not impact fitness when used in moderation and within calorie constraints. As with many phenomena, the reality lies somewhere between these extremes.

It is important to remember that alcohol's effects occur on a spectrum related to level of consumption. The impact of one cocktail per week is going to be different than that of four per night, every week. The more you drink, the larger the effect will be. Body size mediates these effects as well, with larger people being able to drink more than smaller people before experiencing more negative outcomes.

The United States Departments of Health and Agriculture define one alcoholic drink as 12 fl. oz. of approximately 5% alcohol beer, 5 fl. oz. of approximately 12% alcohol wine, or 1.5 fl. oz. of approximately 40% (80 proof) distilled liquor. We will use these definitions of a single alcoholic beverage for this chapter. Keep in mind sex differences in the amounts of enzymes that break down alcohol and average body size mean that men can usually drink on the higher end of any given range, and women should aim for the lower end.

For most people who are not highly competitive athletes, light drinking (1-3 drinks once or twice per week) will not have significant effects on health, body composition, or performance. As we cross over into moderate drinking (3-10 drinks per week), even in small amounts (1-3 drinks per day), small differences in body composition can start to be observed. At this level of drinking, health is not likely to be affected, so the small body composition trade-off is one many people are willing to make in order to be able to have drinks on the weekend or wine with dinner. At four or more drinks per day on average, the effects begin to threaten health and fitness goals more seriously.

DETRIMENTS OF ALCOHOL CONSUMPTION

Blunting of Muscle Growth

Alcohol reduces the rates of muscle growth. Through a variety of pathways, some related to estrogen and testosterone production, the more you drink, the less muscle you are likely to grow.

Muscle Loss

You are not likely to lose muscle on a maintenance or muscle-gain diet when drinking moderately, but alcohol increases the chances of muscle loss when you are hypocaloric. So even if you are fitting your beer calories into your diet, they might be having a more negative effect than other calories would.

Fat Gain

When you consume alcohol, most of your cells prefer to burn it as a fuel source before they switch back to burning their usual mixture of carbs and fats. This means that if you are isocaloric or hypercaloric, your body is not burning the other food calories you are consuming as efficiently, and they are slightly more likely to be stored as fat. When you are hypocaloric, this means that rather than burning your body's fat, cells will preferentially use alcohol calories, pausing your fat-loss progress (and as mentioned, increasing muscle-loss potential—a double whammy). While alcohol does not directly convert to body fat in any meaningful way, it can indirectly increase fat storage or slow fat burning. Add up those missed burn opportunities over the weeks and you have some significant fat gains on an iso- or hypercaloric diet and some missed fat-loss opportunities on a hypocaloric diet.

Fat Gain From Ancillary Alcohol Calories

Although alcohol itself only facilitates added fat storage, the additional sugar in mixed drinks can directly contribute to fat storage, compounding the negative effects of a few drinks. In theory, you can account for calories and still have a few drinks, even on a fat-loss plan. In reality, the number of calories you have to cut from your food to offset even a couple of high-sugar drinks becomes problematic for macro- and micronutrient needs. Most drinks of this kind (margaritas, piña coladas, etc.) contain a very large number of calories, and having just a few can make calorie cuts necessary in the 500 to 1000 range. (The National Institutes of Health has an online alcoholic drink calorie calculator that can be eye opening.) A high-calorie drink might be acceptable as a one-time occurrence on a fat-loss diet, but is not a good habit for fat loss or health and fitness outcomes in general.

Fat Gain From Lapses in Adherence

Unfortunately, the sensible, controlled, forward-thinking required for good diet adherence is dialed down the more alcohol you consume. The more you drink, the more likely you are to simply reach for things that give you immediate pleasure. If you are on a hypocaloric diet, those things tend to be tasty, calorie-dense comfort foods.

Recovery Problems From Toxicity

The number one toxin most people expose themselves to is alcohol. Because it is toxic, alcohol directly reduces the rate and completeness of recovery. This means that the harder you train and the more recovery demand you put on your body, the more notable the negative effects of alcohol will be. So while it might be just fine to have some drinks during lower volume training phases, those same drinks might come at a greater cost during higher volume training phases or hypocaloric diets, when recovery demands are pushed close to threshold levels.

Recovery Problems From Sleep Disruption

Under-sleeping is powerfully related to impediments in fat loss and muscle gain. Alcohol disrupts the normal sleep cycle in part by preventing the normal descent into deep sleep. This impacts recovery in addition to toxin exposure effects. The effect of alcohol on sleep is caused by going to bed intoxicated and can be minimized to some extent by sobering up before trying to fall asleep.

Hydration Problems

Alcohol consumption causes dehydration which can impede recovery and performance when at pronounced levels. You can obviate this process by drinking extra fluids during and after your drinking, but because alcohol is a diuretic, you are going to be making quite a few extra trips to the bathroom.

If you are not opposed to making some trade-offs in body composition and performance for the sake of enjoying alcohol in moderation, you can decrease some of alcohol's negative effects by following some combination of these approaches:

- Do not consume more than two to four drinks at a time, more than a few times a week.
- Stick to drinks with less calories and minimal additional sugar and fat.
- Keep tempting, easy-access comfort food out of reach when drinking.
- Drink less when in high-volume, recovery-demanding training phases.
- Drink less when in hypocaloric diet phases.
- Drink calorie-free fluids between drinks and after drinking to stay hydrated.
- Stop drinking a couple hours before going to bed.

These strategies can be used to minimize alcohol's negative effects, but there are times when abstinence is a better choice. Time your drinking for phases of your diet and training when it will be least impactful. Tactics like not starting your fat-loss diet right before your all-inclusive vacation or a series of bachelor/ette parties and weddings can go a long way toward both your enjoyment of those things and your diet success.

CHAPTER SUMMARY

- The negative effects of alcohol manifest on a dose basis; the more you drink, the worse the effects.
- Alcohol consumption can directly inhibit muscle growth and retention, fat loss, the ability to recover from hard training, the ability to achieve high-quality sleep, and it can lead to dehydration.
- Alcohol consumption during a diet requires a trade-off of body composition and performance for lifestyle enjoyment.

CHAPTER 17

Fads and Fallacies

Unfortunately, wrong approaches to diet are so rampant that by the time we publish this book, there will likely be a number of new fad diets that we were unable cover here. We intend to be as comprehensive as possible in debunking current popular misconceptions and fads. Hopefully, with the knowledge and tools gained from this book, you will be able to identify and debunk new nutrition fads on your own as they arise.

RECENT TRENDS

Butter and Fats Added to Coffee

The trend of adding grass-fed butter or coconut oil to coffee has now circled the world. At the end of the day, there is nothing magic about putting a big slab of saturated fat in your coffee. In the context of an otherwise healthy diet, a little saturated fat in your morning cup of joe is not the end of the world. Our message to you the reader is that there is no substantial health benefit to drinking your fat calories in coffee specifically; you should obtain those calories however you see fit as long as you are sticking to your diet plan and living a healthy lifestyle.

One claim is that this concoction will reduce appetite. Indeed it will, but this is simply the virtue of caffeine and 500 calories worth of fat. Moving those fats to your breakfast meal or adding cream to your coffee would be a tastier alternative with an equally appetite-suppressing effect. Another claim is that by avoiding carbs (and drinking butter coffee instead) when cortisol is higher in the morning, you can prevent fat gain. The problem with this rationale is that carbs *reduce cortisol when they are eaten*, creating a self-solving problem. In fact, if you are eating 500 calories of fat at a time when cortisol levels are high (such as the morning), they have a higher chance of being stored as fat than carbs do. Putting butter in your coffee because you like the taste is a fine choice if you have calories to spare for a beverage, but do not expect that the outcomes will differ from eating butter with your morning meal.

Intermittent Fasting

This strategy involves blocking off long stretches of time in your diet schedule when no eating is allowed and condensing all eating into a short period, usually in the evening. Unfortunately, as we know from the nutrient timing diet principle, this diet structure is not the best option for body composition (muscle retention) or sport performance. Following are assessments of the purported benefits of fasting.

Adherence

While fasting might make temporary adherence to a hypocaloric diet easier for some people, it also has downsides for a long-term healthy lifestyle. Even for adherence, the direct research on fasting does not show any significant increases in adherence compared to consuming a normal number of daily meals (3-5). Some research even shows reduced adherence to fasting protocols and less dietary continuation months after completing a fasting study compared to a calorie restriction study with normal meal spacing. This means that there are few people who see adherence benefits from fasting. For the few people who do adhere better to their calorie and macro allotments using a fasting strategy, adherence will be much more valuable than optimal meal timing but will come at a trade-off where best body composition results are concerned.

Autophagy

Autophagy is the process by which your body destroys its own cells and tissues. This process is critical to health; without it, body structures would wear down and begin to function poorly.

Proponents of fasting often tout this as a benefit of the method. Although fasting does increase autophagy, so does any calorie deficit. Your body must catabolize its own components to fuel basic survival needs when not enough food is being taken in. Hard exercise also significantly boosts autophagy. The only evidence for a special boost to autophagy from intermittent fasting has so far come from studies of starving yeast and remains unproven in humans or mammals.

Growth Hormone Increases/Anabolism

When you fast, your growth hormone (GH) levels increase. This is because GH gives the signal for fat and carbs to be used for fuel instead of being stored in the muscle. When you fast, your body releases GH in order to feed on the stored contents of some of its cells. The purported anabolic effect, however, is not possible under fasting conditions. Growth hormone is only anabolic when there is an abundance of protein and calories. If you fast to raise growth hormone levels, the lack of excess nutrients leaves out the potential muscle growth benefits. If you give this just a bit of thought, it starts to sound absurd—you are supposed to get *bigger* by *not eating* for long periods of time. This is contradicted by the physiological need to supply muscles regularly with amino acids (and the machinery that builds muscle with calories to operate). Although GH levels are increased, the fasting state inhibits their muscle-building effects, and fasting itself creates a catabolic environment, making net muscle loss a more likely outcome.

If you feel you can adhere to your diet program better with fasting, know that you will be trading off maximum muscle retention or growth depending on the diet. Some muscle tissue will inevitably be used for fuel during long periods without eating (especially on a hypocaloric diet). If you would like to keep a diet structure similar to fasting while conserving a bit more muscle than traditional fasting allows, just consume meals comprised of only protein periodically during the "fasting" period and eat the rest of your macros in meals after the "fasting" period.

Intermittent fasting is unlikely to kill you or cause you to lose all your muscle gains, but it is not effective for best performance or body composition changes.

Carb Backloading

Carb backloading refers to eating fewer carbs in the morning and more carbs at night.

Carb backloading claims that because cortisol levels are high and insulin sensitivity is low in the morning, it is best to avoid eating carbs because under these conditions they are more likely to be stored as fat. Eating meals of mostly protein, training midday, and then adding carbs to your meals for the last several meals to get the most muscle and least fat gains is what the carb backloading approach recommends. As mentioned in the critique of butter in coffee, high morning cortisol levels do not actually cause more carbs to be stored as fat; cortisol is reduced by the consumption of carbs. In addition, insulin sensitivity is *higher* in the morning (post all-night fast) than it is in the evening, so that part is simply incorrect. That being said, if you wake up and do not eat carbs for hours, your insulin sensitivity might be higher than normal by the evening due to prolonged time spent without carbs (prolonged time without carbs also increases risk of muscle catabolism due to energy needs and so the purported benefit of this strategy is negated). Regardless of whether you eat your carbs in the AM or PM, the hormone logic does not add up for carb backloading and related diets.

Cleanses and Detoxes

The idea behind a cleanse or a detox is pretty straightforward. You consume only a limited amount of food (or no food at all) and usually drink plenty of a specific kind of low-calorie beverage, whether it be an herbal blend, lemon water, or a mix of certain vegetables or fruits. This hiatus from normal eating is proposed to both stop the influx of foodborne toxins into your body and remove the built-up toxins that are already there. The problem is that there is no practical difference in the amount of toxins that you are consuming during such a cleanse. The most pervasive toxin consumed by humans is probably alcohol, and this is generally done by choice.

Your liver processes most of the toxins out of your body over time, and cleanses and detoxes do not assist or rush this process. Further, while most of the herbs and blends used in detoxes are healthy, they unfortunately do not have any special toxin-removing capabilities. Direct assessments of detox and cleansing diets show the same effect as lowering calories and eating healthy. The downside to longer periods of "detoxing" or "cleansing" is that protocols often lack protein, resulting in muscle loss. Any studies showing evidence of a benefit to detoxing are usually severely lacking in experimental rigor and seldom appear in a peer-reviewed journal (if at all). Any positive outcomes are related to the cessation of the consumption of unhealthy foods. A better choice for health and fitness would be to eat mostly healthy foods and get in plenty of veggies, fruits, and whole grains all the time.

A huge downside of the detox and cleanse paradigm is that it postulates that you can reverse weeks or months of poor eating habits within days of strict adherence to a special dietary and fluid protocol. In order to restore your health to the condition you had before a stint of poor eating practices, you have to eat well for *at least as long* as you ate badly. In some cases, eating badly can do irreversible damage to your health, so buying into quick fixes can be even more dangerous if you have been eating badly for a long time. Though it is tempting to want to believe that just couple of days of special dieting can give you a clean slate, it is not so.

Alkaline/Acidic Diets

A certain class of diets proposes to bring your body's pH into balance. On the face of it, that sounds great, but like cleanses and detoxes, your body is already very good at regulating this. If your blood pH is altered by as little as 0.4 (from its normal range of 7.35-7.45 pH), you will die. For this reason, the body maintains its blood acidity *very* tightly with a host of pH buffers. Certain gut pH levels can affect the microbiome, but the alkalinity of food does not correlate to these changes as they arise from by-products of digestion. Eating alkaline foods or drinking alkaline water will have zero impact on your gut as stomach acid will neutralize whatever small alterations in pH might come from food pH immediately upon contact. The pH of your urine can be altered with foods, but this is due to metabolites produced during the digestion process and has zero impact on blood or cellular pH levels.

Alkaline water and diets are essentially a scam. There is not even a seed of truth to their claims.

Inflammation

Inflammation is often thought to be wholly negative. While it is true that chronic systemic inflammation puts you at higher risk for developing more serious conditions, acute inflammation is also central to the recovery and adaptation process post workout. If body composition and fitness outcomes are a priority, wiping out all inflammation is a bad idea. Instead, we want adequate acute, local inflammation for recovery and adaptation, injury healing, and infection fighting. We want to avoid chronic, systemic inflammation.

Many people claim that particular foods and diets reduce chronic systemic inflammation, but the best intervention for chronic inflammation is just weight loss.

High body fat levels seem to create and reinforce chronic inflammation, so losing fat is the most dependable way to reverse this. Be wary of diets, pills, and specific foods purported to be anti-inflammatory.

Digestive Problems as Causes of Weight Gain

There is no shortage of companies selling digestive enzymes or other pro-digestive supplements with claims that they will help you lose weight. People will often claim that they are not digesting food well and that this is why they are struggling to lose weight.

The problem with this logic is that it is backwards. If you were not digesting all the food you were eating, you ought to be able to eat more food than usual and not gain weight. To be stored as fat, the nutrients you eat must first be digested and absorbed. If they are not, they just pass through. The human body has an incredibly powerful digestive system and can absorb every food you eat in the 95-plus percentile of efficiency. The more efficient your digestion, the more calories you get out of food. It is likely that if you suffer from digestive problems, you will lose weight, and at medically troubling rates. For example, individuals with celiac and Crohn's disease are often very underweight prior to the management of their conditions because their digestive systems have trouble absorbing the food they eat, and thus they lose huge fractions of ingested calories. If you need help *losing* weight, enhancing your digestion is unlikely to help.

Avoiding Hard-to-Pronounce Ingredients

Unfortunately, skipping hard-to-pronounce ingredients will not make you healthier. There will be more of these kinds of words in the ingredient lists of processed foods, which in many cases are less healthy, so in this sense there is some truth to the idea that simpler is better. On the other hand, you would be best served not to skip (5R)-[(1S)-1,2-Dihydroxyethyl]-3,4-dihydroxyfuran-2(5H)-one (ascorbic acid or vitamin C), pantothenic acid (vitamin B5), or eicosapentaenoic acid (EPA, an Omega-3 fatty acid). In fact, these compounds with difficult-to-pronounce names are often found in whole foods that do not even have an ingredient list to read and are added to other food products to make them (at least appear) healthier. The truth is that nutrition is just not that simple—we cannot simply find health and fitness by ruling things out based on name alone; a bit more discernment is required.

Hormones as Causes of Weight Gain

This pervasive myth offers a hugely appealing fantasy that there is nothing wrong with your current diet and exercise routine (or lack thereof) and that all your weight gain or failure to lose is due to your hormones. While hormones do play a role in metabolic rate, a calorie deficit will still result in weight loss. Ironically, one thing that *can* shift your hormones in a way that reduces metabolism is dieting for too long.

Hormones also play a role in body composition at any given weight. With more testosterone and less cortisol, you can gain muscle and lose fat at the same time. If the ratio is the other way around, you can lose muscle and gain fat. Short of huge doses of exogenous hormones, both these cases are extremely rare. Solutions being sold to "fix hormone problems" tend to include herbs and specific food recommendations, neither of which are powerful enough to shift your hormonal profile. If you are over-dieted, take a long break from reduced calorie intake; this will be the most powerful tool you have to bring your hormones back to baseline. Some herbal supplements and specific food items are extremely unlikely to alter your hormone production such that you can lose weight without altering diet and training. Your diet principles and a well-designed training program are science-tested means of getting you to your goal.

Coconut Oil

Coconut oil has gathered quite the reputation in recent years. It is an excellent lubricant, pretty good for your skin and hair when applied externally, a great conditioner, smells great, and it makes the foods you use it in taste better and have better texture. It definitely has its benefits, but claims that this food item has extensive medical health benefits are largely dubious.

Coconut oil is alleged to help with everything from fat loss to cancer. When coconut oil first gained its bump in popularity in the mid-2010s, the volume of research on its health effects was not yet substantial enough to validate these claims. As of this book, the comprehensive literature on the health effects of coconut oil paints a mixed picture, but its high saturated fat content makes it unhealthy in large amounts. Coconut oil is like other saturated fat; just fine in moderation but should be eclipsed in daily consumption amounts by monounsaturated and polyunsaturated fat sources like nuts, avocados, and olive oil.

PERSISTENT OR RECURRING TRENDS

Natural Is Better (The Naturalistic Fallacy)

Also known as the "appeal to nature fallacy," the naturalistic fallacy makes the claim that *because something is natural, it must be good*. The claim within the context of diet is that the more something has been altered by humans, the less healthy and performance-enhancing it is to consume. Under this assumption, eating cookies made with cane sugar and grass-fed butter ought to be better for you than vitamin-fortified, sugar-free meringue cookies made with egg whites and sucralose. If you are on a fat-loss diet, the rationale is reversed—the sugar-free meringue cookies (meringue is made with egg whites) not only have protein, but no added fats or carbohydrates and so will be much lower in calories per unit volume than the "natural" cookies, not to mention they have the added vitamins. For health and fitness, the less natural cookies in this example are better for you.

It is not universally the case that unnatural is better than natural either. There is no general way to use naturalness as a measure for goodness. In nutrition, less processed (more "natural") foods tend to be healthier than more processed (less "natural") foods, but some processed food (like protein powder) is very healthy. During and after hard training, when the digestive burden required by unprocessed food is too great, more processed food is often better for athletic performance. Additionally, for vegan protein sources, processing can make protein more digestible, better absorbed, and can also reduce some "natural" factors such as phytoestrogens in soy that you might want to keep within reasonable daily limits. How natural any food is does not necessarily dictate how good it is for you. Many factors must be assessed in choosing foods for your health and fitness goals, and you should always consider the basic diet principles and food composition when making these choices. Ideally, this book has given you the tools to make these decisions rationally and avoid committing this naturalistic fallacy.

Processed Food

There are certain processing methods and certain categories of processed food that are definitely not ideal for your health. The processing of conventional fats into trans fats is one of the best examples, but the primary reasons that processed foods tend to be less healthy is that they lack micronutrients and are highly palatable (i.e., they promote overeating). In many cases, it is not the processed food that is bad for you as much as it is failing to consume whole foods. The problem with processed foods is that people consume them in place of and in higher quantities than foods with added nutrients and benefits.

Lack of Nutrients/Overeating Processed Foods

When turning whole grains into white flour, most of the fiber, vitamins, minerals, and phytochemicals are removed. While there is nothing wrong with this in and of itself, if you eat exclusively white bread, you will miss out on the nutrients that whole grains, vegetables, and fruits can provide. Processing also usually increases the calorie density of foods and makes them tastier. If your diet is mainly processed foods, you will likely feel less full while consuming more calories than if you were eating a primarily whole-food diet, which has the potential to result in an increase in bodyweight.

Examples of Processing That Makes Food More Healthy

Not all processing methods make food less healthy. For example, processing allows milk fat and carbs to be separated from whey and casein proteins, which are extremely healthy and have some specific fitness benefits when consumed appropriately. Another example is the processing of soy products which not only makes the complete vegan protein found in soy more readily available for absorption by the body, but also provides the benefit of removing phytoestrogens, some of which, when eaten in large amounts, may have adverse endocrine-related effects.

A diet composed of mainly whole foods will provide the fiber and micronutrients for best health and fitness, but some processed food (like protein powders, vegan "meats," etc.) can be beneficial as well. Even less healthy processed foods (such as those containing trans fats) will not have a significant impact on health or fitness if consumed rarely and in very small amounts.

Non-Genetically Modified Food (Non-GMO)

GMOs are foods that have been modified genetically via a more advanced technique than cross-breeding. Intentional human-led crossbreeding of plants has been practiced for thousands of years, but advanced GM technology is only about 40 years old. The first GM crop was invented in 1982, and GM crops first came to market in the US and Europe in 1994. The basic premise of GM crops is that they have genes of other organisms inserted into their genomes, such as a gene for pesticide resistance from a bacterium being inserted into a plant to give it a greater resistance against pests. Since their introduction, GM crops have exploded in use because of their distinct advantages over conventional crops. A huge number of individuals have protested this expansion, fearing health and environmental negatives of GMOs despite a lack of evidence for such things.

You name it, people have accused GMOs of causing it. Cancer, diabetes, neurodegenerative disease, autism; the list goes on. With this much smoke, you would think there must be fire, but the scientific consensus is that GMOs are no more dangerous than unmodified foods. In the published peer-reviewed literature, there is *not a single confirmed case* of GMOs having *any harm to health*. This is after more than 30 years of testing, 20 years of use, and more than 10 years of chronic use by hundreds of millions of people worldwide.

For those skeptical despite this massive accumulation of longitudinal data, consider a quick thought experiment. The avocado evolved in Mexico, Central, and South America. If you trace some of your ancestry to that region, you are in the clear. If not, every time you consume an avocado, you are eating a plant that *your ancestors did not co-evolve with*. If you are really interested in not consuming foods that might be "unnatural" in any scientific basis, then coevolution concerns should come before GM concerns. At least GM foods are tested with cells, animals, and humans for years before they get released as products to the open market.

Organic Foods

In chemistry, "organic" means "carbon based," so both the carbon dioxide we breathe out and the fuel used in gas engines are technically organic. Organic has come to mean something different in the modern food industry—it typically implies lack of synthetic pesticides or fertilizers in the case of produce, and a lack of antibiotic or hormone use in the case of livestock. You might note that organic farmers can use "natural" pesticides and fertilizers, but as we have learned, natural does not always mean safer or better. Organic farmers are also allowed to use synthetic ("unnatural") substances if there is no natural source of the substance available, so even if natural were better, organic farming does not necessarily qualify.

The vast majority of studies have shown no difference in in nutritive value between organic foods and conventional foods. Research on long-term health effects using controlled studies in humans is lacking, and conclusions about any single variable are difficult to draw from cohort studies. Most people do not eat either completely organic or completely conventional all the time and confounding lifestyle factors such as exercise, smoking, and alcohol habits make drawing conclusions complicated. The fact that research shows no significant nutrient differences between organic and conventional foods thus far strongly suggests that, even if there are differences, they are too small to matter.

Troublingly, there is a very well-documented biasing pattern in the research on organic foods, where research by third parties usually finds no differences (sometimes conventional foods are even found to have more nutritive value), but research by organic-advocacy groups and hired scientists find slight advantages for organic foods. Even more troubling, the latter research tends to suffer from obvious and serious flaws in study design. When doing your own reading, look for articles in peer-reviewed journals by scientists with clauses specifying no conflict of interest.

Organic food proponents also claim organic food tastes better. Unfortunately, even that is not true, aside from locally farmed organic food. Fresh foods do taste better, organic or not, to blind taste testers. When equated for freshness, organic does not score better for taste in a blinded experiment. The only verified difference between organic food and conventional food is price.

Eating at Night Makes You Fat

The idea that eating after some time in the evening causes extra fat gains has been around longer than most people have been tabulating the trajectories of diet fads. The direct research on this question comes out almost completely equivocal. Some studies show connections between evening eating and weight gain, most do not show any correlation, and some show the opposite effect, that eating less in the evening causes more fat gain.

Having read this book, you might recall that calorie intake is the biggest determinant of weight change. This probably explains the variety of contradictory results collected when only meal timing is considered. Once calories are equated, eating most of your food at night versus in the morning seems to make little or no difference. This reinforces how much more important calorie totals are compared to nutrient timing. Where differences can be measured is in long-term body composition changes for meals spread throughout the day versus condensed into short periods before or after long fasts, with the former leading to better results.

Breakfast Is the Most Important Meal of the Day

There is a rationale to having some protein shortly after waking to keep the muscles supplied with amino acids after hours of sleep with no protein intake. There does not appear to be any reason that this first-thing protein intake is any more important than any other meal's protein. Further, there is no data suggesting that your first meal needs to be anything more complicated than a protein shake (outside of training-specific meal needs).

Hormones in Food

Some hormones or hormone-like factors found in food occur naturally. The isoflavones in soy, for example, can mimic estrogen in certain body systems. Other hormones found in food are introduced via farming techniques. Cows, for example, are given anabolic or androgenic steroids to increase the amount of meat a single cow can provide. There are those who would be thrilled to be taking free anabolic steroid doses legally via their steak, but those less thrilled at such a prospect can rest easy–these drugs are not transferable. First of all, the actual levels of hormone residue found in meat are physiologically irrelevant. For example, the extra estrogens found in 3 oz of meat treated with hormones can be about 0.5 ng (this is half of one billionth of a gram) more than in untreated meat (which has about 0.75 ng itself from just natural production). To give some perspective, the same amount of eggs has almost 100 ng of estrogenic compounds and peanuts have over 15,0000 ng (not a typo) of phytoestrogens (an estrogen-like compound found in plants).

Second and more importantly, the hormones that are given to cattle are *not orally bioavailable*. The cow's liver breaks down such hormones almost completely, so getting them through the meat that you consume is completely ineffective. When humans are prescribed estrogen, testosterone, or anabolic hormones by a doctor, they must be injected unless they are specially modified, which is expensive and complicated and therefore not used for farm animals. So not only are the hormone levels in animal products inconsequentially small, they are not orally bioavailable either. To put this in context, not a single athlete, in the history of doping control, ever tested positive for any hormone because of the animal products they ate.

(Though more than a few have tried to blame that process in attempts to hide their performance-enhancing drug use).

Tofu has over 15 *million* ng of phytoestrogens per 3-oz serving. While a moderate intake of soy in your diet is not likely to lead to any issues, consistent, very high soy consumption (daily or multiple daily meals) can in fact lead to more estrogenic activity in both males and females. This is usually harmless, though in extreme cases it can slightly affect body composition. There is some evidence that high intake of soy through the lifespan might have some reproductive effects (especially for females), and the use of soy-based baby formula has not been found to be risky but needs considerably more investigation.

In moderation, soy products are almost certainly not going to reduce health, body composition, or performance outcomes. In fact, soy intake is linked with better bone health, the prevention of some cancers, and better heart health. Studies have shown no downsides to soy consumption at just under 20% of your daily protein intake (25 g of protein from soy for an average 150-lb. person), but higher consumption has not been well studied. Some clinical and population studies suggest health benefits for adults when soy is consumed at two to four times the aforementioned amount. If you are a vegan and rely on non-animal proteins for your daily nutrition, varying soy intake with other protein sources like mycoprotein might be a wise move before the weight of the evidence can reveal the proper limits and recommended intakes for soy products, but a couple servings of soy per day are likely more beneficial than not.

Antibiotics in Food

Keeping farm animals healthy involves the use of antibiotics. This is especially true in larger, higher volume farms. So much antibiotic use occurs in farm animals that they are currently the biggest source of antibiotic-resistant bacteria, which is definitely an environmental and health concern in the long term, and steps to address it are underway.

While the development of antibiotic resistance is a serious concern, the presence of antibiotics in meat itself is not a concern. Regulatory agencies do not allow even trace quantities to occur in meat sold in stores. Animals that are being prepared for slaughter have to spend a mandated window of time antibiotic-free to clear all traces from their bodies. Buying animal products from animals not treated with antibiotics makes some sense in the context of global antibiotic effectiveness concerns, but this will not reduce your own intake of antibiotics.

If you would like to purchase healthier animal products and stay science-based, current evidence suggests that grass-fed animal products are slightly, but notably healthier than grain-fed animal products, mostly because they contain higher levels of Omega-3 fats.

Chemicals in Food

It is impossible to avoid eating chemicals because, by definition, all the food you eat is composed of mixtures of chemicals—even fruits and vegetables. So the real claim is generally that man-made chemicals are bad.

There are instances in which the claim that artificial chemicals added to food make it less healthy or worse for body composition is true. For example, the trans fats added to fast foods and baked goods to extend their shelf lives have been shown to be detrimental to health. On the other hand, some natural food ingredients are actually quite harmful. For example, hydrogen cyanide is an extremely toxic chemical found in raw cassava and bamboo as well as the pits of cherries and apricots. With any toxic substance the amount ingested and the sensitivity of the individual will play a role in the response.

The International Agency for Research on Cancer (IARC) evaluates substances to determine how carcinogenic they are. Those most likely to be carcinogenic to humans are classified as Group 1. Of the over 100 substances currently listed as Group 1, more than half are naturally occurring. In fact, most of the carcinogens we get from diet are natural plant compounds probably made by plants to defend themselves. Not that we should avoid plant consumption, this is just to say that natural compounds are not necessarily safer or healthier than artificial ones. We know more about the health effects of most food additives than we do about specific compounds in natural foods, so rejecting man-made chemicals in foods is not a rational rule to live by. Assessing the scientific data regarding the safety of any substance, natural or man-made, makes a great deal more sense.

Artificial Sweeteners

Artificial sweeteners are compounds that taste sweet but have either very low or no calories at all. Technically called non-nutritive sweeteners for this reason, their straightforward appeal is pretty obvious—a sweet taste without all of the calories. Popular social media accounts would have you believe that artificial sweeteners are dangerous, but this is not at all the case.

The safety of aspartame (a commonly vilified sweetener) is asserted by the independent medical governing bodies of more than 90 countries. It has almost unanimous approval for safety by the top medical and drug safety councils in the world. The FDA has pronounced that aspartame is "one of the most thoroughly tested and studied food additives the agency has ever approved." The story is much the same for all other major artificial sweeteners, including sucralose, acesulfame potassium, and saccharin. A large amount of calorie-free sweetener can be consumed before an even mild health risk. The safe amounts are a bit different for each sweetener, but the FDA's maximum safe dose for sucralose, for example, is stated as: "Using the no-observed-effect level of 500 mg/kg/day* and applying a 100-fold safety factor, the agency has determined an ADI (acceptable daily intake) of 5 mg/kg/day for sucralose. This ADI estimate is well above the 90th-percentile EDI (expected dietary intake) for sucralose of 1.6 mg/kg bw/d."

To be very clear before we translate this into real-world terms: The FDA is taking the amount of sucralose at which *no negative health effects were observed*, and then dividing that by 100. So you can likely consume 100 times the recommended maximum intake and still be safe from any negative health effects. For a 150-lb. person, the maximum recommended intake is approximately 338 mg of sucralose (or 56 teaspoons of Splenda brand sweetener) per day—this would be difficult for most to achieve for a single day, much less on a daily basis. Further, this means that no negative health effect should be observed at 33,800 mg (over 5,600 teaspoons of Splenda), which is probably not even a feat that anyone could accomplish. Aspartame has even higher maximums. If you drink regular diet coke or nearly any other common diet soda, just above 20 cans per day would be the equivalent level of safety compared to 56 teaspoons of Splenda. In summary, it is just very difficult to consume enough artificial sweetener to risk any kind of health effects. This is based on hundreds of studies on individual cells, animals, and humans.

What about all those cancer studies in rats? The first study that initiated this scare was done in the 1970s, and saccharin at high doses was found to cause bladder cancer in rats. Pretty scary, except that in the early 2000s, it was shown that this reaction to saccharin was unique to rats and mechanistically impossible in humans. To illustrate the point, it has also been shown that vitamin C increases tumor growth in rats and mice, but does not seem to have tumor growth effects in humans. The second incident of carcinogenicity of artificial sweeteners in rodent studies was from a group of studies published by the European Ramazzini Foundation of Oncology and Environmental Sciences, known collectively as the Ramazzini studies. These studies concluded that rats were getting higher rates of cancer from low-level aspartame exposure. This was of course alarming, so much of the rest of the toxicology community wanted more information. Upon closer inspection, the Ramazzini studies were rife with the kinds of errors that normally preclude publication altogether. Some of these errors include using older rats for the aspartame group and younger rats for the control group, lack of randomization, and potentially carcinogenic animal living conditions, among many other issues. Upon requests for raw data (the actual study results prior to interpretation), the foundation provided only some of the data, which in the practice of science is unacceptable. Perhaps the most telling feature of this episode is that no other laboratories have managed to replicate the findings of this lab.

So yes, even the oft-vilified aspartame is almost certainly safe at anything approaching reasonable intakes. You can rest easy that your calorie-free sweeteners will not give you cancer or do any serious health damage, but there are downsides to these sweeteners. While sweeteners can be a great way to skip calories and enjoy something sweet while dieting, they *do not reduce hunger*. When you eat a full-sugar dessert, you get the sugar fix *and* the hunger-suppressing calories that go with it. With artificial sweeteners, you only get the mental sugar fix.

Almost all direct studies of replacing sugar in controlled diets with artificial sweeteners show fat and weight loss for those consuming the sugar-free sweeteners in place of sugar. In contrast, cross-sectional studies of individuals running their own diets show more artificial sweetener consumption is correlated with obesity. Many have interpreted this result to mean that sugar-free sweeteners cause obesity, but this conclusion assumes that correlation means causation. Because a wealth of other, more controlled research has shown weight loss with artificial sweeteners and because they do not contain calories, concluding that they cause weight gain makes little sense. It is much more likely that overweight people are more likely to be dieting to try to lose weight and therefore consuming more diet foods including artificial sweeteners. Obese individuals are also more likely to have bariatric surgery, but we do not conclude that bariatric surgery causes obesity because the two are correlated.

Considering the possible mechanisms by which artificial sweeteners could cause long-term fat gain while causing fat loss in controlled studies further rules out this conclusion. Very limited research has shown some effect on gut bacteria (but the direct link between these changes and weight gain or loss has yet to be established). Because no studies have directly shown weight gain in humans due to alterations in gut bacteria, this does not explain the observation. It might be that sweeteners provide a sweet taste without the filling calories, which spurs people to eat even more. However, higher hunger levels have not been reported in the human studies, so it seems unlikely. Insulin secretion caused by the ingestion of artificial sweeteners was a potential factor but has been ruled out in humans through multiple studies.

Since the direct experimental studies show weight loss with no complications from sweeteners, and this is what mechanism-based theory would predict, we can recommend their use within the safety margins described earlier. They are almost certainly not carcinogenic or dangerous in any notable way. That being said, they are not all-powerful and are only a single, very limited tool in the fat-loss arsenal we can potentially employ.

Turning Fat Into Muscle

An old, but still startlingly common, belief is that if you gain weight quickly and then retain the excess weight for longer, you can "harden up" and a higher percentage of that weight will become muscle. Unfortunately, this is completely false. The nutritional variable that powers muscle growth is the *hypercaloric condition*. If you are maintaining weight, then logically you must be in an isocaloric condition. In this state, there is no process for your body to simply "convert" your extra fat tissue to muscle; the fat must be lost in a hypocaloric period or stay where it resides. The presence of fat negatively affects the P-Ratio and thus decreases the likelihood of muscle gain. If it were efficient to put on muscle in this way, going on an all-fast-food binge diet for a couple weeks and then simply maintaining after could get you new muscle. Alas, gaining muscle at the best rates without gaining added fat requires logical calculation, self-control, and quite a bit of patience—behaviors that are good for a lot of beneficial outcomes related to body composition alteration and performance enhancement.

Juicing

We do not mean juicing as in slang for the use of anabolic and other performance enhancing substances, but rather the practice of extracting and drinking juice from vegetables or fruits with the expectation of health and fitness benefits. Ironically, many proponents of juicing are also proponents of whole, natural food diets and opposed to sugar–forgetting that juicing is a means of "processing" food that turns fruits especially into higher glycemic sugar drinks.

Juicing is so popular in the diet industry that a video or picture of someone blending or squeezing their own juice is almost synonymous with the concepts health and fitness in advertising. While fresh juice does contain plenty of micronutrients, juicing removes all the fiber from fruits and vegetables. Part of the reason fruits and veggies are good for your health is that they are high in fiber; juicing reduces this and thus removes the health benefits as well as the high volume which would reduce hunger. Adding whole fruits and veggies to your meals is in most cases a healthier, better option than juicing. Once exception might be during hypocaloric diets. Because liquid food makes calorie consumption easier, juicing can help you get more micronutrients and calories without feeling as full as you would after eating the whole food counterparts. Blending fruit when making smoothies is less of an issue because, when blended, the fruit retain more of their slow-digesting properties.

Mistaking Thirst for Hunger

The tiny bit of truth to this claim is that drinking a high volume of fluid rapidly does actually stretch the stomach and reduce your hunger levels. In this instance, your body is mistaking being full of fluid with being full of calories, which is not the same thing as mistaking thirst for hunger. Not only is there no evidence to suggest that people mistake thirst for hunger and thus overeat when they could have simply had a glass of water, the evolutionary likelihood of such critical senses being easily confused is low.

Hyperhydration Extremism

Since its peak popularity in the mid-2000s, many individuals are nothing short of *obsessed* with their hydration. The good news is that your thirst response will make you very clearly aware that you need water long before your health is remotely in danger. In some special situations such as rapid onset of activity and high sweat rates, thirst lags behind dehydration (the kind that meaningfully impacts your performance). Planning ahead for periods of activity in intense heat is advisable, but these are not normal conditions. On a day-to-day basis, drinking to thirst and regularly checking that your urine is pale yellow will keep you as hydrated as you need to be.

Dieting to Come Off of All Prescription Drugs

One of the huge benefits to dieting, especially fat- and weight-loss dieting for individuals who are overweight, is that health usually improves drastically when weight is lost and body composition improved. Health can often improve so much in some body systems that certain prescription drugs an individual used to take are no longer needed. For example, after losing 40 lb. of fat over a year, someone who formerly took medication for high blood pressure might be able to drop the dose or discontinue altogether. This is not always going to be the case and should be done under the supervision of a physician. Some issues requiring medication are not improved with increased leanness or fitness. Others can be improved in some individuals but not in everyone. It is absolutely fine to be dieting with the goal of improving your health, but dieting to come off of all prescription drugs might not be a realistic pursuit. Your doctor can help you determine if and when it is safe to come off any of your medications. The point of dieting for health is to get healthy, not to swear off medications on principle.

Gaining Weight From Undereating

In the diet world, some people will claim that they are not losing weight because they are undereating. First things first: the First Law of Thermodynamics cannot be violated. There is no way to *gain tissue in a calorie deficit*, but there are reasons that people might have this misconception that are worth discussing.

Post-Diet Rebound

Sometimes when people say that low calories made them gain weight, they mean that they gained weight after a diet, from a rebound weight gain effect. While the number of calories they were consuming immediately post diet may not have been very high compared to their pre-diet norms, at the end of the diet, with lower metabolism, lower NEAT, and hormonal changes from the diet, it takes fewer calories to create a surplus. A calorie surplus still caused the weight gain, but the surplus still felt like very few calories at the time. In the literal sense, it is the overeating after the diet that caused the weight gain, but the excessive deficit of the undereating did potentiate it. Not a mystery of thermodynamics, but definitely supports the need for diets to be moderate in daily deficit and duration and have a maintenance plan in place for after the diet.

Diet Fatigue and Water Weight

Your diet fatigue increases across a hypocaloric phase. This fatigue includes the rise of chronically expressed stress hormones, such as cortisol. Hormones like these and other factors caused by long-term, large deficits can cause the body to retain more water than normal.

Sometimes the amount of water can be so large that no apparent weight loss is seen on the scale for weeks. If you eat a salty meal toward the end of a deficit period, your total bodyweight can even increase, explaining how some would come to suspect that undereating is causing weight gain. In a sense, it is causing gain, but it is water weight and not tissue weight gain. At the end of a diet when you transition to maintenance intelligently, you will lose all that water weight in several days or weeks and end up lighter during maintenance than you ever were during the diet. This may cause the misinterpretation that increased calories caused the weight loss, furthering incorrect assumptions about the relationship between calories and tissue change.

Underreported Calories

On average, people underreport the number of daily calories they are consuming. Not only do they underreport the size of their meals, they often forget to count some or even most of their bites and snacks between meals. When someone says they have been eating 900 calories per day and are still gaining weight, they have more than likely been miscalculating.

Overestimated Activity

Much as with underreporting calories, people often overestimate physical activity. From daily activity to exercise, the average person will think they are doing more than they really are. Cardio machines and other devices that calculate calories burned tend to overstate amounts, so weight change is usually a better measure of actual daily calorie expenditure.

Changes in Calorie Expenditure

Decreased NEAT, altered hormones, and lowered metabolism from a hypocaloric diet (especially a harsh or prolonged diet) result in lower daily calorie needs. Even your output on exercise efforts will decrease as you become more fatigued on a diet. A combination of this and underreporting calories means weight gain is likely the result of being in a calorie surplus, albeit one that feels like a deficit. When a calorie surplus is feeling like a deficit, it is probably time for a long overdue and extended break from fat-loss dieting.

Diet/Binge Cycles

Diet and binging cycles are all too common. Individuals will diet hard for months, lose weight, but then fail to take maintenance breaks. Instead they push as hard as they can for as long as they can. Diet fatigue builds up, tissue loss slows, and water weight drifts up, resulting in weight change stalls on the scale. The constant restriction and hunger *without any decreases in scale weight* are simply too frustrating, and they crack and spend a week or so binge-eating. The calorie surplus, lower metabolism, and lower NEAT result in tissue gain; the salt and carbs from the extra food add substantial water weight, so the scale tips up dramatically. Fueled by regret and renewed fire to get the weight back off, they jump back into a diet. Having failed to alleviate any real diet fatigue due to the short duration of the binge, diet fatigue is as high as ever, and scale weight stops declining not long after the diet is reinitiated. Frustrations mount, another binging episode follows, and the cycle continues. Suffering through the hard work of a diet for no net loss in weight over weeks, and possibly a net gain if your binges are big enough, is not productive or motivating. This situation also often leads to the false conclusion that "undereating" is causing weight gain, when really it is the binge-eating under conditions of decreased calorie expenditure.

To exit this nasty cycle, the hypocaloric diet needs to come to a temporary end. By focusing on eating at maintenance, you can get stronger, become more aerobically fit, and *give your body and mind the time they need to heal* from all those many months of yo-yo dieting. Those who are particularly burned out on the dieting process (perhaps after years of yo-yo dieting) might consider a full diet reset. During this period, you might move away from all counting and tracking of macros and calories and eat what sounds good for a period. Then, over months, ease back into formal dieting. You can eventually get back into a hypocaloric diet, but one that is constrained to 12 weeks or less and 0.5 to 1% of bodyweight loss per week. If you have a history with yo-yo dieting, it is better to start with a slower loss rate and a shorter duration diet. After this diet, you would move on to an adequately long maintenance phase to recover from the diet, and so on.

Negative Calorie Foods

The claim of these foods is that they require more calories to chew and digest than they contain. In other words, if you ate only these foods you should be in a greater calorie deficit the more you ate. Sadly, there are no such foods.

Empty Calories

The term "empty calories" is usually meant to describe foods lacking in micronutrients. The fallacy here is the belief that consuming such foods at any time is a bad idea. While consuming foods devoid of micronutrients as your sole source of calories would be very unhealthy, so-called "empty calorie" foods have a place in a healthy diet. The Gatorade you drink during your workout could be described as "empty calories," but it has a benefit to your fitness development that other options cannot provide.

Superfoods

Superfoods are supposed to have so many nutrients in them that they can wildly affect your health by themselves. It is true that some foods really are packed with more nutrients than others on average. Brightly colored fruits and deeply colored vegetables likely top the list, and even whole eggs could be classified as nutrient dense. Nutrient density is not always desirable. Consider fat-soluble vitamins, for example. These can be stored in body fat and if chronically overeaten can cause health problems. While it is unlikely that you will overeat "superfoods" to the point of danger, their benefits are also greatly overstated. Unless you are deficient in certain nutrients (which is very rare in the Western world, even with a poor diet), nutrient-dense foods are not mandatory. A normal, varied intake of healthy foods will give you the doses of micronutrients needed—beyond this no added benefits exist for ingesting extra nutrients.

Dietary vs. Serum Cholesterol

Despite many claims to the contrary, serum cholesterol (the readings you get at the doctor's office) does in fact correlate with health outcomes. The lower your LDL ("bad" cholesterol) and the higher your HDL ("good" cholesterol), the less likely you are to suffer from cardiovascular disease down the road. Being leaner and active and eating healthy are the best ways of altering these measures. But where does dietary cholesterol fit in? After all, most animal products have some amount of cholesterol. In the 1980s, the dogma was (without much evidence) that eating dietary cholesterol would raise your bad cholesterol levels. Subsequently, in study after study, individuals who ate high amounts of dietary cholesterol from seafood sources failed to display higher serum cholesterol profiles. When the data on cholesterol intake were examined more closely, excess calories were *definitely* associated with poorer cholesterol profiles and excess saturated fats were less impactful, but still reliably correlated with poorer cholesterol results.

When saturated fat and calorie data were factored out, dietary cholesterol had a very weak relationship with serum cholesterol values. If your cholesterol is very high, decreasing dietary cholesterol might be necessary. If your serum cholesterol levels are good, there is generally no reason to worry about dietary intake.

DIETING STYLES AND STRATEGIES

Veganism as the Only Way to Health

Veganism is one of many ways to eat healthy and perform at a high level with the added and laudable intention of reducing animal suffering. However, the notion that you *must be vegan* to be healthy is fallacious. Many vegans and non-vegans assume that animal products are inherently unhealthy. Such people can give up altogether in their attempts at healthy eating because they lack the willpower or circumstances to commit to a vegan lifestyle. Vegan diets *with the proper supplementation and precautions* produce some of the healthiest outcomes consistently, but similar results are seen with diets containing animal products that also constrain the eater to mostly whole foods and a high number of veggies, fruits, grains, and monounsaturated fats. As long as calories, food composition, and macros are in their healthy ranges, a wide variety of plant and animal products are conducive to health.

On the performance side, it does seem that vegans will have a slightly harder time putting on muscle and perhaps even performing at the highest levels in some sports. Most of this can be mitigated with proper organization of the diet and proper supplementation. Getting most fats from plants and most protein from lean animal products is likely the easiest way to maximize health and fitness outcomes in the context of well-programmed, mainly whole-food diets, but abandoning veganism for an easier option is not always necessary. For those concerned with animal suffering, the trade-off of having to more carefully supplement and plan your diet is worthwhile.

If you choose to be vegan, do so for environmental and ethical reasons, knowing that it will require more work for best outcomes and will not automatically improve health or fitness. With the growing popularity of veganism, the food industry now produces plenty of junk food options. These days one can easily be vegan and still eat terribly. Products like Mycoprotein (fungus-based complete protein that is digested and absorbed as well as any animal protein) and nutritional yeast (another source of complete vegan protein that is well absorbed) are upsides to this food development. In addition, vegan supplements (such as vitamin D3 from fungus rather than animal products) exist. Although it is easier to be an unhealthy vegan these days, it is also much easier to be a healthy, fit one.

In what seems to be a reaction to the growing popularity of veganism, some have adopted the position that in order to be your leanest, fittest, and most muscular, you must eat meat. You can certainly get as lean with veganism as you can with a diet that includes animal products, but the performance and muscle growth side is a bit less clear. As of this book, it is not definitive whether properly supplemented veganism can match a diet in animal products in its muscle-building and peak-performance-enhancing potential. The current best guess from our team is that it is possible but much more difficult to maximize these potentials on a vegan diet. The big take-home point: Being vegan for the environment, for animal welfare, and for health are all completely rational and very good ideas. The idea that you cannot be healthy or perform highly without cutting out all animal products is just not true. There is a chance that your top-end potential for muscularity might be slightly reduced—though more by practical rather than theoretical limitations because of the increased difficulty of maintaining a nutritionally optimal and consistent vegan diet.

Excess Protein Concerns

There are three distinct claims about the supposed dangers of overeating protein that are currently popular. The first notion is that protein intake above the minimum (greater than 0.3 g per pound of bodyweight per day) is bad for the kidneys. As discussed in chapter 3, the literature on protein consumption in healthy individuals is very clear that even huge amounts of protein (2 g per pound per day) do not have any sort of disruptive effect on the kidneys, even when consumed in this amount for months on end. The epidemiological data is also absent of any indication of negative impacts on the kidneys of otherwise healthy individuals.

The book, based in part on the famous "China Study" which shares its name, would have you believe that meat causes cancer and a host of other diseases. The China Study itself, when the huge bulk of data are analyzed, shows more correlation between plant protein intake and cancer than meat intake and cancer–though correlation does not equal causation, and it would not be logical to conclude that plant protein causes cancer based on these data either. The animal studies cited in this book are also troublesome. Though they did observe increased tumor growth in a rat group consuming casein, those rats (along with all rat groups in the study) were being administered a life-threatening amount of tumor growth factor. The rats in the non-casein group, although their tumors were smaller, were *dying*. So the conclusion that casein causes cancer is only true insofar as the rats in the casein group were still alive to have their tumors measured. A follow-up study done in monkeys and using a more reasonable dosage of tumor-causing toxins showed cancer prevention in animals fed casein protein compared to the low-protein group.

There is *some* evidence that higher protein intake might lead to a very slight decline in longevity, but high levels of exercise do that, too. It seems fitness, in general, shortens life to a very small extent, but arguably sweetens life to a much larger extent. To complicate matters, while lower protein in the middle age has been correlated to slightly longer lifespans, *higher* protein intake in the elderly has been correlated with *increased* longevity. All this being said, protein is *not unhealthy* in any special way when eaten in larger amounts, and you might only bump into a small negative effect when pushing extreme longevity.

Other protein claims include the notion that athletes do not need much more protein than the minimum outlined for health in this book. This view was prevalent even in mainstream clinical nutrition up to the 1990s. Today, the volume of research on protein's beneficial effects on performance and body composition is enormous, comprehensive, and unambiguous.

Keto/Anti-Carb Diets

There are three alleged culprits as far as those in support of the anti-carb movement are concerned. The first is carbs themselves, the second is sugar, more specifically, and the third is insulin, the hormone that is allegedly responsible for all the negative effects of the aforementioned two.

Carbs

Anti-carb diets assert that carbohydrates are especially obesogenic and cause diabetes if overconsumed. In actuality, consumed fats can be stored as body fat very readily without any conversion and are more obesogenic than carbs. On the diabetes front, carbs do have a very small role to play but are outranked by much more salient risk factors. The number one risk factor for developing Type II Diabetes is genetics. The next most important factor is body fat percentage and to some degree bodyweight in general. The higher your body fat and weight are, the more likely you are to become diabetic. The third factor is your level of physical activity. The more physically active you are, the less likely you are to become diabetic. Perhaps only after all these factors are accounted for, leaving something like 5% or less of the chance of getting Type 2 Diabetes unexplained, the percentage of carbs in your diet might play a role. In most animal studies in which the researches *purposefully give animals Type 2 Diabetes,* scientists rely on overfeeding the animals with fat, not carbs, to cause the diabetic condition. Cutting carbs without attending to body fat percentage and exercise as a means of reducing your chances of developing diabetes is like altering creatine intake as a way to gain muscle. Without fine tuning the main diet principles for a hypercaloric diet and getting consistent training, some creatine will not have a significant effect. Likewise, lowering carb intake is unlikely to have a notable effect on your chances of developing diabetes without a decrease in body fat percentage and physical activity. Because we know that reducing carbs on a hypocaloric diet is less muscle-sparing than reducing fat, it follows that even low-carb dieting for the sake of improved body fat percentage is not the most efficient way to make such a change.

Sugars

Because the data on carbs and poor health does not support the causal nature of carbs, some anti-carb proponents turn the spotlight instead onto sugars. By doing so, anti-carb advocates garner quite a bit more support in the general population—lies with a hint of truth are always more believable. Excess sugar consumption is in fact a risk factor for dental health and can be problematic for individuals with certain gastrointestinal or health conditions. Outside of those effects, it is by no means clear that sugar is unilaterally bad for health. In fact, fruits are packed with sugar but, as shown in nearly every one of the countless studies performed, are also directly associated with *better* health. Some sources of high amounts of sugar are junk food desserts (think gas station pastry options, candy, and such). These foods–outside of moderate consumption–can lead to an accidental hypercaloric diet and, all things considered, are not the healthiest. The reason for this has much more to do with lacking fiber, micronutrients, and easily consumed excess calories than with sugar itself.

Insulin

The health of fruits and whole grains is too well established to argue with. Nutrients from whole grains release slowly into the bloodstream and do not cause large insulin spikes. Fruits are not only composed of the very insulinogenic glucose sugar, but also of the very low glycemic index fructose and fiber that turns whole fruits into very low glycemic foods. Higher glycemic sugar sources, especially the fast-digesting kind, cause rapid insulin elevations, and this is supposedly the real culprit. When squaring this view with the evidence, some serious problems emerge.

First of all, some foods that have been shown repeatedly to promote health and leanness are very insulinergic (i.e., causative of high insulin secretion), such as low-fat milk and other dairy products like Greek yogurt. Secondly, higher fat diets are less insulinergic than higher carb diets (because fats do not cause any insulin secretion when consumed), but they are more obesogenic. Lastly, though insulin secretion has been hypothesized to increase rebound-appetite after the consumption of a meal, direct research into has produced conflicting results, with some evidence that insulin secretion actually *lowers* post-eating appetite.

We can also ask whether people who eat more carbs experience all the proposed negative side effects of carbs on average more than other people. When looking at that data, there is no compelling correlation between carbs and the suggested negative outcomes. A second and rather powerful trend in the data is that vegans and vegetarians consume up to 80% of their daily calories from carbs, often racking up an impressive sugar intake within that carb consumption and are among the healthiest individuals ever studied. They have by far the lowest obesity rates, and no evidence whatsoever of any carb-induced maladies despite their above-average carb consumption.

Athletic Performance

Various claims that carbs are not needed for athletic performance have been made. These claims hold the most merit in the lowest intensity, highest duration sporting events, such as ultra-endurance races (such as 50-mile trail running races), though even in these circumstances, additional carbs tend to increase average performances. In nearly every other setting, carb intake has been undeniably shown to have performance-enhancing effects. To drive the point home, the counter studies show that reducing carb consumption below a certain point unequivocally results in loss of performance.

Low-Fat Guidelines and the Obesity Epidemic

In the 1980s and 1990s, the United States government actively promoted a higher carb, lower fat diet. It was even reflected in the now-comical food guide pyramid. After decades of advocacy, obesity actually increased. This led many to believe that carbs were playing a role in obesity, but it turns out that what the government advocated and what people actually did were significantly different. In basic terms, the government advocated *decreasing fats* while keeping carb intakes high, but the vast majority of people who gained weight during these times simply added carbs *on top of their already high-fat and high-carb diets*. This, of course, shot calories through the roof, and probably strongly contributed to the increase in obesity. In essence, the dietary advice of eating carbs was taken, but the part of the advice about cutting fats or cutting calories was not.

The fundamental cause of obesity is the mismatch between activity and diet that results in a chronic hypercaloric condition. Factors contributing to this mismatch during the 80s and 90s might include increased mechanization of the work environment (and thus a decline in physical activity during work hours), the increase in per-capita wealth and decrease in the relative cost of food that makes overeating easier, and very importantly, the development and increasing popularity of foods that are convenient, delicious, and affordable, known to most of us as "junk foods."

Low-Fat Diets

For the better part of two decades, dietary fat was demonized. Every single disease was seemingly caused in part by dietary fat; foods were termed "fattening," which usually meant they had a lot of fat in them; and everyone was sure that the less fat you ate, the better. The very idea of "eating healthy" precluded the consumption of even moderately fatty foods. Yet, even in those dark days for dietary fat fans, there was discord between evidence and popular thought. Even in the beginning of the anti-fat crusade, there was a pretty well-documented aberration: nuts. Nuts were of course understood to have very high levels of fat, but they never could be pinned to obesity or even to unhealthy outcomes. Through the early 1990s and beyond, the evidence that nuts were in fact quite healthy began to mount rapidly.

The incongruity between nuts and the supposed negatives of dietary fat intake set the stage for the popularity of the Mediterranean Diet in the 1990s. Here was a diet that advocated relatively lower carb consumption, lots of greens and fish, and most interestingly, a whole lot of nuts, seeds, and olive oil–all the latter being very high in fat. Not only was the Mediterranean Diet gaining popularity, increasing research validated components of its health-promoting nature. All of a sudden there was a popular and scientifically supported diet that advocated much higher fat intake. Further, as olive oil was being linked to new health benefits, anti-fat crusaders shifted their messaging from "eat very little fat" to "eat very little saturated fat." It simply became untenable to argue that all fat was unhealthy.

For the early part of the 2000s, it was tentatively accepted in popular diet culture that unsaturated fats were okay, but that saturated fats were negative for health. Upon a reanalysis of old studies, especially with more advanced statistical techniques, and the integration of new, more savvy studies on the varieties and sources of fat available, an interesting trend emerged. It looked like *where* you got your fats from mattered, even if they were saturated. For example, the saturated fats in many dairy products like milk and yogurt were being shown to have beneficial properties for health, so many that at least one review found more health benefits from full-fat dairy than from fat-free dairy. Egg yolks, the victims of decades of demonization, were at least partially vindicated, and the relationship of grass-fed meats and health risks was shown to be more unclear than previously thought.

As many revolutions do, the saturated fat revolution went a bit too far for a time. People were saying that bacon was healthy and were putting coconut oil (a saturated fat) into almost everything. It turned out that preserved meats and the saturated fats in them might not be the healthiest things in large quantities, and that coconut oil was in fact unhealthy in large quantities. Today, the best evidence we have gives us the perspective that, first and foremost, calories must be kept within appropriate ranges to support a healthy weight. Once calorie intake is equated, the would-be downsides of almost any kinds of fats fall drastically. Secondly, if enough (minimum for health) protein and carbs are being consumed, the negatives of high fat intake again shrink. Lastly, if most of your fats are monounsaturated and polyunsaturated, and the minority of your fats (though it can still be up to one-third) are saturated (with zero or minimal trans fats), the health negatives of fats pretty much disappear.

Eat Fat to Burn Fat

When you eat a lot of fat, your body actually starts burning more fat. This is a factual statement. This sets up an exciting prospect, but unfortunately the additional fat you are burning comes from the additional fat you are eating, and *not your body fat*. This leaves you no leaner than you were, and if you eat enough fat in addition to your other macros to be hypercaloric, you just gain fat on the net balance. On a deficit, increasing or decreasing fat calories while keeping total calories constant will not have an impact on body fat loss.

Gluten-Free/Anti-Grain Diets

A noteworthy variation of the anti-carb movement labels grains or gluten (a protein found in wheat) the cause of obesity, inflammation leading to health problems, and digestive issues. The truth behind this fallacy is that some individuals are sensitive to the various ingredients in certain grains. Most notably are individuals with celiac disease, who are intolerant of wheat gluten. About 1% of the population has celiac disease. This serious disease aside, some people still report digestive discomfort when consuming gluten. At this juncture, scientists are not sure if any gluten sensitivities outside of the disease exist. Studies directly examining this have yielded mostly negative results. In one famous study, non-celiac individuals reported equivalent gastrointestinal distress to foods they were told contained gluten, whether or not any gluten was present in the food, suggesting that non-celiac sensitivities are often psychosomatic.

Discomfort, whether generated by food or imagined, is still discomfort, and we do not recommend eating anything that makes you feel unwell, regardless of whether your reaction can be classified. That said, the fact that some individuals do not tolerate certain grains well neither indicates that grains are bad for everyone or that individuals sensitive to certain grains must avoid *all* grains. There is probably not a single food to which no one has a negative reaction, so individual reactions should be taken into account only in individual cases.

In large collections of studies, whole grains have been shown to promote a huge number of healthy outcomes, such as the reduction of risk factors for heart disease, the lowering of blood pressure, and decreases in chronic systemic inflammation. The body of research on whole grains can in no way be construed to conclude that grains are in any unique way fat-promoting, performance-inhibiting, or negative for health. If you are not sensitive to grains or gluten, there is no good reason to categorically exclude them from your diet and plenty of good reasons to include them.

Anti-Dairy

The summary of the anti-dairy fallacy is similar to the anti-grain fallacy. Some individuals have allergies to dairy, lactose intolerance, or digestive trouble with certain dairy products. These issues are not due to any inherent property of dairy products, but rather to individuals' lack of enzymes needed to digest dairy or specific immune reactions. The fact that *some people* do not tolerate a certain food group is not a reason to label it patently unhealthy for everyone. The balance of the evidence from scientific research on dairy consumption suggests a net positive for health and fitness in controlled trials and epidemiological studies (where scientists examine massive datasets about people's health and dietary habits and draw correlations). For those not sensitive to dairy, there is no cogent argument against the consumption of dairy products from the perspectives of health, performance, or body composition. If you happen to be lactose intolerant, lactose-free dairy products are available as are lactose pills that can make your intolerance a non-issue. There has been some research correlating increased dairy intake to increased outbreaks in those suffering from acne. For those who are acne prone, experimenting with reducing dairy consumption might be prudent.

Genetic Diets

The idea behind genetic testing for diet design is perfectly sound. Use information about your genetics to prescribe a type of diet that best fits you individually. Someday in the future, companies will possess the analytical technologies and algorithms to make sound, accurate diet recommendations based on genetics (though even then we predict the overall effect will be minimal compared to the main diet principles).

It is currently impossible to write diets based on genetic testing that will be better in any reliable way than basing intake on size and activity level. Even recent successes in related pursuits have seen mixed results. In one study, it was possible to test individual glycemic responses to foods, but in a later study, researchers used that data to prescribe individual diet recommendations to one group of dieters and gave another group non-individualized diets. The two groups lost the same amount of weight and fat. Ironically, this could have been predicted from the start of the experiment, because we already know that the glycemic index of foods only accounts for a very small percentage of a diet's effect–small enough that when both groups eat in a similarly healthy manner, precise glycemic matching is not powerful enough to be statistically detectable.

Everyone must reduce the number of calories in their diet to lose fat; everyone has to eat more to gain muscle. Carbs still act as fuel; protein is still needed for muscle maintenance. If and when genetic diets do inform diet decisions, they will likely be at the margins. Such advice would be "eat just a bit more carbs than a formula would predict" or "diet for longer than 12 weeks because you have genetic diet resiliency." It is unlikely to lead to magic-pill solutions such "so long as you stay away from XYZ foods, you will not gain weight."

Blood-Type Dieting

There are two means of testing blood which claim to provide information pertaining to nutritional recommendations. The first is a legitimate test to gain an understanding of nutrient deficiencies or excesses. This should be done with the help of a registered dietician or medical doctor so that proper interpretation can occur and recommended courses of action be taken. Because most people do not have serious deficiencies or excesses, such a practice is by no means something that the average dieter needs to engage in at all. The second blood-based nutritional recommendations come from what is often called "blood-type dieting." The latter is where your blood type (the information you fill out on your blood donor card) is used to prescribe a diet that is supposed to be best suited for your health and performance. This idea is completely unsubstantiated by evidence, contradicted by all available studies, and is very weak on theoretical grounds. In other words, it is a scam. Your blood type has no significant bearing on what or how much you should eat nor your potential outcomes based on different diets.

Elimination Diets

There are two types of elimination diets. One is a legitimate part of a diagnostic process in the medical field. This type of prescribed diet eliminates whole classes of foods (grains, for example) to try to isolate which foods are causing an allergic response in the patient.

The second type of elimination diet is one that cuts out an entire food group as a strategy for weight loss. While some people might lose some weight by cutting an entire food group out if they had previously relied on it for a significant portion of daily calories, this strategy is arbitrary at best. Most data show that people will quickly replace the eliminated food group with other calorie sources and regain the weight *or* simply revert back to eating the forbidden food.

Elimination diets of this kind do not work for most people, especially long term. There are instances where this strategy can be helpful for some individuals. Some people do better with abstaining completely from some junk foods, for example, because they find it difficult to eat them in moderation. If addictive behaviors around certain foods plague you, abstinence can be a good option. This type of diet is not a cure-all or logical strategy for weight loss as it does not allow progressive decrease and increase of calories across weight loss and maintenance.

Single-Food Diets

You may have heard of the "Grapefruit Diet" or the "Cabbage Soup Diet" and other plans where you temporarily eat a massive amount of one particular food. This is effective in the sense that it reduces your calories from other foods by quite a bit and so can work well in the short term for making scale weight move down. The foods recommended on these diets are low calorie, are often low on the FPRH scale, and high on the satiety index, making it hard to overeat them.

How much cabbage soup are you really going to eat? How much do you *crave* cabbage soup? These diets also give a structure to follow, keeping you from a whole lot of other high-calorie food options.

There are many problems with this type of diet. First, it often leads to a severe drop in protein which means you are likely to lose some muscle. Second, when you come off the diet, you will likely replace the specific food with foods from your old habits since this diet has not taught you any sustainable strategies or healthy diet habits. Finally, the combination of these problems means that you will have rebound weight gain, and this gain is likely to be fat and not muscle, leaving you with worse body composition than when you started.

Clean Eating

The term "clean eating" has waned in popularity, but it is still used enough to warrant some discussion. Clean eating gained a lot of traction in bodybuilding circles and was generally defined as a diet low in fat, salt, glycemic carbs, and processed foods with a tendency toward low palatability. While there are certainly variations of this definition, this is the basic idea.

As you can probably see, this diet (provided protein and calories are set intelligently) is a template for an effective fat-loss diet. It is probably not a sustainable diet or a good option for a muscle-gain diet. Unfortunately, numerous people believe they need to eat as clean as possible during all phases of diet for their best results. Limiting salt and especially limiting fat and tasty foods on a muscle-gain diet needlessly limits people from fitting real-world foods into their real-world lives and reduces adherence.

If you ate all processed junk foods but hit your macro and calorie targets, switching to a mostly healthy, whole-food diet with the same calories and macros would result in at most a 5% difference in fitness outcomes per the total influence of the food composition principle. If the latter plan is temporary for the gain phase and improves your adherence, it is likely the better choice to achieve your goals. The ideal scenario is probably somewhere in between, where you eat plenty of healthy foods, but achieve some of the more difficult calorie increases with tastier processed foods. The important thing to understand is that muscle gain on a 100% "clean" diet might be unnecessarily difficult and can only improve results by a very small margin.

Intuitive Eating

The term "intuitive eating" has some real value. When you are making the choice between one healthy, balanced option and another, choose the one that "feels" better. You might well be craving a micronutrient your body needs. Further, for those who have been dieting and assessing macros and calories for a long time, the extensive practice might allow them to eyeball and intuit portion sizes, macro, and calorie content in order to stay isocaloric.

The problem with intuitive eating is that it often works completely in reverse of fitness and health goals. Thanks to evolution, most people's bodies *intuit* that they should be putting on fat when food is plentiful, preparing via evolutionary design for the inevitable famine to come. Our intuition simply did not evolve in the modern world, and in terms of food-consumption behaviors, is largely misaligned with it. It is not an overstatement to say that the vast majority of obese people got that way from following their intuition to some extent. It just feels good to eat lots of tasty food and take it easy. Ideally, we should use the vast amount of data and knowledge we have about what foods and strategies that are best for our health, fitness, and physique goals and only within that framework allow intuitive choices to be made.

Lifestyle Change Versus Formal Dieting

The seemingly sage advice to "make healthy lifestyle changes rather than dieting," like most advice, is very well intentioned. Individuals who hop from one fad diet to the next and never develop sound eating habits to support and maintain their goals are certainly missing the lifestyle element (to their own detriment). The reality is that, while lifestyle changes can initiate some progress and are certainly important for sustaining changes, substantial fitness and physique development will require some periods of focused dieting. Lifestyle changes do not have the power to change your physique and performance like formal diets do, but formal diets are not sustainable in the long term. There is no need to choose between healthy lifestyles *or* formal diets—both can be used at appropriate times to achieve goals and live a balanced, healthy life.

Fast Weight Loss for the Very Obese

This is the notion that because obese people have a lot of weight to lose, they should be programmed to lose it at a very fast rate. Up to 2% per week is not an uncommon suggestion. To put this in context, it means that individuals weighing 300 lb. might be advised, or themselves decide, to lose up to 6 lb. *per week*. There are advantages and disadvantages to this approach. The advantages are twofold. First, the obese person becomes rapidly less obese. Excess fat reduces lifespan, so the sooner weight is lost, the more time is added to your life and the better your long-term health. The second advantage is that rapid weight loss is visible on the scale, in the mirror, and in how clothes fit, which is highly motivating.

Unfortunately, the disadvantages are powerful enough to outweigh all the advantages combined. Very fast weight loss results in severe daily physical and mental energy deficits and severe hunger. This all adds up to a very high rate of failure due to falling off the wagon and even higher rates of rebound weight gain (often to a heavier weight). Losing weight at paces over 1% bodyweight per week is such a dependable contributor to rebound gain that the concept of the mini-cut was designed to take advantage of this for the explicit purpose of facilitating weight gain in those seeking to push the limits of muscle growth. Not exceeding 1% of weight loss per week is perhaps *especially important* for the obese. Obese populations are precisely the people who have been the *most* unsuccessful with dieting over the years. The people who are the *most* predisposed to the rebound effect. The people who will most benefit from slower, controlled diets that teach them a lifestyle of healthy eating.

SUPPLEMENT FADS

Testosterone Boosters

There is only one class of drugs that can reliably boost natural testosterone production in healthy individuals. Aromatase inhibitors boost testosterone production by inhibiting the enzyme that converts testosterone to estrogen; inhibiting this process leaves more circulating testosterone. These drugs do not increase muscularity on their own because estrogen is also needed at certain levels for muscle growth.

If only aromatase inhibitors can actually boost testosterone levels, you might be wondering what the active ingredients in prohormones and other such supposed testosterone-boosting supplements could be. Typical supplements either contain a blend of herbs and substances that will have no effect on testosterone or muscle whatsoever, anabolic steroids, or both. In short, if your testosterone booster works really well, it contains steroids–steroids boost muscle growth while shutting down your natural testosterone production. You can boost testosterone within normal ranges by getting proper sleep, rest, and nutrition, but to get more than that, your only option is anabolic steroids and all the health, moral, and legal ramifications they bring.

Nutrient Partitioning Agents

The story of "nutrient partitioning agents," which claim to shuttle more of your eaten food into muscle and less into fat, is similar to testosterone boosters. Outside of very powerful steroids and other hormonal substances such as injectable growth hormone, there is no supplemental way to boost nutrient partitioning. Hard training, proper diet, adequate rest, and sleep are your best bet.

Selective Androgen Receptor Modulators (SARMs)

SARMs are a class of designer drug that turns on the androgen receptor in cells, causing mostly the same effects as anabolic steroids. SARMs are more advanced than steroids and predominantly target the androgen receptors in skeletal muscle tissues while interacting much less with other tissues. This gives SARMs the ability to cause increased muscle growth while minimizing side effects.

Currently SARMs are legal in most countries and can be purchased online. The problem is that real SARMs are complex drugs that are expensive to manufacture. In recent surveys, the vast majority of drugs sold online claiming to be or to contain SARMs simply did not have any actual SARMs in them. Some had trace amounts, others had just regular oral steroids, and still others had seemingly no active ingredients at all. In fact, "SARMs" were being sold online before their proprietary formulas had been published. Your chance of getting SARMs when you purchase something labeled as such is not great at present. If you have the means, getting any supplements labeled as SARMs lab tested is a good idea. Please remember that these are powerful drugs with unique side effects of their own and should not be used without medical supervision and definitely not used in sports federations in which they are banned.

That Hot New Supplement

Testosterone boosters and SARMs are just two currently prominent examples in a seemingly endless line of supplements claiming impressive, but unverified effects. When new supplements come out, they can get enough media attention and anecdotal notoriety (despite not doing what they are advertised to do) that even skeptical people start to wonder if there is anything to the claims. Since less than 10 of the thousands available made our list of effective supplements in chapter 6, your continued skepticism is encouraged.

Cleverness as Diet Wisdom

In the fitness industry, how clever or unconventional your claim sounds is often very predictive of how much attention it will get in the social sphere and the media, and how many people will actually attempt to heed your advice, no matter how wrong it is. "Burn fat by eating dessert foods!" "Lose weight by eating more!" "One quick trick to lose belly fat..." All these claims eternally pop up on social media platforms. This phenomenon occurs because *we want to believe* that clever, quirky, or counterintuitive approaches will allow fitness to be quickly and easily ours.

Fitness can be yours, but it is not going to be yours through hacks, shortcuts, or clever tricks. It will be yours only through the application of sound scientific principles and hard work, commitment, and patience.

CHAPTER SUMMARY

- New fads, trends, ideologies, and "old wives' tales" in nutrition come and go faster than we can keep up with.
- The overwhelming majority of new trends or nutritional "bio-hacks" have little to no support or merit and often falsely advertise that they somehow circumvent the basic principles discussed in this book.
- Many trends appeal to logical fallacies, which may sound initially intriguing, however fall apart when analyzed through a principled approach.
- There is simply no substitute for a scientifically based diet paired with hard work and consistency.

Bibliography

CHAPTER 2

Baker B. Weight loss and diet plans. Am J Nurs. 2006 Jun;106(6):52-9; quiz 60. Review.

Blundell JE, King NA. Overconsumption as a cause of weight gain: behavioural-physiological interactions in the control of food intake (appetite). Ciba Found Symp. 1996;201:138-54; discussion 154-8, 188-93. Review.

Bray GA. Lifestyle and pharmacological approaches to weight loss: efficacy and safety. J Clin Endocrinol Metab. 2008 Nov;93(11 Suppl 1):S81-8. doi: 10.1210/jc.2008-1294. Review. Erratum in: J Clin Endocrinol Metab. 2009 Jan;94(1):324.

Davis RB, Turner LW. A review of current weight management: research and recommendations. J Am Acad Nurse Pract. 2001 Jan;13(1):15-9; quiz 20-1. Review.

Drenowatz C. Reciprocal Compensation to Changes in Dietary Intake and Energy Expenditure within the Concept of Energy Balance. Adv Nutr. 2015 Sep 15;6(5):592-9. Print 2015 Sep. Review.

Economos CD, Bortz SS, Nelson ME. Nutritional practices of elite athletes. Practical recommendations. Sports Med. 1993 Dec;16(6):381-99. Review.

Finer N. Low-calorie diets and sustained weight loss. Obes Res. 2001 Nov;9 Suppl 4:290S-294S. Review.

Fleming JA, Kris-Etherton PM. Macronutrient Content of the Diet: What Do We Know About Energy Balance and Weight Maintenance? Curr Obes Rep. 2016 Jun;5(2):208- 13.

Garthe I, Raastad T, Refsnes PE, Koivisto A, Sundgot- Borgen J. Effect of two different weight-loss rates on body composition and strength and power-related performance in elite athletes. Int J Sport Nutr Exerc Metab. 2011Apr;21(2):97-104.

Gerrior, S., Juan, W., & Peter, B. (2006). An Easy Approach to Calculating Estimated Energy Requirements. Preventing Chronic Disease, 3(4), A129.

Guyenet, S. J., & Schwartz, M. W. (2012). Regulation of Food Intake, Energy Balance, and Body Fat Mass: Implications for the Pathogenesis and Treatment of Obesity. The Journal of Clinical Endocrinology and Metabolism, 97(3), 745–755.

Hall, K. D., Heymsfield, S. B., Kemnitz, J. W., Klein, S., Schoeller, D. A., & Speakman, J. R. (2012). Energy balance and its components: implications for body weight regulation. The American Journal of Clinical Nutrition, 95(4), 989–994.

Helms, E. R., Aragon, A. A., & Fitschen, P. J. (2014). Evidence-based recommendations for natural bodybuilding contest preparation: nutrition and supplementation. Journal of the International Society of Sports Nutrition, 11, 20.

Heydenreich, J., Kayser, B., Schutz, Y., & Melzer, K. (2017). Total Energy Expenditure, Energy Intake, and Body Composition in Endurance Athletes Across the Training Season: A Systematic Review. Sports Medicine - Open, 3, 8.

Hill JO, Drougas H, Peters JC. Obesity treatment: can diet composition play a role? Ann Intern Med. 1993 Oct 1;119(7 Pt 2):694-7. Review.

Hill, J. O., Wyatt, H. R., & Peters, J. C. (2012). Energy Balance and Obesity. Circulation, 126(1), 126–132.

Hopkins M, Blundell JE. Energy balance, body composition, sedentariness and appetite regulation: pathways to obesity. Clin Sci (Lond). 2016 Sep 1;130(18):1615-28.

Kreider, R. B., Wilborn, C. D., Taylor, L., Campbell, B., Almada, A. L., Collins, R., ... Antonio, J. (2010). ISSN exercise & sport nutrition review: research & recommendations. Journal of the International Society of Sports Nutrition, 7, 7.

Kushner RF, Ryan DH. Assessment and lifestyle management of patients with obesity: clinical recommendations from systematic reviews. JAMA. 2014 Sep 3;312(9):943-52.

Laddu D, Dow C, Hingle M, Thomson C, Going S. A review of evidence-based strategies to treat obesity in adults. Nutr Clin Pract. 2011 Oct;26(5):512-25.

Langeveld M, DeVries JH. The long-term effect of energy restricted diets for treating obesity. Obesity (Silver Spring). 2015 Aug;23(8):1529-38.

Longland TM, Oikawa SY, Mitchell CJ, Devries MC, Phillips SM. Higher compared with lower dietary protein during an energy deficit combined with intense exercise promotes greater lean mass gain and fat mass loss: a randomized trial. Am J Clin Nutr. 2016 Mar;103(3):738-46.

Malik VS, Hu FB. Popular weight-loss diets: from evidence to practice. Nat Clin Pract Cardiovasc Med. 2007 Jan;4(1):34-41. Review.

Manore MM. Weight management in the performance athlete. Nestle Nutr Inst Workshop Ser. 2013;75:123-33.

Manore, M. M. (2015). Weight Management for Athletes and Active Individuals: A Brief Review. Sports Medicine (Auckland, N.z.), 45(Suppl 1), 83–92.

McMillan-Price J, Brand-Miller J. Dietary approaches to overweight and obesity. Clin Dermatol. 2004 Jul- Aug;22(4):310-4. Review.

Mielgo-Ayuso J, Maroto-Sánchez B, Luzardo-Socorro R, Palacios G, Palacios Gil-Antuñano N, González-Gross M; EXERNET Study Group. Evaluation of nutritional status and energy expenditure in athletes. Nutr Hosp. 2015 Feb 26;31 Suppl3:227-36.

Morton, R. W., McGlory, C., & Phillips, S. M. (2015). Nutritional interventions to augment resistance training- induced skeletal muscle hypertrophy. Frontiers in Physiology, 6, 245.

Phillips SM. The science of muscle hypertrophy: making dietary protein count. Proc Nutr Soc. 2011 Feb;70(1):100-3. Epub 2010 Nov 22. Review.

Poehlman ET. A review: exercise and its influence on resting energy metabolism in man. Med Sci Sports Exerc. 1989 Oct;21(5):515-25. Review.

Pramuková, B., Szabadosová, V., & Šoltésová, A. (2011). Current knowledge about sports nutrition. The Australasian Medical Journal, 4(3), 107–110.

Purcell, L. K., & Canadian Paediatric Society, Paediatric Sports and Exercise Medicine Section. (2013). Sport nutrition for young athletes. Paediatrics & Child Health, 18(4), 200–202.

Romieu, I., Dossus, L., Barquera, S., Blottière, H. M., Franks, P. W., Gunter, M., ... On behalf of the IARC working group on Energy Balance and Obesity. (2017). Energy balance and obesity: what are the main drivers? Cancer Causes & Control, 28(3), 247–258.

Schoeller DA. The energy balance equation: looking back and looking forward are two very different views. Nutr Rev. 2009 May;67(5):249-54.

Schutz Y. Macronutrients and energy balance in obesity. Metabolism. 1995 Sep;44(9 Suppl 3):7-11. Review.

Stark, M., Lukaszuk, J., Prawitz, A., & Salacinski, A. (2012). Protein timing and its effects on muscular hypertrophy and strength in individuals engaged in weight- training. Journal of the International Society of Sports Nutrition, 9, 54.

Steinbeck K. Obesity: the science behind the management. Intern Med J. 2002 May-Jun;32(5-6):237-41. Review.

Tangney CC, Gustashaw KA, Stefan TM, Sullivan C, Ventrelle J, Filipowski CA, Heffernan AD, Hankins J; Clinical Nutrition Department at Rush University Medical Center. A review: which dietary plan is best for your patients seeking weight loss and sustained weight management? Dis Mon. 2005 May;51(5):284-316. Review.

Thomas, D. M., Bouchard, C., Church, T., Slentz, C., Kraus, W. E., Redman, L. M., ... Heymsfield,

S. B. (2012). Why do individuals not lose more weight from an exercise intervention at a defined dose? An energy balance analysis. Obesity Reviews : An Official Journal of the International Association for the Study of Obesity, 13(10), 835–847.

Volek JS, Vanheest JL, Forsythe CE. Diet and exercise for weight loss: a review of current issues. Sports Med. 2005;35(1):1-9. Review.

Weigle DS. Modified macronutrient diets and weight loss– are food choice and variety more important than caloric restriction? Nat Clin Pract Endocrinol Metab.2007 Nov;3(11):728-9. Epub 2007 Sep 4. Review.

Weinheimer EM, Sands LP, Campbell WW. A systematic review of the separate and combined effects of energy restriction and exercise on fat-free mass in middle-aged and older adults: implications for sarcopenic obesity. Nutr Rev. 2010 Jul;68(7):375-88.

Westerterp KR. Control of Energy Expenditure in Humans. [Updated 2016 Nov 11]. In: De Groot LJ, Chrousos G, Dungan K, et al., editors. Endotext [Internet]. South Dartmouth (MA): MDText.com, Inc.; 2000.0

Westerterp KR. Exercise, energy expenditure and energy balance, as measured with doubly labelled water. Proc Nutr Soc. 2018 Feb;77(1):4-10. Epub 2017 Jul 20.

Westerterp, K. R. (2013). Physical activity and physical activity induced energy expenditure in humans: measurement, determinants, and effects. Frontiers in Physiology, 4, 90.

CHAPTER 3

Abdulla H, Smith K, Atherton PJ, Idris I. Role of insulin in the regulation of human skeletal muscle protein synthesis and breakdown: a systematic review and meta-analysis. Diabetologia. 2016 Jan;59(1):44-55.

Acheson KJ, Schutz Y, Bessard T, Flatt JP, Jéquier E. Carbohydrate metabolism and de novo lipogenesis in human obesity. Am J Clin Nutr. 1987 Jan;45(1):78-85.

Adeva-Andany, M. M., González-Lucán, M., Donapetry- García, C., Fernández-Fernández, C., & Ameneiros- Rodríguez, E. (2016). Glycogen metabolism in humans. BBA Clinical, 5, 85–100.

Aranceta J, Pérez-Rodrigo C. Recommended dietary reference intakes, nutritional goals and dietary guidelines for fat and fatty acids: a systematic review. Br J Nutr. 2012 Jun;107 Suppl 2:S8-22.

Artioli, G. G., Bertuzzi, R. C., Roschel, H., Mendes, S. H., Lancha, A. H., & Franchini, E. (2012). Determining the Contribution of the Energy Systems During Exercise. Journal of Visualized Experiments : JoVE, (61), 3413. Advance online publication.

Ascherio A, Willett WC. Health effects of trans fatty acids. Am J Clin Nutr. 1997 Oct;66(4 Suppl):1006S-1010S. Review.

Astrup, A., Raben, A., & Geiker, N. (2015). The role of higher protein diets in weight control and obesity-related comorbidities. International Journal of Obesity (2005), 39(5), 721–726.

Aune, D., Keum, N., Giovannucci, E., Fadnes, L. T., Boffetta, P., Greenwood, D. C., ... Norat, T. (2016). Whole grain consumption and risk of cardiovascular disease, cancer, and all cause and cause specific mortality: systematic review and dose-response meta-analysis of prospective studies. The BMJ, 353, i2716.

Aune, D., Keum, N., Giovannucci, E., Fadnes, L. T., Boffetta, P., Greenwood, D. C., ... Norat, T. (2016). Whole grain consumption and risk of cardiovascular disease, cancer, and all cause and cause specific mortality: systematic review and dose-response meta-analysis of prospective studies. The BMJ, 353, i2716.

Aune, D., Keum, N., Giovannucci, E., Fadnes, L. T., Boffetta, P., Greenwood, D. C., Tonstad, S., Vatten, L. J., Riboli, E., ... Norat, T. (2016). Whole grain consumption and risk of cardiovascular disease, cancer, and all cause and cause specific mortality: systematic review and dose-response meta-analysis of prospective studies. BMJ (Clinical research ed.), 353, i2716.

Baker, J. S., McCormick, M. C., & Robergs, R. A. (2010). Interaction among Skeletal Muscle Metabolic Energy Systems during Intense Exercise. Journal of Nutrition and Metabolism, 2010, 905612.

Barba CV, Cabrera MI. Recommended energy and nutrient intakes for Filipinos 2002. Asia Pac J Clin Nutr. 2008;17 Suppl 2:399-404.

Beck, K. L., Thomson, J. S., Swift, R. J., & von Hurst, P. R. (2015). Role of nutrition in performance enhancement and postexercise recovery. Open Access Journal of Sports Medicine, 6, 259–267.

Berg JM, Tymoczko JL, Stryer L. Biochemistry. 5th edition. New York: W H Freeman; 2002. Section 30.4, Fuel Choice During Exercise Is Determined by Intensity and Duration of Activity.

Bilsborough S, Mann N. A review of issues of dietary protein intake in humans. Int J Sport Nutr Exerc Metab. 2006 Apr;16(2):129-52. Review.

Biolo G, Williams BD, Fleming RY, Wolfe RR. Insulin action on muscle protein kinetics and amino acid transport during recovery after resistance exercise. Diabetes. 1999 May;48(5):949-57.

Bonjour JP. Protein intake and bone health. Int J Vitam Nutr Res. 2011 Mar;81(2-3):134-42.

Børsheim E, Cree MG, Tipton KD, Elliott TA, Aarsland A, Wolfe RR. Effect of carbohydrate intake on net muscle protein synthesis during recovery from resistance exercise. J Appl Physiol (1985). 2004 Feb;96(2):674-8. Epub 2003 Oct 31.

Bosse JD, Dixon BM. Dietary protein to maximize resistance training: a review and examination of protein spread and change theories. J Int Soc Sports Nutr. 2012 Sep 8;9(1):42.

Bosse, J. D., & Dixon, B. M. (2012). Dietary protein to maximize resistance training: a review and examination of protein spread and change theories. Journal of the International Society of Sports Nutrition, 9, 42.

Brown, J. (1960). FAT AND CARBOHYDRATE METABOLISM IN HUMANS–A Study of Nutritional and Hormonal Effects. California Medicine, 93(3), 132–136.

Burke LM, Hawley JA, Wong SH, Jeukendrup AE. Carbohydrates for training and competition. J Sports Sci. 2011;29 Suppl 1:S17-27.

Burke LM, Millet G, Tarnopolsky MA; International Association of Athletics Federations. Nutrition for distance events. J Sports Sci. 2007;25 Suppl 1:S29-38. Review. Erratum in: J Sports Sci. 2009 Apr;27(6):667.

Stellingwerff T, Boit MK, Res PT; International Association of Athletics Federations. Nutritional strategies to optimize training and racing in middle-distance athletes. J Sports Sci. 2007;25 Suppl 1:S17-28. Review. Erratum in: J Sports Sci. 2009 Apr;27(6):667.

Saunders MJ. Coingestion of carbohydrate-protein during endurance exercise: influence on performance and recovery. Int J Sport Nutr Exerc Metab. 2007 Aug;17 Suppl:S87-103. Review.

Robins A. Nutritional recommendations for competing in the Ironman triathlon. Curr Sports Med Rep. 2007 Jul;6(4):241-8. Review.

Jeukendrup AE, Jentjens RL, Moseley L. Nutritional considerations in triathlon. Sports Med. 2005;35(2):163-81. Review.

Coyle EF. Fluid and fuel intake during exercise. J Sports Sci. 2004 Jan;22(1):39-55. Review.

Burke LM, Kiens B, Ivy JL. Carbohydrates and fat for training and recovery. J Sports Sci. 2004 Jan;22(1):15-30. Review

Burke, L. M. (2015). Re-Examining High-Fat Diets for Sports Performance: Did We Call the "Nail in the Coffin" Too Soon? Sports Medicine (Auckland, N.z.), 45(Suppl 1), 33–49.

Burke, L. M. (2015). Re-Examining High-Fat Diets for Sports Performance: Did We Call the "Nail in the Coffin" Too Soon? Sports Medicine (Auckland, N.z.), 45(Suppl 1), 33–49.

Chen GC, Tong X, Xu JY, Han SF, Wan ZX, Qin JB, Qin LQ. Whole-grain intake and total, cardiovascular, and cancer mortality: a systematic review and meta-analysis of prospective studies. Am J Clin Nutr. 2016 Jul;104(1):164-72. Epub 2016 May 25. Review.

Chow LS, Albright RC, Bigelow ML, Toffolo G, Cobelli C, Nair KS. Mechanism of insulin's anabolic effect on muscle: measurements of muscle protein synthesis and breakdown using aminoacyl-tRNA and other surrogate measures. Am J Physiol Endocrinol Metab. 2006 Oct;291(4):E729-36. Epub 2006 May 16.

Churchward-Venne, T. A., Burd, N. A., & Phillips, S. M. (2012). Nutritional regulation of muscle protein synthesis with resistance exercise: strategies to enhance anabolism. Nutrition & Metabolism, 9, 40.

Clase, C. M., & Smyth, A. (2015). Chronic kidney disease: diet. BMJ Clinical Evidence, 2015, 2004.

Colombani, P. C., Mannhart, C., & Mettler, S. (2013). Carbohydrates and exercise performance in non-fasted athletes: A systematic review of studies mimicking real-life. Nutrition Journal, 12, 16.

Connor WE, Duell PB, Connor SL. Benefits and hazards of dietary carbohydrate. Curr Atheroscler Rep. 2005 Nov;7(6):428-34. Review. PubMed PMID: 16256000.Hu FB. Protein, body weight, and cardiovascular health. Am J Clin Nutr. 2005 Jul;82(1 Suppl):242S-247S. Review.

Costill DL. Carbohydrate for athletic training and performance. Bol Asoc Med P R. 1991 Aug;83(8):350-3. Review.

Cunnane, S., Nugent, S., Roy, M., Courchesne-Loyer, A., Croteau, E., Tremblay, S., ... Rapoport, S. (2011). BRAIN FUEL METABOLISM, AGING AND ALZHEIMER'S DISEASE. Nutrition (Burbank, Los Angeles County, Calif.), 27(1), 3–20.

Cunningham W, Hyson D. The skinny on high-protein, low-carbohydrate diets. Prev Cardiol. 2006 Summer;9(3):166-71; quiz 172-3. Review.

Das UN. Essential Fatty acids - a review. Curr Pharm Biotechnol. 2006 Dec;7(6):467-82. Review.

Dashti, H. M., Mathew, T. C., Hussein, T., Asfar, S. K., Behbahani, A., Khoursheed, M. A., ... Al-Zaid, N. S. (2004). Long-term effects of a ketogenic diet in obese patients. Experimental & Clinical Cardiology, 9(3), 200– 205.

Dashty M. A quick look at biochemistry: carbohydrate metabolism. Clin Biochem. 2013 Oct;46(15):1339-52.

Davis JM, Bailey SP. Possible mechanisms of central nervous system fatigue during exercise. Med Sci Sports Exerc. 1997 Jan;29(1):45-57. Review.

De Feo P. Hormonal regulation of human protein metabolism. Eur J Endocrinol. 1996 Jul;135(1):7-18. Review.

Deldicque, L., & Francaux, M. (2015). Recommendations for Healthy Nutrition in Female Endurance Runners: An Update. Frontiers in Nutrition, 2, 17.

Dimitriadis G, Mitrou P, Lambadiari V, Maratou E, Raptis SA. Insulin effects in muscle and adipose tissue. Diabetes Res Clin Pract. 2011 Aug;93 Suppl 1:S52-9.

Dong JY, Zhang ZL, Wang PY, Qin LQ. Effects of high- protein diets on body weight, glycaemic control, blood lipids and blood pressure in type 2 diabetes: meta-analysis of randomised controlled trials. Br J Nutr. 2013 Sep 14;110(5):781-9.

Elango R, Ball RO, Pencharz PB. Individual amino acid requirements in humans: an update. Curr Opin Clin Nutr Metab Care. 2008 Jan;11(1):34-9. Review.

Elango R, Ball RO, Pencharz PB. Individual amino acid requirements in humans: an update. Curr Opin Clin Nutr Metab Care. 2008 Jan;11(1):34-9. Review.

Elango R, Humayun MA, Ball RO, Pencharz PB. Evidence that protein requirements have been significantly underestimated. Curr Opin Clin Nutr Metab Care. 2010 Jan;13(1):52-7.

ESCOBAR, K. A., MORALES, J., & VANDUSSELDORP, T. A. (2016). The Effect of a Moderately Low and High Carbohydrate Intake on Crossfit Performance. International Journal of Exercise Science, 9(4), 460–470.

Falkowska, A., Gutowska, I., Goschorska, M., Nowacki, P., Chlubek, D., & Baranowska-Bosiacka, I. (2015).

Energy Metabolism of the Brain, Including the Cooperation between Astrocytes and Neurons, Especially in the Context of Glycogen Metabolism. International Journal of Molecular Sciences, 16(11), 25959–25981.

Ferrando, A. A., Chinkes, D. L., Wolf, S. E., Matin, S., Herndon, D. N., & Wolfe, R. R. (1999). A submaximal dose of insulin promotes net skeletal muscle protein synthesis in patients with severe burns. Annals of Surgery, 229(1), 11–18.

Ferruzzi, M. G., Jonnalagadda, S. S., Liu, S., Marquart, L., McKeown, N., Reicks, M., ... Webb, D. (2014). Developing a Standard Definition of Whole-Grain Foods for Dietary Recommendations: Summary Report of a Multidisciplinary Expert Roundtable Discussion. Advances in Nutrition, 5(2), 164–176.

Fryburg, D. A., Jahn, L. A., Hill, S. A., Oliveras, D. M., & Barrett, E. J. (1995). Insulin and insulin-like growth factor-I enhance human skeletal muscle protein anabolism during hyperaminoacidemia by different mechanisms. Journal of Clinical Investigation, 96(4), 1722–1729.

Fujita, S., Rasmussen, B. B., Cadenas, J. G., Grady, J. J., & Volpi, E. (2006). Effect of insulin on human skeletal muscle protein synthesis is modulated by insulin-induced changes in muscle blood flow and amino acid availability. American Journal of Physiology. Endocrinology and Metabolism, 291(4), E745–E754.

Gaesser GA. Carbohydrate quantity and quality in relation to body mass index. J Am Diet Assoc. 2007 Oct;107(10):1768-80. Review.

Galgani, J., & Ravussin, E. (2008). Energy metabolism, fuel selection and body weight regulation. International Journal of Obesity (2005), 32(Suppl 7), S109–S119.

Gastin PB. Energy system interaction and relative contribution during maximal exercise. Sports Med. 2001;31(10):725-41. Review.

Geser CA. Hormonal interactions in carbohydrate metabolism. Int Z Vitam Ernahrungsforsch Beih. 1976;15:58-65..

Glynn, E. L., Fry, C. S., Drummond, M. J., Dreyer, H. C., Dhanani, S., Volpi, E., & Rasmussen, B. B. (2010). Muscle protein breakdown has a minor role in the protein anabolic response to essential amino acid and carbohydrate intake following resistance exercise. American Journal of Physiology - Regulatory, Integrative and Comparative Physiology, 299(2), R533–R540.

Hargreaves M. Interactions between muscle glycogen and blood glucose during exercise. Exerc Sport Sci Rev. 1997;25:21-39. Review.

Hauner H, Bechthold A, Boeing H, Brönstrup A, Buyken A, Leschik-Bonnet E, Linseisen J, Schulze M, Strohm D, Wolfram G; German Nutrition Society. Evidence-based guideline of the German Nutrition Society: carbohydrate intake and prevention of nutrition-related diseases. Ann Nutr Metab. 2012;60 Suppl 1:1-58.

Hawley JA, Leckey JJ. Carbohydrate Dependence During Prolonged, Intense Endurance Exercise. Sports Med. 2015 Nov;45 Suppl 1:S5-12.

Jeukendrup A. A step towards personalized sports nutrition: carbohydrate intake during exercise. Sports Med. 2014 May;44 Suppl 1:S25-33.

Cermak NM, van Loon LJ. The use of carbohydrates during exercise as an ergogenic aid. Sports Med. 2013 Nov;43(11):1139-55.

Maughan RJ, Burke LM. Practical nutritional recommendations for the athlete. Nestle Nutr Inst Workshop Ser. 2011;69:131-49.

Stellingwerff T, Maughan RJ, Burke LM. Nutrition for power sports: middle-distance running, track cycling, rowing, canoeing/kayaking, and swimming. J Sports Sci. 2011;29 Suppl 1:S79-89.

Health Benefits of Dietary Whole Grains: An Umbrella Review of Meta-analyses. (2016). Journal of chiropractic medicine, 16(1), 10-18.

Helms ER, Zinn C, Rowlands DS, Brown SR. A systematic review of dietary protein during caloric restriction in resistance trained lean athletes: a case for higher intakes. Int J Sport Nutr Exerc Metab. 2014 Apr;24(2):127-38.

Heydenreich, J., Kayser, B., Schutz, Y., & Melzer, K. (2017). Total Energy Expenditure, Energy Intake, and Body Composition in Endurance Athletes Across the Training Season: A Systematic Review. Sports Medicine - Open, 3, 8.

Hirsch J. Role and benefits of carbohydrate in the diet: key issues for future dietary guidelines. Am J Clin Nutr. 1995 Apr;61(4 Suppl):996S-1000S. Review.

Horowitz JF, Klein S. Lipid metabolism during endurance exercise. Am J Clin Nutr. 2000 Aug;72(2 Suppl):558S-63S. Review.

Ivy JL. Muscle glycogen synthesis before and after exercise. Sports Med. 1991 Jan;11(1):6-19. Review.

Jacobs DR Jr, Gallaher DD. Whole grain intake and cardiovascular disease: a review. Curr Atheroscler Rep. 2004 Nov;6(6):415-23. Review.

Jensen, J., Rustad, P. I., Kolnes, A. J., & Lai, Y.-C. (2011). The Role of Skeletal Muscle Glycogen Breakdown for Regulation of Insulin Sensitivity by Exercise. Frontiers in Physiology, 2, 112.

Jéquier E. Response to and range of acceptable fat intake in adults. Eur J Clin Nutr. 1999 Apr;53 Suppl 1:S84-8; discussion S88-93. Review.

Jeukendrup AE, Saris WH, Wagenmakers AJ. Fat metabolism during exercise: a review. Part I: fatty acid mobilization and muscle metabolism. Int J Sports Med. 1998 May;19(4):231-44. Review.

Jeukendrup AE, Saris WH, Wagenmakers AJ. Fat metabolism during exercise: a review--part II: regulation of metabolism and the effects of training. Int J Sports Med. 1998 Jul;19(5):293-302. Review.

Jeukendrup AE, Saris WH, Wagenmakers AJ. Fat metabolism during exercise: a review--part III: effects of nutritional interventions. Int J Sports Med. 1998 Aug;19(6):371-9. Review.

Jeukendrup AE. Nutrition for endurance sports: marathon, triathlon, and road cycling. J Sports Sci. 2011;29 Suppl 1:S91-9.

Jeukendrup, A. E. (2017). Periodized Nutrition for Athletes. Sports Medicine (Auckland, N.z.), 47(Suppl 1), 51–63.

Jonnalagadda, S. S., Harnack, L., Hai Liu, R., McKeown, N., Seal, C., Liu, S., & Fahey, G. C. (2011). Putting the Whole Grain Puzzle Together: Health Benefits Associated with Whole Grains—Summary of American Society for Nutrition 2010 Satellite Symposium. The Journal of Nutrition, 141(5), 1011S–1022S.

Jonnalagadda, S. S., Harnack, L., Liu, R. H., McKeown, N., Seal, C., Liu, S., & Fahey, G. C. (2011). Putting the whole grain puzzle together: health benefits associated with whole grains--summary of American Society for Nutrition 2010 Satellite Symposium. The Journal of nutrition, 141(5), 1011S-22S.

Kamper AL, Strandgaard S. Long-Term Effects of High- Protein Diets on Renal Function. Annu Rev Nutr. 2017 Aug 21;37:347-369.

Ko GJ, Obi Y, Tortorici AR, Kalantar-Zadeh K. Dietary protein intake and chronic kidney disease. Curr Opin Clin Nutr Metab Care. 2017 Jan;20(1):77-85. Review.

Aparicio M. Protein intake and chronic kidney disease: literature review, 2003 to 2008. J Ren Nutr. 2009 Sep;19(5 Suppl):S5-8.

Friedman AN. High-protein diets: potential effects on the kidney in renal health and disease. Am J Kidney Dis. 2004 Dec;44(6):950-62. Review.

Kelly, C. L., Sünram-Lea, S. I., & Crawford, T. J. (2015). The Role of Motivation, Glucose and Self-Control in the Antisaccade Task. PLoS ONE, 10(3), e0122218.

Kerstetter JE, Kenny AM, Insogna KL. Dietary protein and skeletal health: a review of recent human research. Curr Opin Lipidol. 2011 Feb;22(1):16-20.

Kiens B, Astrup A. Ketogenic Diets for Fat Loss and Exercise Performance: Benefits and Safety? Exerc Sport Sci Rev. 2015 Jul;43(3):109.

Knechtle B, Boutellier U. [Nutrition in long physical endurance events]. Praxis (Bern 1994). 2000 Dec 7;89(49):2051-62. Review. German.

Pendergast DR, Leddy JJ, Venkatraman JT. A perspective on fat intake in athletes. J Am Coll Nutr. 2000 Jun;19(3):345-50. Review.

Jacobs KA, Sherman WM. The efficacy of carbohydrate supplementation and chronic high- carbohydrate diets for improving endurance performance. Int J Sport Nutr. 1999 Mar;9(1):92-115. Review.

Hawley JA, Schabort EJ, Noakes TD, Dennis SC. Carbohydrate-loading and exercise performance. An update. Sports Med. 1997 Aug;24(2):73-81. Review.

Walberg-Rankin J. Dietary carbohydrate as an ergogenic aid for prolonged and brief competitions in sport. Int J Sport Nutr. 1995 Jun;5 Suppl:S13-28. Review.

Applegate EA. Nutritional considerations for ultraendurance performance. Int J Sport Nutr. 1991 Jun;1(2):118-26. Review.

Coggan AR, Coyle EF. Carbohydrate ingestion during prolonged exercise: effects on metabolism and performance. Exerc Sport Sci Rev. 1991;19:1-40. Review.

Hargreaves M. Carbohydrates and exercise. J Sports Sci. 1991 Summer;9 Spec No:17-28. Review.

Brotherhood JR. Nutrition and sports performance. Sports Med. 1984 Sep-Oct;1(5):350-89. Review.

Knuiman, P., Hopman, M. T. E., & Mensink, M. (2015). Glycogen availability and skeletal muscle adaptations with endurance and resistance exercise. Nutrition & Metabolism, 12, 59.

Koh-Banerjee P, Rimm EB. Whole grain consumption and weight gain: a review of the epidemiological evidence, potential mechanisms and opportunities for future research. Proc Nutr Soc. 2003 Feb;62(1):25-9. Review.

Kosinski, C., & Jornayvaz, F. R. (2017). Effects of Ketogenic Diets on Cardiovascular Risk Factors: Evidence from Animal and Human Studies. Nutrients, 9(5), 517.

Kreider, R. B., Earnest, C. P., Lundberg, J., Rasmussen, C., Greenwood, M., Cowan, P., & Almada, A. L. (2007). Effects of ingesting protein with various forms of carbohydrate following resistance-exercise on substrate availability and markers of anabolism, catabolism, and immunity. Journal of the International Society of Sports Nutrition, 4, 18.

Kremmyda LS, Tvrzicka E, Stankova B, Zak A. Fatty acids as biocompounds: their role in human metabolism, health and disease: a review. part 2: fatty acid physiological roles and applications in human health and disease. Biomed Pap Med Fac Univ Palacky Olomouc Czech Repub. 2011 Sep;155(3):195-218.

Kyrø, C., & Tjønneland, A. (2016). Whole grains and public health. The BMJ, 353, i3046.

Kyrø, C., & Tjønneland, A. (2016). Whole grains and public health. BMJ (Clinical research ed.), 353, i3046.

Lambert EV, Goedecke JH. The role of dietary macronutrients in optimizing endurance performance. Curr Sports Med Rep. 2003 Aug;2(4):194-201. Review.

Brown RC. Nutrition for optimal performance during exercise: carbohydrate and fat. Curr Sports Med Rep. 2002 Aug;1(4):222-9. Review.

Peters EM. Nutritional aspects in ultra-endurance exercise. Curr Opin Clin Nutr Metab Care. 2003 Jul;6(4):427-34. Review.

Burke LM. Energy needs of athletes. Can J Appl Physiol. 2001;26 Suppl:S202-19. Review.

Lands, B. (2012). Consequences of Essential Fatty Acids. Nutrients, 4(9), 1338-1357.

Lange KH. Fat metabolism in exercise—with special reference to training and growth hormone administration. Scand J Med Sci Sports. 2004 Apr;14(2):74-99. Review.

Layman DK, Clifton P, Gannon MC, Krauss RM, Nuttall FQ. Protein in optimal health: heart disease and type 2 diabetes. Am J Clin Nutr. 2008 May;87(5):1571S-1575S. Review.

Leidy HJ, Carnell NS, Mattes RD, Campbell WW. Higher protein intake preserves lean mass and satiety with weight loss in pre-obese and obese women. Obesity (Silver Spring). 2007 Feb;15(2):421-9.

Leidy HJ, Clifton PM, Astrup A, Wycherley TP, Westerterp-Plantenga MS, Luscombe-Marsh ND, Woods SC, Mattes RD. The role of protein in weight loss and maintenance. Am J Clin Nutr. 2015 Apr 29. pii: ajcn084038. [Epub ahead of print]

Astrup A, Raben A, Geiker N. The role of higher protein diets in weight control and obesity-related comorbidities. Int J Obes (Lond). 2015 May;39(5):721-6.

Westerterp-Plantenga MS, Lemmens SG, Westerterp KR. Dietary protein - its role in satiety, energetics, weight loss and health. Br J Nutr. 2012 Aug;108 Suppl 2:S105-12.

Lemon PW, Proctor DN. Protein intake and athletic performance. Sports Med. 1991 Nov;12(5):313-25. Review.

Li, B., Zhang, G., Tan, M., Zhao, L., Jin, L., Tang, X., ... Zhong, K. (2016). Consumption of whole grains in relation to mortality from all causes, cardiovascular disease, and diabetes: Dose–response meta-analysis of prospective cohort studies. Medicine, 95(33), e4229.

Lichtenstein AH, Kennedy E, Barrier P, Danford D, Ernst ND, Grundy SM, Leveille GA, Van Horn L, Williams CL, Booth SL. Dietary fat consumption and health. Nutr Rev. 1998 May;56(5 Pt 2):S3-19; discussion S19-28. Review.

Ma, X., Tang, W.-G., Yang, Y., Zhang, Q.-L., Zheng, J.-L., & Xiang, Y.-B. (2016). Association between whole grain intake and all-cause mortality: a meta-analysis of cohort studies. Oncotarget, 7(38), 61996–62005.

Manninen, A. H. (2006). Very-low-carbohydrate diets and preservation of muscle mass. Nutrition & Metabolism, 3, 9.

Martens EA, Westerterp-Plantenga MS. Protein diets, body weight loss and weight maintenance. Curr Opin Clin Nutr Metab Care. 2014 Jan;17(1):75-9.

Martin, W. F., Armstrong, L. E., & Rodriguez, N. R. (2005). Dietary protein intake and renal function. Nutrition & Metabolism, 2, 25.

Matsui, T., Soya, S., Okamoto, M., Ichitani, Y., Kawanaka, K., & Soya, H. (2011). Brain glycogen decreases during prolonged exercise. The Journal of Physiology, 589(Pt 13), 3383–3393.

McRae, M. P. (2017). Health Benefits of Dietary Whole Grains: An Umbrella Review of Meta-analyses. Journal of Chiropractic Medicine, 16(1), 10–18.

Mergenthaler, P., Lindauer, U., Dienel, G. A., & Meisel, A. (2013). Sugar for the brain: the role of glucose in physiological and pathological brain function. Trends in Neurosciences, 36(10), 587–597.

Miller SL, Tipton KD, Chinkes DL, Wolf SE, Wolfe RR. Independent and combined effects of amino acids and glucose after resistance exercise. Med Sci Sports Exerc. 2003 Mar;35(3):449-55.

Mitchell, W. K., Wilkinson, D. J., Phillips, B. E., Lund, J. N., Smith, K., & Atherton, P. J. (2016). Human Skeletal Muscle Protein Metabolism Responses to Amino Acid Nutrition. Advances in Nutrition, 7(4), 828S–838S.

Montfort-Steiger, V., & Williams, C. A. (2007). Carbohydrate Intake Considerations for Young Athletes. Journal of Sports Science & Medicine, 6(3), 343–352.

Morris AA. Cerebral ketone body metabolism. J Inherit Metab Dis. 2005;28(2):109-21. Review.

Mul, J. D., Stanford, K. I., Hirshman, M. F., & Goodyear, L. (2015). Exercise and Regulation of Carbohydrate Metabolism. Progress in Molecular Biology and Translational Science, 135, 17–37.

Naseeb MA, Volpe SL. Protein and exercise in the prevention of sarcopenia and aging. Nutr Res. 2017 Apr;40:1-20.

Noland RC. Exercise and Regulation of Lipid Metabolism. Prog Mol Biol Transl Sci. 2015;135:39-74.

Nowson C, O'Connell S. Protein Requirements and Recommendations for Older People: A Review. Nutrients. 2015 Aug 14;7(8):6874-99.

Nybo L. CNS fatigue and prolonged exercise: effect of glucose supplementation. Med Sci Sports Exerc. 2003 Apr;35(4):589-94.

Ørtenblad, N., Westerblad, H., & Nielsen, J. (2013). Muscle glycogen stores and fatigue. The Journal of Physiology, 591(Pt 18), 4405–4413.

Ørtenblad, N., Westerblad, H., & Nielsen, J. (2013). Muscle glycogen stores and fatigue. The Journal of Physiology, 591(Pt 18), 4405–4413.

Paoli, A. (2014). Ketogenic Diet for Obesity: Friend or Foe? International Journal of Environmental Research and Public Health, 11(2), 2092–2107.

Paoli, A., Rubini, A., Volek, J. S., & Grimaldi, K. A. (2013). Beyond weight loss: a review of the therapeutic uses of very-low-carbohydrate (ketogenic) diets. European Journal of Clinical Nutrition, 67(8), 789–796.

Pasiakos SM. Metabolic advantages of higher protein diets and benefits of dairy foods on weight management, glycemic regulation, and bone. J Food Sci. 2015 Mar;80 Suppl 1:A2-7.

Pedersen, A. N., Kondrup, J., & Børsheim, E. (2013). Health effects of protein intake in healthy adults: a systematic literature review. Food & Nutrition Research, 57, 10.3402/fnr.v57i0.21245.

Pesta, D. H., & Samuel, V. T. (2014). A high-protein diet for reducing body fat: mechanisms and possible caveats. Nutrition & Metabolism, 11, 53.

Peters, S. J., & LeBlanc, P. J. (2004). Metabolic aspects of low carbohydrate diets and exercise. Nutrition & Metabolism, 1, 7.

Phillips SK, Wiseman RW, Woledge RC, Kushmerick MJ. The effect of metabolic fuel on force production and resting inorganic phosphate levels in mouse skeletal muscle. J Physiol. 1993 Mar;462:135-46.

Phillips SM, Van Loon LJ. Dietary protein for athletes: from requirements to optimum adaptation. J Sports Sci. 2011;29 Suppl 1:S29-38.

Phillips SM, Van Loon LJ. Dietary protein for athletes: from requirements to optimum adaptation. J Sports Sci. 2011;29 Suppl 1:S29-38.

Phillips SM. Protein requirements and supplementation in strength sports. Nutrition. 2004 Jul-Aug;20(7-8):689-95. Review.

Phillips, S. M. (2014). A Brief Review of Higher Dietary Protein Diets in Weight Loss: A Focus on Athletes. Sports Medicine (Auckland, N.z.), 44(Suppl 2), 149–153.

Phinney, S. D. (2004). Ketogenic diets and physical performance. Nutrition & Metabolism, 1, 2.

Pinckaers, P. J. M., Churchward-Venne, T. A., Bailey, D., & van Loon, L. J. C. (2017). Ketone Bodies and Exercise Performance: The Next Magic Bullet or Merely Hype? Sports Medicine (Auckland, N.z.), 47(3), 383–391.

Pöchmüller, M., Schwingshackl, L., Colombani, P. C., & Hoffmann, G. (2016). A systematic review and meta- analysis of carbohydrate benefits associated with randomized controlled competition-based performance trials. Journal of the International Society of Sports Nutrition, 13, 27.

Proud CG. Regulation of protein synthesis by insulin. Biochem Soc Trans. 2006 Apr;34(Pt 2):213-6. Review.

Ranallo RF, Rhodes EC. Lipid metabolism during exercise. Sports Med. 1998 Jul;26(1):29-42. Review.

Rao J, Oz G, Seaquist ER. Regulation of cerebral glucose metabolism. Minerva Endocrinol. 2006 Jun;31(2):149-58. Review.

Rasmussen BB, Tipton KD, Miller SL, Wolf SE, Wolfe RR. An oral essential amino acid-carbohydrate supplement enhances muscle protein anabolism after resistance exercise. J Appl Physiol (1985). 2000 Feb;88(2):386-92.

Rebello CJ, Greenway FL, Finley JW. Whole grains and pulses: a comparison of the nutritional and health benefits. J Agric Food Chem. 2014 Jul 23;62(29):7029-49.

Röhling, M., Herder, C., Stemper, T., & Müssig, K. (2016). Influence of Acute and Chronic Exercise on Glucose Uptake. Journal of Diabetes Research, 2016, 2868652.

Schönfeld, P., & Reiser, G. (2013). Why does brain metabolism not favor burning of fatty acids to provide energy? - Reflections on disadvantages of the use of free fatty acids as fuel for brain. Journal of Cerebral Blood Flow & Metabolism, 33(10), 1493–1499.

Schwingshackl, L., & Hoffmann, G. (2014). Comparison of High vs. Normal/Low Protein Diets on Renal Function in Subjects without Chronic Kidney Disease: A Systematic Review and Meta-Analysis. PLoS ONE, 9(5), e97656.

Simopoulos AP. Essential fatty acids in health and chronic disease. Am J Clin Nutr. 1999 Sep;70(3 Suppl):560S- 569S. Review.

Sinclair HM. Essential fatty acids in perspective. Hum Nutr Clin Nutr. 1984 Jul;38(4):245-60.

Skerrett, P. J., & Willett, W. C. (2010). Essentials of Healthy Eating: A Guide. Journal of Midwifery & Women's Health, 55(6), 492–501.

Slavin J. Whole grains and human health. Nutr Res Rev. 2004 Jun;17(1):99-110.

Slavin J. Why whole grains are protective: biological mechanisms. Proc Nutr Soc. 2003 Feb;62(1):129-34. Review.

Slavin JL, Jacobs D, Marquart L, Wiemer K. The role of whole grains in disease prevention. J Am Diet Assoc. 2001 Jul;101(7):780-5. Review.

Smith, C. E., & Tucker, K. L. (2011). Health benefits of cereal fibre: a review of clinical trials. Nutrition Research Reviews, 24(1), 118–131.

Soenen S, Westerterp-Plantenga MS. Proteins and satiety: implications for weight management. Curr Opin Clin Nutr Metab Care. 2008 Nov;11(6):747-51.

Veldhorst M, Smeets A, Soenen S, Hochstenbach-Waelen A, Hursel R, Diepvens K, Lejeune M, Luscombe-Marsh N, Westerterp-Plantenga M. Protein-induced satiety: effects and mechanisms of different proteins. Physiol Behav. 2008 May 23;94(2):300-7.

Halton TL, Hu FB. The effects of high protein diets on thermogenesis, satiety and weight loss: a critical review. J Am Coll Nutr. 2004 Oct;23(5):373-85. Review.

Spriet, L. L. (2014). New Insights into the Interaction of Carbohydrate and Fat Metabolism During Exercise. Sports Medicine (Auckland, N.z.), 44(Suppl 1), 87–96.

Stark, M., Lukaszuk, J., Prawitz, A., & Salacinski, A. (2012). Protein timing and its effects on muscular hypertrophy and strength in individuals engaged in weight- training. Journal of the International Society of Sports Nutrition, 9, 54.

Sünram-Lea SI, Foster JK, Durlach P, Perez C. Glucose facilitation of cognitive performance in healthy young adults: examination of the influence of fast-duration, time of day and pre-consumption plasma glucose levels.Psychopharmacology (Berl). 2001 Aug;157(1):46- 54.

Kaplan RJ, Greenwood CE, Winocur G, Wolever TM. Cognitive performance is associated with glucose regulation in healthy elderly persons and can be enhanced with glucose and dietary carbohydrates. Am J Clin Nutr. 2000 Sep;72(3):825-36.

Owens DS, Benton D. The impact of raising blood glucose on reaction times. Neuropsychobiology. 1994;30(2-3):106- 13.

Te Morenga L, Mann J. The role of high-protein diets in body weight management and health. Br J Nutr. 2012 Aug;108 Suppl 2:S130-8.

Thyfault JP, Carper MJ, Richmond SR, Hulver MW, Potteiger JA. Effects of liquid carbohydrate ingestion on markers of anabolism following high-intensity resistance exercise. J Strength Cond Res. 2004 Feb;18(1):174-9.

Tvrzicka E, Kremmyda LS, Stankova B, Zak A. Fatty acids as biocompounds: their role in human metabolism, health and disease--a review. Part 1: classification, dietary sources and biological functions. Biomed Pap Med Fac Univ Palacky Olomouc Czech Repub. 2011 Jun;155(2):117-30. Review.

van der Zwaluw NL, van de Rest O, Kessels RP, de Groot LC. Short-term effects of glucose and sucrose on cognitive performance and mood in elderly people. J Clin Exp Neuropsychol. 2014;36(5):517-27.

Owen L, Sunram-Lea SI. Metabolic agents that enhance ATP can improve cognitive functioning: a review of the evidence for glucose, oxygen, pyruvate, creatine, and L- carnitine. Nutrients. 2011 Aug;3(8):735-55.

Greenwood CE. Dietary carbohydrate, glucose regulation, and cognitiveperformance in elderly persons. Nutr Rev. 2003 May;61(5 Pt 2):S68-74. Review.

Volpi E, Lucidi P, Cruciani G, Monacchia F, Reboldi G, Brunetti P, Bolli GB, De Feo P. Contribution of amino acids and insulin to protein anabolism during meal absorption. Diabetes. 1996 Sep;45(9):1245-52.

Weinert, D. J. (2009). Nutrition and muscle protein synthesis: a descriptive review. The Journal of the Canadian Chiropractic Association, 53(3), 186–193.

Westerterp-Plantenga MS, Lemmens SG, Westerterp KR. Dietary protein - its role in satiety, energetics, weight loss and health. Br J Nutr. 2012 Aug;108 Suppl 2:S105-12.

Abou-Samra R, Keersmaekers L, Brienza D, Mukherjee R, Macé K. Effect of different protein sources on satiation and short-term satiety when consumed as a starter. Nutr J. 2011 Dec 23;10:139.

Westerterp-Plantenga MS, Nieuwenhuizen A, Tomé D, Soenen S, Westerterp KR. Dietary protein, weight loss, and weight maintenance. Annu Rev Nutr. 2009;29:21-41.

Westerterp-Plantenga MS. The significance of protein in food intake and body weight regulation. Curr Opin Clin Nutr Metab Care. 2003 Nov;6(6):635-8. Review.

Williams, C., & Rollo, I. (2015). Carbohydrate Nutrition and Team Sport Performance. Sports Medicine (Auckland, N.z.), 45(Suppl 1), 13–22.

Wilson PB. Does Carbohydrate Intake During Endurance Running Improve Performance? A Critical Review. J Strength Cond Res. 2016 Dec;30(12):3539-3559. Review.

Williams C, Rollo I. Carbohydrate Nutrition and Team Sport Performance. Sports Med. 2015 Nov;45 Suppl 1:S13-22.

Beelen M, Cermak NM, van Loon LJ. [Performance enhancement by carbohydrate intake during sport: effects of carbohydrates during and after high-intensity exercise]. Ned Tijdschr Geneeskd. 2015;159:A7465. Review. Dutch.

Cermak NM, van Loon LJ. The use of carbohydrates during exercise as an ergogenic aid. Sports Med. 2013 Nov;43(11):1139-55.

Burke LM, Hawley JA, Wong SH, Jeukendrup AE. Carbohydrates for training and competition. J Sports Sci. 2011;29 Suppl 1:S17-27.

Jeukendrup AE. Carbohydrate intake during exercise and performance. Nutrition. 2004 Jul-Aug;20(7-8):669-77. Review.

Burke LM, Cox GR, Culmmings NK, Desbrow B. Guidelines for daily carbohydrate intake: do athletes achieve them? Sports Med. 2001;31(4):267-99. Review.

Witard, O. C., Wardle, S. L., Macnaughton, L. S., Hodgson, A. B., & Tipton, K. D. (2016). Protein Considerations for Optimising Skeletal Muscle Mass in Healthy Young and Older Adults. Nutrients, 8(4), 181.

Wolfe RR. Effects of insulin on muscle tissue. Curr Opin Clin Nutr Metab Care. 2000 Jan;3(1):67-71. Review.

Wolfe RR. Fat metabolism in exercise. Adv Exp Med Biol. 1998;441:147-56. Review.

Wu G. Dietary protein intake and human health. Food Funct. 2016 Mar;7(3):1251-65.

Yu, H., Fujii, N. L., Toyoda, T., An, D., Farese, R. V., Leitges, M., ... Goodyear, L. J. (2015). Contraction stimulates muscle glucose uptake independent of atypical PKC . Physiological Reports, 3(11), e12565.

Zaj c, A., Chalimoniuk, M., Maszczyk, A., Goła , A., & Lngfort, J. (2015). Central and Peripheral Fatigue During Resistance Exercise – A Critical Review. Journal of Human Kinetics, 49, 159–169.

Zajac, A., Poprzecki, S., Maszczyk, A., Czuba, M., Michalczyk, M., & Zydek, G. (2014). The Effects of a Ketogenic Diet on Exercise Metabolism and Physical Performance in Off-Road Cyclists. Nutrients, 6(7), 2493– 2508.

Zhang B, Zhao Q, Guo W, Bao W, Wang X. Association of whole grain intake with all-cause, cardiovascular, and cancer mortality: a systematic review and dose-response meta-analysis from prospective cohort studies. Eur J Clin Nutr. 2018 Jan;72(1):57-65. doi: 10.1038/ejcn.2017.149. Epub 2017 Nov 1. Review. PubMed PMID: 29091078.

Zhang Y, Kuang Y, LaManna JC, Puchowicz MA. Contribution of brain glucose and ketone bodies to oxidative metabolism. Adv Exp Med Biol. 2013;765:365- 370.

Zierler K. Whole body glucose metabolism. Am J Physiol. 1999 Mar;276(3 Pt1):E409-26. Review.

CHAPTER 4

Aragon AA, Schoenfeld BJ. Nutrient timing revisited: is there a post-exercise anabolic window? J Int Soc Sports Nutr. 2013 Jan 29;10(1):5.

Araya H, Pak N, Vera G, Alviña M. Digestion rate of legume carbohydrates and glycemic index of legume- based meals. Int J Food Sci Nutr. 2003 Mar;54(2):119-26.

Baker, L. B., Rollo, I., Stein, K. W., & Jeukendrup, A. E. (2015). Acute Effects of Carbohydrate Supplementation on Intermittent Sports Performance. Nutrients, 7(7), 5733–5763.

Bellisle F, McDevitt R, Prentice AM. Meal frequency and energy balance. Br J Nutr. 1997 Apr;77 Suppl 1:S57-70. Review..

Boirie Y, Guillet C. Fast digestive proteins and sarcopenia of aging. Curr Opin Clin Nutr Metab Care. 2018 Jan;21(1):37-41.

Boirie, Y., Dangin, M., Gachon, P., Vasson, M.-P., Maubois, J.-L., & Beaufrère, B. (1997). Slow and fast dietary proteins differently modulate postprandial protein accretion. Proceedings of the National Academy of Sciences of the United States of America, 94(26), 14930– 14935.

Burke LM, Hawley JA, Wong SH, Jeukendrup AE. Carbohydrates for training and competition. J Sports Sci. 2011;29 Suppl 1:S17-27.

Burke LM, Hawley JA, Wong SH, Jeukendrup AE. Carbohydrates for training and competition. J Sports Sci. 2011;29 Suppl 1:S17-27.

Burke LM, Kiens B, Ivy JL. Carbohydrates and fat for training and recovery. J Sports Sci. 2004 Jan;22(1):15-30. Review.

Candow DG, Chilibeck PD. Timing of creatine or protein supplementation and resistance training in the elderly. Appl Physiol Nutr Metab. 2008 Feb;33(1):184-90.

Coyle EF. Carbohydrate supplementation during exercise. J Nutr. 1992 Mar;122(3Suppl):788-95. Review.

Coyle EF. Timing and method of increased carbohydrate intake to cope with heavy training, competition and recovery. J Sports Sci. 1991 Summer;9 Spec No:29-51; discussion 51-2. Review.

Cribb PJ, Hayes A. Effects of supplement timing and resistance exercise on skeletal muscle hypertrophy. Med Sci Sports Exerc. 2006 Nov;38(11):1918-25.

Doo, H., Chun, H., & Doo, M. (2016). Associations of daily sleep duration and dietary macronutrient consumption with obesity and dyslipidemia in Koreans: A cross-sectional study. Medicine, 95(45), e5360.

Esfahani A, Wong JM, Mirrahimi A, Villa CR, Kendall CW. The application of the glycemic index and glycemic load in weight loss: A review of the clinical evidence. IUBMB Life. 2011 Jan;63(1):7-13.

Foltz M, Maljaars J, Schuring EA, van der Wal RJ, Boer T, Duchateau GS, Peters HP, Stellaard F, Masclee AA. Intragastric layering of lipids delays lipid absorption and increases plasma CCK but has minor effects on gastric emptying and appetite. Am J Physiol Gastrointest Liver Physiol. 2009 May;296(5):G982-91.

Friedman JE, Neufer PD, Dohm GL. Regulation of glycogen resynthesis following exercise. Dietary considerations. Sports Med. 1991 Apr;11(4):232-43. Review.

Garaulet M, Gómez-Abellán P. Timing of food intake and obesity: a novel association. Physiol Behav. 2014 Jul;134:44-50.

Grandner, M. A., Jackson, N., Gerstner, J. R., & Knutson, L. (2013). Dietary nutrients associated with short and long sleep duration. Data from a nationally representative sample. Appetite, 64, 71–80.

Haff GG, Lehmkuhl MJ, McCoy LB, Stone MH. Carbohydrate supplementation and resistance training. J Strength Cond Res. 2003 Feb;17(1):187-96. Review.

Hawley JA, Burke LM. Effect of meal frequency and timing on physical performance. Br J Nutr. 1997 Apr;77 Suppl 1:S91-103. Review.

Hoffman, J. R., & Falvo, M. J. (2004). Protein – Which is Best? Journal of Sports Science & Medicine, 3(3), 118– 130.

Holmes, R. (1971). Carbohydrate digestion and absorption. Journal of Clinical Pathology. Supplement (Royal College of Pathologists)., 5, 10–13.

Horne BD, Muhlestein JB, Anderson JL. Health effects of intermittent fasting: hormesis or harm? A systematic review. Am J Clin Nutr. 2015 Aug;102(2):464-70.

Hutchison AT, Heilbronn LK. Metabolic impacts of altering meal frequency and timing – Does when we eat matter? Biochimie. 2016 May;124:187-97.

Institute of Medicine (US) Committee on Military Nutrition Research; Marriott BM, editor. Fluid Replacement and Heat Stress. Washington (DC): National Academies Press (US); 1994. 5, Carbohydrate Supplements During and Immediately Post Exercise.

Ivy, J. L. (2004). Regulation of Muscle Glycogen Repletion, Muscle Protein Synthesis and Repair Following Exercise. Journal of Sports Science & Medicine, 3(3), 131–138.

Jenkins DJ, Jenkins AL, Wolever TM, Collier GR, Rao AV, Thompson LU. Starchy foods and fiber: reduced rate of digestion and improved carbohydrate metabolism. Scand J Gastroenterol Suppl. 1987;129:132-41. Review.

Jeukendrup AE. Carbohydrate and exercise performance: the role of multiple transportable carbohydrates. Curr Opin Clin Nutr Metab Care. 2010 Jul;13(4):452-7.

Jeukendrup AE. Carbohydrate intake during exercise and performance. Nutrition. 2004 Jul-Aug;20(7-8):669-77. Review.

Jeukendrup, A. (2014). A Step Towards Personalized Sports Nutrition: Carbohydrate Intake During Exercise. Sports Medicine (Auckland, N.z.), 44(Suppl 1), 25–33.

Johnstone A. Fasting for weight loss: an effective strategy or latest dieting trend? Int J Obes (Lond). 2015 May;39(5):727-33.

Julia M. W. Wong, David J. A. Jenkins; Carbohydrate Digestibility and Metabolic Effects, The Journal of Nutrition, Volume 137, Issue 11, 1 November 2007, Pages 2539S–2546S,

Kerksick C, Harvey T, Stout J, Campbell B, Wilborn C, Kreider R, Kalman D, Ziegenfuss T, Lopez H, Landis J, Ivy JL, Antonio J. International Society of Sports Nutrition position stand: nutrient timing. J Int Soc Sports Nutr. 2008 Oct 3;5:17. Erratum in: J Int Soc Sports Nutr. 2008;5:18.

Kinsey, A. W., & Ormsbee, M. J. (2015). The health impact of nighttime eating: old and new perspectives. Nutrients, 7(4), 2648-62.

Kirk TR. Role of dietary carbohydrate and frequent eating in body-weight control. Proc Nutr Soc. 2000 Aug;59(3):349-58. Review.

Knuiman, P., Hopman, M. T. E., & Mensink, M. (2015). Glycogen availability and skeletal muscle adaptations with endurance and resistance exercise. Nutrition & Metabolism, 12, 59.

Koletzko B, Toschke AM. Meal patterns and frequencies: do they affect body weight in children and adolescents? Crit Rev Food Sci Nutr. 2010 Feb;50(2):100-5.

La Bounty PM, Campbell BI, Wilson J, Galvan E, Berardi J, Kleiner SM, Kreider RB, Stout JR, Ziegenfuss T, Spano M, Smith A, Antonio J. International Society of Sports Nutrition position stand: meal frequency. J Int Soc Sports Nutr. 2011 Mar 16;8:4.

Lattimer, J. M., & Haub, M. D. (2010). Effects of Dietary Fiber and Its Components on Metabolic Health. Nutrients, 2(12), 1266–1289.

Lemon PW, Berardi JM, Noreen EE. The role of protein and amino acid supplements in the athlete's diet: does type or timing of ingestion matter? Curr Sports Med Rep. 2002 Aug;1(4):214-21. Review.

Lindseth, G., & Murray, A. (2016). Dietary Macronutrients and Sleep. Western Journal of Nursing Research, 38(8), 938–958.

Longo VD, Mattson MP. Fasting: molecular mechanisms and clinical applications. Cell Metab. 2014 Feb 4;19(2):181-92.

Longo, V. D., & Mattson, M. P. (2014). Fasting: Molecular Mechanisms and Clinical Applications. Cell Metabolism, 19(2), 181–192.

Louise M. Burke, John A. Hawley, Stephen H. S. Wong & Asker E. Jeukendrup (2011) Carbohydrates for training and competition, Journal of Sports Sciences, 29:sup1, S17-S27.

Louis-Sylvestre J, Lluch A, Neant F, Blundell JE. Highlighting the positive impact of increasing feeding frequency on metabolism and weight management. Forum Nutr. 2003;56:126-8. Review.

Mamerow, M. M., Mettler, J. A., English, K. L., Casperson, S. L., Arentson-Lantz, E., Sheffield-Moore, M., ... Paddon- Jones, D. (2014). Dietary Protein Distribution Positively Influences 24-h Muscle Protein Synthesis in Healthy Adults. The Journal of Nutrition, 144(6), 876–880.

Mattson MP, Longo VD, Harvie M. Impact of intermittent fasting on health and disease processes. Ageing Res Rev. 2017 Oct;39:46-58.

Mattson MP. Energy intake, meal frequency, and health: a neurobiological perspective. Annu Rev Nutr. 2005;25:237-60. Review.

McCartney D, Desbrow B, Irwin C. Post-exercise Ingestion of Carbohydrate, Protein and Water: A Systematic Review and Meta-analysis for Effects on Subsequent Athletic Performance. Sports Med. 2018 Feb;48(2):379-408.

McCrory MA, Shaw AC, Lee JA. Energy and Nutrient Timing for Weight Control: Does Timing of Ingestion Matter? Endocrinol Metab Clin North Am. 2016 Sep;45(3):689-718.

Millard-Stafford M, Childers WL, Conger SA, Kampfer AJ, Rahnert JA. Recovery nutrition: timing and composition after endurance exercise. Curr Sports Med Rep. 2008 Jul-Aug;7(4):193-201.

Mosoni L, Mirand PP. Type and timing of protein feeding to optimize anabolism. Curr Opin Clin Nutr Metab Care. 2003 May;6(3):301-6. Review.

Mota J, Fidalgo F, Silva R, Ribeiro JC, Santos R, Carvalho J, Santos MP. Relationships between physical activity, obesity and meal frequency in adolescents. Ann Hum Biol. 2008 Jan-Feb;35(1):1-10.

Nybo L. CNS fatigue and prolonged exercise: effect of glucose supplementation. Med Sci Sports Exerc. 2003 Apr;35(4):589-94.

Ormsbee, M. J., Bach, C. W., & Baur, D. A. (2014). Pre- Exercise Nutrition: The Role of Macronutrients, Modified Starches and Supplements on Metabolism and Endurance Performance. Nutrients, 6(5), 1782–1808.

Ørtenblad, N., Westerblad, H., & Nielsen, J. (2013). Muscle glycogen stores and fatigue. The Journal of Physiology, 591(Pt 18), 4405–4413.

Patterson RE, Sears DD. Metabolic Effects of Intermittent Fasting. Annu Rev Nutr. 2017 Aug 21;37:371-393.

Patterson, R. E., Laughlin, G. A., Sears, D. D., LaCroix, A. Z., Marinac, C., Gallo, L. C., ... Villaseñor, A. (2015). INTERMITTENT FASTING AND HUMAN METABOLIC HEALTH. Journal of the Academy of Nutrition and Dietetics, 115(8), 1203–1212.

Pöchmüller, M., Schwingshackl, L., Colombani, P. C., & Hoffmann, G. (2016). A systematic review and meta- analysis of carbohydrate benefits associated with randomized controlled competition-based performance trials. Journal of the International Society of Sports Nutrition, 13, 27.

Poole, C., Wilborn, C., Taylor, L., & Kerksick, C. (2010). The Role of Post-Exercise Nutrient Administration on Muscle Protein Synthesis and Glycogen Synthesis.
Journal of Sports Science & Medicine, 9(3), 354–363.

Samra RA. Fats and Satiety. In: Montmayeur JP, le Coutre J, editors. Fat Detection: Taste, Texture, and Post Ingestive Effects. Boca Raton (FL): CRC Press/Taylor & Francis; 2010. Chapter 15.

Schoenfeld BJ, Aragon AA, Krieger JW. The effect of protein timing on muscle strength and hypertrophy: a meta-analysis. J Int Soc Sports Nutr. 2013 Dec 3;10(1):53.

Schoenfeld, B. J., & Aragon, A. A. (2018). How much protein can the body use in a single meal for muscle- building? Implications for daily protein distribution. Journal of the International Society of Sports Nutrition, 15, 10.

Schoenfeld, B. J., Aragon, A., Wilborn, C., Urbina, S. L., Hayward, S. E., & Krieger, J. (2017). Pre- versus post- exercise protein intake has similar effects on muscular adaptations. PeerJ, 5, e2825.

Stark M, Lukaszuk J, Prawitz A, Salacinski A. Protein timing and its effects on muscular hypertrophy and strength in individuals engaged in weight-training. J Int Soc Sports Nutr. 2012 Dec 14;9(1):54.

Stark, M., Lukaszuk, J., Prawitz, A., & Salacinski, A. (2012). Protein timing and its effects on muscular hypertrophy and strength in individuals engaged in weight- training. Journal of the International Society of Sports Nutrition, 9, 54.

Stearns RL, Emmanuel H, Volek JS, Casa DJ. Effects of ingesting protein in combination with carbohydrate during exercise on endurance performance: a systematic review with meta-analysis. J Strength Cond Res. 2010 Aug;24(8):2192-202.

Stellingwerff T, Cox GR. Systematic review: Carbohydrate supplementation on exercise performance or capacity of varying durations. Appl Physiol Nutr Metab. 2014 Sep;39(9):998-1011. Epub 2014 Mar 25. Review.

Stephens BR, Braun B. Impact of nutrient intake timing on the metabolic response to exercise. Nutr Rev. 2008 Aug;66(8):473-6.

St-Onge MP, Mikic A, Pietrolungo CE. Effects of Diet on Sleep Quality. Adv Nutr. 2016 Sep 15;7(5):938-49. Print 2016 Sep. Review.

Timlin MT, Pereira MA. Breakfast frequency and quality in the etiology of adult obesity and chronic diseases. Nutr Rev. 2007 Jun;65(6 Pt 1):268-81. Review.

Tinsley GM, La Bounty PM. Effects of intermittent fasting on body composition and clinical health markers in humans. Nutr Rev. 2015 Oct;73(10):661-74.

Tipton KD. Role of protein and hydrolysates before exercise. Int J Sport Nutr Exerc Metab. 2007 Aug;17 Suppl:S77-86. Review..

Williams, C., & Rollo, I. (2015). Carbohydrate Nutrition and Team Sport Performance. Sports Medicine (Auckland, N.z.), 45(Suppl 1), 13–22.

Wilson PB. Does Carbohydrate Intake During Endurance Running Improve Performance? A Critical Review. J Strength Cond Res. 2016 Dec;30(12):3539-3559. Review.

Zarrinpar A, Chaix A, Panda S. Daily Eating Patterns and Their Impact on Health and Disease. Trends Endocrinol Metab. 2016 Feb;27(2):69-83.

CHAPTER 5

Aguilera CM, Ramírez-Tortosa MC, Mesa MD, Gil A. [Protective effect of monounsaturated and polyunsaturated fatty acids on the development of cardiovascular disease]. Nutr Hosp. 2001 May-Jun;16(3):78-91. Review. Spanish.

Akhondzadeh S, Gerbarg PL, Brown RP. Nutrients for prevention and treatment of mental health disorders. Psychiatr Clin North Am. 2013 Mar;36(1):25-36.

Willett WC, Stampfer MJ. Current evidence on healthy eating. Annu Rev Public Health. 2013;34:77-95.

Lambrinoudaki I, Ceasu I, Depypere H, Erel T, Rees M, Schenck-Gustafsson K, Simoncini T, Tremollieres F, van der Schouw YT, Pérez-López FR. EMAS position statement: Diet and health in midlife and beyond. Maturitas. 2013 Jan;74(1):99-104.

Yusof AS, Isa ZM, Shah SA. Dietary patterns and risk of colorectal cancer: a systematic review of cohort studies (2000-2011). Asian Pac J Cancer Prev. 2012;13(9):4713-7. Review.

Mosby TT, Cosgrove M, Sarkardei S, Platt KL, Kaina B. Nutrition in adult and childhood cancer: role of carcinogens and anti-carcinogens. Anticancer Res. 2012 Oct;32(10):4171-92. Review.

Kumar V, Sinha AK, Makkar HP, de Boeck G, Becker K. Dietary roles of non-starch polysaccharides in human nutrition: a review. Crit Rev Food Sci Nutr. 2012;52(10):899-935.

McKeag NA, McKinley MC, Woodside JV, Harbinson MT, McKeown PP. The role of micronutrients in heart failure. J Acad Nutr Diet. 2012 Jun;112(6):870-86.

Sánchez-Muniz FJ. Dietary fibre and cardiovascular health. Nutr Hosp. 2012 Jan-Feb;27(1):31-45.

Lattimer JM, Haub MD. Effects of dietary fiber and its components on metabolic health. Nutrients. 2010 Dec;2(12):1266-89. doi: 10.3390/nu2121266. Epub 2010 Dec 15. Review.

Lee MS, Huang YC, Su HH, Lee MZ, Wahlqvist ML. A simple food quality index predicts mortality in elderly Taiwanese. J Nutr Health Aging. 2011 Dec;15(10):815-21.

Olsen A, Egeberg R, Halkjær J, Christensen J, Overvad K, Tjønneland A. Healthy aspects of the Nordic diet are related to lower total mortality. J Nutr. 2011 Apr 1;141(4):639-44.

Okarter N, Liu RH. Health benefits of whole grain phytochemicals. Crit Rev Food Sci Nutr. 2010 Mar;50(3):193-208.

Hauner H, Hauner D. The Impact of Nutrition on the Development and Prognosis of Breast Cancer. Breast Care (Basel). 2010;5(6):377-381. Epub 2010 Dec 8.

Mello VD, Laaksonen DE. [Dietary fibers: current trends and health benefits in the metabolic syndrome and type 2 diabetes]. Arq Bras Endocrinol Metabol. 2009 Jul;53(5):509-18. Review. Portuguese.

Manach C, Hubert J, Llorach R, Scalbert A. The complex links between dietary phytochemicals and human health deciphered by metabolomics. Mol Nutr Food Res. 2009 Oct;53(10):1303-15.

Babio N, Bulló M, Salas-Salvadó J. Mediterranean diet and metabolic syndrome: the evidence. Public Health Nutr. 2009 Sep;12(9A):1607-17.

Lutsey PL, Steffen LM, Stevens J. Dietary intake and the development of the metabolic syndrome: the Atherosclerosis Risk in Communities study. Circulation. 2008 Feb 12;117(6):754-61.

Rochfort S, Panozzo J. Phytochemicals for health, the role of pulses. J Agric Food Chem. 2007 Oct 3;55(20):7981-94. Epub 2007 Sep 5. Review.

Stevenson DE, Hurst RD. Polyphenolic phytochemicals– just antioxidants or much more? Cell Mol Life Sci. 2007 Nov;64(22):2900-16. Review.

Huskisson E, Maggini S, Ruf M. The role of vitamins and minerals in energy metabolism and well-being. J Int Med Res. 2007 May-Jun;35(3):277-89. Review.

Bourre JM. Effects of nutrients (in food) on the structure and function of the nervous system: update on dietary requirements for brain. Part

1: micronutrients. J Nutr Health Aging. 2006 Sep-Oct;10(5):377-85. Review.

Shenkin A. Micronutrients in health and disease. Postgrad Med J. 2006 Sep;82(971):559-67. Review.

Giugliano D, Ceriello A, Esposito K. The effects of diet on inflammation: emphasis on the metabolic syndrome. J Am Coll Cardiol. 2006 Aug 15;48(4):677-85. Epub 2006 Jul 24. Review.

Nieves JW. Osteoporosis: the role of micronutrients. Am J Clin Nutr. 2005 May;81(5):1232S-1239S. Review.

Liu RH. Potential synergy of phytochemicals in cancer prevention: mechanism of action. J Nutr. 2004 Dec;134(12 Suppl):3479S-3485S. Review.

Higgins JA. Resistant starch: metabolic effects and potential health benefits. J AOAC Int. 2004 May- Jun;87(3):761-8. Review.

Steffen LM, Jacobs DR Jr, Stevens J, Shahar E, Carithers T, Folsom AR. Associations of whole-grain, refined-grain, and fruit and vegetable consumption with risks of all-cause mortality and incident coronary artery disease and ischemic stroke: the Atherosclerosis Risk in Communities (ARIC) Study. Am J Clin Nutr. 2003 Sep;78(3):383-90.

Bloch AS. Nutrition for health promotion: phytochemicals, functional foods, and alternative approaches to combat obesity. Dent Clin North Am. 2003 Apr;47(2):411-23, viii-ix. Review.

Hu FB, Willett WC. Optimal diets for prevention of coronary heart disease. JAMA. 2002 Nov 27;288(20):2569-78. Review.

Michels KB, Wolk A. A prospective study of variety of healthy foods and mortality in women. Int J Epidemiol. 2002 Aug;31(4):847-54.

Bendich A. Micronutrients in women's health and immune function. Nutrition. 2001 Oct;17(10):858-67. Review.

Aguilera CM, Ramírez-Tortosa MC, Mesa MD, Gil A. [Protective effect of monounsaturated and polyunsaturated fatty acids on the development of cardiovascular disease]. Nutr Hosp. 2001 May-Jun;16(3):78-91. Review. Spanish.

Anderson JW, Smith BM, Gustafson NJ. Health benefits and practical aspects of high-fiber diets. Am J Clin Nutr. 1994 May;59(5 Suppl):1242S-1247S. Review.

Liu K, Stamler J, Trevisan M, Moss D. Dietary lipids, sugar, fiber and mortality from coronary heart disease. Bivariate analysis of international data. Arteriosclerosis. 1982 May-Jun;2(3):221-7.

Probst, Y. C., Guan, V. X., & Kent, K. (2017). Dietary phytochemical intake from foods and health outcomes: a systematic review protocol and preliminary scoping. BMJ Open, 7(2), e013337.

Howes MJ, Simmonds MS. The role of phytochemicals as micronutrients in health and disease. Curr Opin Clin Nutr Metab Care. 2014 Nov;17(6):558-66.

Krzyzanowska J, Czubacka A, Oleszek W. Dietary phytochemicals and human health. Adv Exp Med Biol. 2010;698:74-98. Review.

Alonso A, Ruiz-Gutierrez V, Martínez-González MA. Monounsaturated fatty acids, olive oil and blood pressure: epidemiological, clinical and experimental evidence. Public Health Nutr. 2006 Apr;9(2):251-7. Review.

Ascherio A, Willett WC. Health effects of trans fatty acids. Am J Clin Nutr. 1997 Oct;66(4 Suppl):1006S-1010S. Review.

Balk EM, Lichtenstein AH. Omega-3 Fatty Acids and Cardiovascular Disease: Summary of the 2016 Agency of Healthcare Research and Quality Evidence Review. Nutrients. 2017 Aug 11;9(8). pii: E865.

Bendsen NT, Christensen R, Bartels EM, Astrup A. Consumption of industrial and ruminant trans fatty acids and risk of coronary heart disease: a systematic review and meta-analysis of cohort studies. Eur J Clin Nutr. 2011 Jul;65(7):773-83.

Calder PC, Yaqoob P. Omega-3 polyunsaturated fatty acids and human health outcomes. Biofactors. 2009 May- Jun;35(3):266-72.

Calder PC, Yaqoob P. Omega-3 polyunsaturated fatty acids and human health outcomes. Biofactors. 2009 May- Jun;35(3):266-72.

Calton, J. B. (2010). Prevalence of micronutrient deficiency in popular diet plans. Journal of the International Society of Sports Nutrition, 7, 24.

Clarys, P., Deliens, T., Huybrechts, I.,

Deriemaeker, P., Vanaelst, B., De Keyzer, W., ... Mullie, P. (2014). Comparison of Nutritional Quality of the Vegan, Vegetarian, Semi-Vegetarian, Pesco-Vegetarian and Omnivorous Diet. Nutrients, 6(3), 1318–1332.

Clifton PM, Keogh JB. A systematic review of the effect of dietary saturated and polyunsaturated fat on heart disease. Nutr Metab Cardiovasc Dis. 2017 Dec;27(12):1060-1080.

Das UN. Essential Fatty acids - a review. Curr Pharm Biotechnol. 2006 Dec;7(6):467-82. Review.

de Souza RJ, Mente A, Maroleanu A, Cozma AI, Ha V, Kishibe T, Uleryk E, Budylowski P, Schünemann H, Beyene J, Anand SS. Intake of saturated and trans unsaturated fatty acids and risk of all cause mortality, cardiovascular disease, and type 2 diabetes: systematic review and meta-analysis of observational studies. BMJ. 2015 Aug 11;351:h3978.

de Souza RJ, Mente A, Maroleanu A, Cozma AI, Ha V, Kishibe T, Uleryk E, Budylowski P, Schünemann H, Beyene J, Anand SS. Intake of saturated and trans unsaturated fatty acids and risk of all cause mortality, cardiovascular disease, and type 2 diabetes: systematic review and meta-analysis of observational studies. BMJ. 2015 Aug 11;351:h3978.

De Souza, R. J., Mente, A., Maroleanu, A., Cozma, A. I., Ha, V., Kishibe, T., ... Anand, S. S. (2015). Intake of saturated and trans unsaturated fatty acids and risk of all cause mortality, cardiovascular disease, and type 2 diabetes: systematic review and meta-analysis of observational studies. The BMJ, 351, h3978.

De Souza, R. J., Mente, A., Maroleanu, A., Cozma, A. I., Ha, V., Kishibe, T., ... Anand, S. S. (2015). Intake of saturated and trans unsaturated fatty acids and risk of all cause mortality, cardiovascular disease, and type 2 diabetes: systematic review and meta-analysis of observational studies. The BMJ, 351, h3978.

Dhaka, V., Gulia, N., Ahlawat, K. S., & Khatkar, B. S. (2011). Trans fats–sources, health risks and alternative approach - A review. Journal of Food Science and Technology, 48(5), 534–541.

Donaldson CM, Perry TL, Rose MC. Glycemic index and endurance performance. Int J Sport Nutr Exerc Metab. 2010 Apr;20(2):154-65. Review. Erratum in: Int J Sport Nutr Exerc Metab. 2011 Jun;21(3):262-4.

Drewnowski A, Fulgoni VL 3rd. Nutrient density: principles and evaluation tools. Am J Clin Nutr. 2014 May;99(5 Suppl):1223S-8S.

Dyall, S. C. (2015). Long-chain omega-3 fatty acids and the brain: a review of the independent and shared effects of EPA, DPA and DHA. Frontiers in Aging Neuroscience, 7, 52.

Ganguly R, Pierce GN. The toxicity of dietary trans fats. Food Chem Toxicol. 2015 Apr;78:170-6.

Gardner, C. D., Kim, S., Bersamin, A., Dopler-Nelson, M., Otten, J., Oelrich, B., & Cherin, R. (2010). Micronutrient quality of weight-loss diets that focus on macronutrients: results from the A TO Z study. The American Journal of Clinical Nutrition, 92(2), 304–312.

Garg A, Bonanome A, Grundy SM, Zhang ZJ, Unger RH. Comparison of a high-carbohydrate diet with a high- monounsaturated-fat diet in patients with non-insulin- dependent diabetes mellitus. N Engl J Med. 1988 Sep 29;319(13):829-34.

Garg A. High-monounsaturated-fat diets for patients with diabetes mellitus: a meta-analysis. Am J Clin Nutr. 1998 Mar;67(3 Suppl):577S-582S.

Haag M. Essential fatty acids and the brain. Can J Psychiatry. 2003 Apr;48(3):195-203. Review.

Hoffman JR, Falvo MJ. Protein – Which is Best? J Sports Sci Med. 2004 Sep 1;3(3):118-30. eCollection 2004 Sep. Review.

Hoffman, J. R., & Falvo, M. J. (2004). Protein – Which is Best? Journal of Sports Science & Medicine, 3(3), 118–130. Sarwar G. Digestibility of protein and bioavailability of amino acids in foods. Effects on protein quality assessment. World Rev Nutr Diet. 1987;54:26-70. Review.

Huang S, Wang LM, Sivendiran T, Bohrer BM. Review: Amino acid concentration of high protein food products and an overview of the current methods used to determine protein quality. Crit Rev Food Sci Nutr. 2017 Dec 4:1-6.

Iqbal, M. P. (2014). Trans fatty acids – A risk factor for cardiovascular disease. Pakistan Journal of Medical Sciences, 30(1), 194–197.

Katan MB, Zock PL, Mensink RP. Trans fatty acids and their effects on lipoproteins in humans. Annu Rev Nutr. 1995;15:473-93. Review.

Khandelwal, S., Kelly, L., Malik, R., Prabhakaran, D., & Reddy, S. (2013). Impact of omega-6 fatty acids on cardiovascular outcomes: A review. Journal of Preventive Cardiology, 2(3), 325–336.

Khodarahmi, M., & Azadbakht, L. (2014). The Association Between Different Kinds of Fat Intake and Breast Cancer Risk in Women. International Journal of Preventive Medicine, 5(1), 6–15.

Kiefer, D., & Pantuso, T. (2012). Omega-3 fatty acids: An update emphasizing clinical use. Agro Food Industry Hi- Tech, 23(4), 10–13.

Kris-Etherton PM, Pearson TA, Wan Y, Hargrove RL, Moriarty K, Fishell V, Etherton TD. High-monounsaturated fatty acid diets lower both plasma cholesterol and triacylglycerol concentrations. Am J Clin Nutr. 1999 Dec;70(6):1009-15.

Kris-Etherton, P. M. (2010). Trans-Fats and Coronary Heart Disease. Critical Reviews in Food Science and Nutrition, 50(s1), 29–30.

Lands, B. (2012). Consequences of Essential Fatty Acids. Nutrients, 4(9), 1338–1357.

Menaa F, Menaa A, Menaa B, Tréton J. Trans-fatty acids, dangerous bonds for health? A background review paper of their use, consumption, health implications and regulation in France. Eur J Nutr. 2013 Jun;52(4):1289-302.

Micha R, Mozaffarian D. Trans fatty acids: effects on metabolic syndrome, heart disease and diabetes. Nat Rev Endocrinol. 2009 Jun;5(6):335-44.

Millward DJ. The nutritional value of plant-based diets in relation to human amino acid and protein requirements. Proc Nutr Soc. 1999 May;58(2):249-60. Review.

Moughan PJ. Dietary protein quality in humans–an overview. J AOAC Int. 2005 May-Jun;88(3):874-6. Review.

Nettleton, J. A., Brouwer, I. A., Geleijnse, J. M., & Hornstra, G. (2017). Saturated Fat Consumption and Risk of Coronary Heart Disease and Ischemic Stroke: A Science Update. Annals of Nutrition & Metabolism, 70(1), 26–33.

New SA. Bone health: the role of micronutrients. Br Med Bull. 1999;55(3):619-33. Review.

O'Reilly J, Wong SH, Chen Y. Glycaemic index, glycaemic load and exercise performance. Sports Med. 2010 Jan 1;40(1):27-39.

Otles S, Ozgoz S. Health effects of dietary fiber. Acta Sci Pol Technol Aliment. 2014 Apr-Jun;13(2):191-202. Review.

Reedy J, Krebs-Smith SM, Miller PE, Liese AD, Kahle LL, Park Y, Subar AF. Higher diet quality is associated with decreased risk of all-cause, cardiovascular disease, and cancer mortality among older adults. J Nutr. 2014 Jun;144(6):881-9.

Mudgil D, Barak S. Composition, properties and health benefits of indigestible carbohydrate polymers as dietary fiber: a review. Int J Biol Macromol. 2013 Oct;61:1-6.

Hoeft B, Weber P, Eggersdorfer M. Micronutrients – a global perspective on intake, health benefits and economics. Int J Vitam Nutr Res. 2012 Oct;82(5):316-20.

eft B, Weber P, Eggersdorfer M. Micronutrients - a global perspective on intake, health benefits and economics. Int J Vitam Nutr Res. 2012 Oct;82(5):316-20.

Mursu J, Steffen LM, Meyer KA, Duprez D, Jacobs DR Jr. Diet quality indexes and mortality in postmenopausal women: the Iowa Women's Health Study. Am J Clin Nutr. 2013 Aug;98(2):444-53.

Mursu, J., Steffen, L. M., Meyer, K. A., Duprez, D., & Jacobs, D. R. (2013). Diet quality indexes and mortality in postmenopausal women: the Iowa Women's Health Study. The American Journal of Clinical Nutrition, 98(2), 444– 453.

Abdull Razis AF, Noor NM. Cruciferous vegetables: dietary phytochemicals for cancer prevention. Asian Pac J Cancer Prev. 2013;14(3):1565-70. Review.

Qian, F., Korat, A. A., Malik, V., & Hu, F. B. (2016). Metabolic Effects of Monounsaturated

Fatty Acid– Enriched Diets Compared With Carbohydrate or Polyunsaturated Fatty Acid–Enriched Diets in Patients With Type 2 Diabetes: A Systematic Review and Meta- analysis of Randomized Controlled Trials. Diabetes Care, 39(8), 1448–1457.

Rangel-Huerta OD, Aguilera CM, Mesa MD, Gil A. Omega-3 long-chain polyunsaturated fatty acids supplementation on inflammatory biomakers: a systematic review of randomised clinical trials. Br J Nutr. 2012 Jun;107 Suppl 2:S159-70.

Remig V, Franklin B, Margolis S, Kostas G, Nece T, Street JC. Trans fats in America: a review of their use, consumption, health implications, and regulation.
J Am Diet Assoc. 2010 Apr;110(4):585-92.

Rogerson, D. (2017). Vegan diets: practical advice for athletes and exercisers. Journal of the International Society of Sports Nutrition, 14, 36.

Ruxton CH, Reed SC, Simpson MJ, Millington KJ. The health benefits of omega-3 polyunsaturated fatty acids: a review of the evidence. J Hum Nutr Diet. 2004 Oct;17(5):449-59.

Ruxton CH, Reed SC, Simpson MJ, Millington KJ. The health benefits of omega-3 polyunsaturated fatty acids: a review of the evidence. J Hum Nutr Diet. 2004 Oct;17(5):449-59.

Ruxton CH, Reed SC, Simpson MJ, Millington KJ. The health benefits of omega-3 polyunsaturated fatty acids: a review of the evidence. J Hum Nutr Diet. 2004 Oct;17(5):449-59. Review.

Sahan C, Sozmen K, Unal B, O'Flaherty M, Critchley J. Potential benefits of healthy food and lifestyle policies for reducing coronary heart disease mortality in Turkish adults by 2025: a modelling study. BMJ Open. 2016 Jul 7;6(7):e011217.

Fung TT, Pan A, Hou T, Mozaffarian D, Rexrode KM, Willett WC, Hu FB. Food quality score and the risk of coronary artery disease: a prospective analysis in 3 cohorts. Am J Clin Nutr. 2016 Jul;104(1):65-72.

De Smet S, Vossen E. Meat: The balance between nutrition and health. A review. Meat Sci. 2016 Oct;120:145-56.

Bourassa MW, Alim I, Bultman SJ, Ratan RR. Butyrate, neuroepigenetics and the gut microbiome: Can a high fiber diet improve brain health? Neurosci Lett. 2016 Jun 20;625:56-63.

Schoenaker DA, Mishra GD, Callaway LK, Soedamah- Muthu SS. The Role of Energy, Nutrients, Foods, and Dietary Patterns in the Development of Gestational Diabetes Mellitus: A Systematic Review of Observational Studies. Diabetes Care. 2016 Jan;39(1):16-23. d

Sijtsma FP, Soedamah-Muthu SS, de Goede J, Oude Griep LM, Geleijnse JM, Giltay EJ, de Boer MJ, Jacobs DR Jr, Kromhout D. Healthy eating and lower mortality risk in a large cohort of cardiac patients who received state-of-the-art drug treatment. Am J Clin Nutr. 2015 Dec;102(6):1527-33.

Shi Z, Zhang T, Byles J, Martin S, Avery JC, Taylor AW. Food Habits, Lifestyle Factors and Mortality among Oldest Old Chinese: The Chinese Longitudinal Healthy Longevity Survey (CLHLS). Nutrients. 2015 Sep 9;7(9):7562-79.

Ruxton CH, Derbyshire E, Toribio-Mateas M. Role of fatty acids and micronutrients in healthy ageing: a systematic review of randomised controlled trials set in the context of European dietary surveys of older adults. J Hum Nutr Diet. 2016 Jun;29(3):308-24.

Park K. Role of micronutrients in skin health and function. Biomol Ther (Seoul). 2015 May;23(3):207-17. doi: 10.4062/biomolther.2015.003. Epub 2015 May 1. Review.

Hariharan D, Vellanki K, Kramer H. The Western Diet and Chronic Kidney Disease. Curr Hypertens Rep. 2015 Mar;17(3):16.

Ardisson Korat AV, Willett WC, Hu FB. Diet, lifestyle, and genetic risk factors for type 2 diabetes: a review from the Nurses' Health Study, Nurses' Health Study 2, and Health Professionals' Follow-up Study. Curr Nutr Rep. 2014 Dec 1;3(4):345-354.

Howes MJ, Simmonds MS. The role of phytochemicals as micronutrients in health and disease. Curr Opin Clin Nutr Metab Care. 2014 Nov;17(6):558-66.

Gupta C, Prakash D. Phytonutrients as therapeutic agents. J Complement Integr Med. 2014 Sep;11(3):151-

69. Review. PubMed PMID: 25051278.

George SM, Ballard-Barbash R, Manson JE, Reedy J, Shikany JM, Subar AF, Tinker LF, Vitolins M, Neuhouser ML. Comparing indices of diet quality with chronic disease mortality risk in postmenopausal women in the Women's Health Initiative Observational Study: evidence to inform national dietary guidance. Am J Epidemiol. 2014 Sep 15;180(6):616-25.

Ley SH, Hamdy O, Mohan V, Hu FB. Prevention and management of type 2 diabetes: dietary components and nutritional strategies. Lancet. 2014 Jun 7;383(9933):1999-2007.

Sarwar G, McDonough FE. Evaluation of protein digestibility-corrected amino acid score method for assessing protein quality of foods. J Assoc Off Anal Chem. 1990 May-Jun;73(3):347-56. Review.

Schwingshackl, L., & Hoffmann, G. (2014). Monounsaturated fatty acids, olive oil and health status: a systematic review and meta-analysis of cohort studies.
Lipids in Health and Disease, 13, 154.

Siri-Tarino PW, Sun Q, Hu FB, Krauss RM. Saturated fat, carbohydrate, and cardiovascular disease. Am J Clin Nutr. 2010 Mar;91(3):502-9.

Siri-Tarino, P. W., Chiu, S., Bergeron, N., & Krauss, R. M. (2015). Saturated Fats Versus Polyunsaturated Fats Versus Carbohydrates for Cardiovascular Disease Prevention and Treatment. Annual Review of Nutrition, 35, 517–543.

Slavin, J., & Carlson, J. (2014). Carbohydrates. Advances in Nutrition, 5(6), 760–761.

Svendsen, K., Arnesen, E., & Retterstøl, K. (2017). Saturated fat –a never ending story? Food & Nutrition Research, 61(1), 1377572.

Swanson, D., Block, R., & Mousa, S. A. (2012). Omega-3 Fatty Acids EPA and DHA: Health Benefits Throughout Life. Advances in Nutrition, 3(1), 1–7.

Szostak-Wegierek D, Kłosiewicz-Latoszek L, Szostak WB, Cybulska B. The role of dietary fats for preventing cardiovascular disease. A review. Rocz Panstw Zakl Hig. 2013;64(4):263-9. Review.

Teegala SM, Willett WC, Mozaffarian D. Consumption and health effects of trans fatty acids: a review. J AOAC Int. 2009 Sep-Oct;92(5):1250-7. Review.

Teegala SM, Willett WC, Mozaffarian D. Consumption and health effects of trans fatty acids: a review. J AOAC Int. 2009 Sep-Oct;92(5):1250-7. Review.

Thomas DE, Brotherhood JR, Brand JC. Carbohydrate feeding before exercise: effect of glycemic index. Int J Sports Med. 1991 Apr;12(2):180-6.

Tome D. Criteria and markers for protein quality assessment – a review. Br J Nutr. 2012 Aug;108 Suppl 2:S222-9.

Valenzuela A, Morgado N. Trans fatty acid isomers in human health and in the food industry. Biol Res. 1999;32(4):273-87. Review.

van Vliet S, Burd NA, van Loon LJ. The Skeletal Muscle Anabolic Response to Plant- versus Animal-Based Protein Consumption. J Nutr. 2015 Sep;145(9):1981-91.

Walton P, Rhodes EC. Glycaemic index and optimal performance. Sports Med. 1997 Mar;23(3):164-72. Review.

Wanders, A. J., Zock, P. L., & Brouwer, I. A. (2017). Trans Fat Intake and Its Dietary Sources in General Populations Worldwide: A Systematic Review. Nutrients, 9(8), 840.

Wolk A, Bergström R, Hunter D, Willett W, Ljung H, Holmberg L, Bergkvist L, Bruce A, Adami HO. A prospective study of association of monounsaturated fat and other types of fat with risk of breast cancer. Arch Intern Med. 1998 Jan 12;158(1):41-5.

Yashodhara BM, Umakanth S, Pappachan JM, Bhat SK, Kamath R, Choo BH. Omega-3 fatty acids: a comprehensive review of their role in health and disease. Postgrad Med J. 2009 Feb;85(1000):84-90.

Young VR, Pellett PL. Plant proteins in relation to human protein and amino acid nutrition. Am J Clin Nutr. 1994 May;59(5 Suppl):1203S-1212S. Review.

CHAPTER 6

Alexander DD, Weed DL, Chang ET, Miller PE, Mohamed MA, Elkayam L. A systematic review of multivitamin- multimineral use and cardiovascular disease and cancer incidence and total mortality. J Am Coll Nutr. 2013;32(5):339-54.

American Dietetic Association. Position of the American Dietetic Association: fortification and nutritional supplements. J Am Diet Assoc. 2005 Aug;105(8):1300-11.

Angelo G, Drake VJ, Frei B. Efficacy of Multivitamin/mineral Supplementation to Reduce Chronic Disease Risk: A Critical Review of the Evidence from Observational Studies and Randomized Controlled Trials. Crit Rev Food Sci Nutr. 2015;55(14):1968-91.

ANTONIO, J., ELLERBROEK, A., PEACOCK, C., & SILVER, T. (2017). Casein Protein Supplementation in Trained Men and Women: Morning versus Evening. International Journal of Exercise Science, 10(3), 479–486.

Babault, N., Deley, G., Le Ruyet, P., Morgan, F., & Allaert, F. A. (2014). Effects of soluble milk protein or casein supplementation on muscle fatigue following resistance training program: a randomized, double-blind, and placebo-controlled study. Journal of the International Society of Sports Nutrition, 11, 36.

Bemben MG, Lamont HS. Creatine supplementation and exercise performance: recent findings. Sports Med. 2005;35(2):107-25. Review.

Bird, S. P. (2003). Creatine Supplementation and Exercise Performance: A Brief Review. Journal of Sports Science & Medicine, 2(4), 123–132.

Bird, S. P. (2003). Creatine Supplementation and Exercise Performance: A Brief Review. Journal of Sports Science & Medicine, 2(4), 123–132.

Branch JD. Effect of creatine supplementation on body composition and performance: a meta-analysis. Int J Sport Nutr Exerc Metab. 2003 Jun;13(2):198-226.

Buford, T. W., Kreider, R. B., Stout, J. R., Greenwood, M., Campbell, B., Spano, M., ... Antonio, J. (2007). International Society of Sports Nutrition position stand: creatine supplementation and exercise. Journal of the International Society of Sports Nutrition, 4, 6.

Burke, L. M. (2017). Practical Issues in Evidence-Based Use of Performance Supplements: Supplement Interactions, Repeated Use and Individual Responses. Sports Medicine (Auckland, N.z.), 47(Suppl 1), 79–100.

Calder PC, Yaqoob P. Omega-3 polyunsaturated fatty acids and human health outcomes. Biofactors. 2009 May- Jun;35(3):266-72.

Chia JS, Barrett LA, Chow JY, Burns SF. Effects of Caffeine Supplementation on Performance in Ball Games. Sports Med. 2017 Dec;47(12):2453-2471.

Chilibeck, P. D., Kaviani, M., Candow, D. G., & Zello, G. A. (2017). Effect of creatine supplementation during resistance training on lean tissue mass and muscular strength in older adults: a meta-analysis. Open Access Journal of Sports Medicine, 8, 213–226.

Clark, J. F. (1997). Creatine and Phosphocreatine: A Review of Their Use in Exercise and Sport. Journal of Athletic Training, 32(1), 45–51.

Cooper, R., Naclerio, F., Allgrove, J., & Jimenez, A. (2012). Creatine supplementation with specific view to exercise/sports performance: an update. Journal of the International Society of Sports Nutrition, 9, 33.

Coyle EF. Carbohydrate supplementation during exercise. J Nutr. 1992 Mar;122(3 Suppl):788-95. Review.

Nybo L. CNS fatigue and prolonged exercise: effect of glucose supplementation. Med Sci Sports Exerc. 2003 Apr;35(4):589-94.

Institute of Medicine (US) Committee on Military Nutrition Research; Marriott BM, editor. Fluid Replacement and Heat Stress. Washington (DC): National Academies Press (US); 1994. 5, Carbohydrate Supplements During and Immediately Post Exercise.

Stellingwerff T, Cox GR. Systematic review: Carbohydrate supplementation on exercise performance or capacity of varying durations. Appl Physiol Nutr Metab. 2014 Sep;39(9):998-1011.

Haff GG, Lehmkuhl MJ, McCoy LB, Stone MH. Carbohydrate supplementation and resistance training. J Strength Cond Res. 2003 Feb;17(1):187-96. Review.

Baker, L. B., Rollo, I., Stein, K. W., & Jeukendrup, A. E. (2015). Acute Effects of Carbohydrate Supplementation on Intermittent Sports Performance. Nutrients, 7(7), 5733–5763.

Jeukendrup, A. (2014). A Step Towards Personalized Sports Nutrition: Carbohydrate Intake During Exercise. Sports Medicine (Auckland, N.z.), 44(Suppl 1), 25–33.

Burke LM, Hawley JA, Wong SH, Jeukendrup AE. Carbohydrates for training and competition. J Sports Sci. 2011;29 Suppl 1:S17-27.

Jeukendrup AE. Carbohydrate and exercise performance: the role of multiple transportable carbohydrates. Curr Opin Clin Nutr Metab Care. 2010 Jul;13(4):452-7.

Wilson PB. Does Carbohydrate Intake During Endurance Running Improve Performance? A Critical Review. J Strength Cond Res. 2016 Dec;30(12):3539-3559.Review.

Daniels, M. C., & Popkin, B. M. (2010). The impact of water intake on energy intake and weight status: a systematic review. Nutrition Reviews, 68(9), 505–521.

Demant TW, Rhodes EC. Effects of creatine supplementation on exercise performance. Sports Med. 1999 Jul;28(1):49-60. Review.

Domröse U, Heinz J, Westphal S, Luley C, Neumann KH, Dierkes J. Vitamins are associated with survival in patients with end-stage renal disease: a 4-year prospective study. Clin Nephrol. 2007 Apr;67(4):221-9.

Dong JY, Iso H, Kitamura A, Tamakoshi A; Japan Collaborative Cohort Study Group. Multivitamin use and risk of stroke mortality: the Japan collaborative cohort study. Stroke. 2015 May;46(5):1167-72.

Dyall SC. Long-chain omega-3 fatty acids and the brain: a review of the independent and shared effects of EPA, DPA and DHA. Front Aging Neurosci. 2015 Apr 21;7:52.

Ferreira-Pêgo, C., Guelinckx, I., Moreno, L. A., Kavouras, S. A., Gandy, J., Martinez, H., … Salas-Salvadó, J. (2015). Total fluid intake and its determinants: cross- sectional surveys among adults in 13 countries worldwide. European Journal of Nutrition, 54(Suppl 2), 35–43.

Fletcher RH, Fairfield KM. Vitamins for chronic disease prevention in adults: clinical applications. JAMA. 2002 Jun 19;287(23):3127-9.

Gandy, J. (2015). Water intake: validity of population assessment and recommendations. European Journal of Nutrition, 54(Suppl 2), 11–16.

Gao, H., Geng, T., Huang, T., & Zhao, Q. (2017). Fish oil supplementation and insulin sensitivity: a systematic review and meta-analysis. Lipids in Health and Disease, 16, 131.

Ghasemi Fard S, Wang F, Sinclair AJ, Elliott G, Turchini GM. How does high DHA fish oil affect health? A systematic review of evidence. Crit Rev Food Sci Nutr. 2018 Mar 1:1-44.

Goldstein, E. R., Ziegenfuss, T., Kalman, D., Kreider, R., Campbell, B., Wilborn, C., … Antonio, J. (2010). International society of sports nutrition position stand: caffeine and performance. Journal of the International Society of Sports Nutrition, 7, 5.

Grgic, J., Trexler, E. T., Lazinica, B., & Pedisic, Z. (2018). Effects of caffeine intake on muscle strength and power: a systematic review and meta-analysis. Journal of the International Society of Sports Nutrition, 15, 11.

Harris WS. Fish oil supplementation: evidence for health benefits. Cleve Clin J Med. 2004 Mar;71(3):208-10, 212, 215-8 passim. Review.

Hayes A, Cribb PJ. Effect of whey protein isolate on strength, body composition and muscle hypertrophy during resistance training. Curr Opin Clin Nutr Metab Care. 2008 Jan;11(1):40-4. Review.

Dangin M, Boirie Y, Guillet C, Beaufrère B. Influence of the protein digestion rate on protein turnover in young and elderly subjects. J Nutr. 2002 Oct;132(10):3228S-33S. Review.

Hein, Darren, et al. "The impact of whey protein supplementation on muscle strength and body composition: a systematic review and meta-analysis." PHARMACOTHERAPY. Vol. 33. No.

10. 111 RIVER ST, HOBOKEN 07030-5774, NJ USA: WILEY-BLACKWELL, 2013.

de Santana, Davi Alves. "Effects of whey protein supplementation during strength training in lean mass: a systematic review/ Efeitos da suplementacao de whey protein durante o treinamento de forca a massa magra: uma revisao sistematica." Revista Brasileira de Prescrição e Fisiologia do Exercício 8.43 (2014): 68-80.

Hoffman, J. R., & Falvo, M. J. (2004). Protein – Which is Best? Journal of Sports Science & Medicine, 3(3), 118– 130.

Huang HY, Caballero B, Chang S, Alberg A, Semba R, Schneyer C, Wilson RF, Cheng TY, Prokopowicz G, Barnes GJ 2nd, Vassy J, Bass EB. Multivitamin/mineral supplements and prevention of chronic disease. Evid Rep Technol Assess (Full Rep). 2006 May;(139):1-117. Review.

Jäger, R., Kerksick, C. M., Campbell, B. I., Cribb, P. J., Wells, S. D., Skwiat, T. M., ... Antonio, J. (2017). International Society of Sports Nutrition Position Stand: protein and exercise. Journal of the International Society of Sports Nutrition, 14, 20.

Jain AP, Aggarwal KK, Zhang PY. Omega-3 fatty acids and cardiovascular disease. Eur Rev Med Pharmacol Sci. 2015;19(3):441-5. Review.

Jakubowicz D, Froy O. Biochemical and metabolic mechanisms by which dietary whey protein may combat obesity and Type 2 diabetes. J Nutr Biochem. 2013 Jan;24(1):1-5.

Graf S, Egert S, Heer M. Effects of whey protein supplements on metabolism: evidence from human intervention studies. Curr Opin Clin Nutr Metab Care. 2011 Nov;14(6):569-80.

Sundell J, Hulmi J, Rossi J. [Whey protein and creatine as nutritional supplements]. Duodecim. 2011;127(7):700-5. Review. Finnish.

Kantha, S. S. (1987). Dietary effects of fish oils on human health: a review of recent studies. The Yale Journal of Biology and Medicine, 60(1), 37–44.

Kim, J., Lee, J., Kim, S., Yoon, D., Kim, J., & Sung, D. J. (2015). Role of creatine supplementation in exercise- induced muscle damage: A mini review. Journal of Exercise Rehabilitation, 11(5), 244–250.

Kreider RB. Effects of creatine supplementation on performance and training adaptations. Mol Cell Biochem. 2003 Feb;244(1-2):89-94. Review.

Kreider, R. B., Kalman, D. S., Antonio, J., Ziegenfuss, T. N., Wildman, R., Collins, R., ... Lopez, H. L. (2017). International Society of Sports Nutrition position stand: safety and efficacy of creatine supplementation in exercise, sport, and medicine. Journal of the International Society of Sports Nutrition, 14, 18.

Li K, Kaaks R, Linseisen J, Rohrmann S. Vitamin/mineral supplementation and cancer, cardiovascular, and all- cause mortality in a German prospective cohort (EPIC- Heidelberg). Eur J Nutr. 2012 Jun;51(4):407-13.

McGregor, R. A., & Poppitt, S. D. (2013). Milk protein for improved metabolic health: a review of the evidence. Nutrition & Metabolism, 10, 46.

Messerer M, Håkansson N, Wolk A, Akesson A. Dietary supplement use and mortality in a cohort of Swedish men. Br J Nutr. 2008 Mar;99(3):626-31. Epub 2007 Sep 3.

Miller, Paige E., Dominik D. Alexander, and Vanessa Perez. "Effects of whey protein and resistance exercise on body composition: a meta-analysis of randomized controlled trials." Journal of the American College of Nutrition 33.2 (2014): 163-175.

Mitchell, C. J., McGregor, R. A., D'Souza, R. F., Thorstensen, E. B., Markworth, J. F., Fanning, A. C., ... Cameron-Smith, D. (2015). Consumption of Milk Protein or Whey Protein Results in a Similar Increase in Muscle Protein Synthesis in Middle Aged Men. Nutrients, 7(10), 8685– 8699.

More J. Who needs vitamin supplements? J Fam Health Care. 2007;17(2):57-60. Review.

Naclerio F, Larumbe-Zabala E. Effects of Whey Protein Alone or as Part of a Multi-ingredient Formulation on Strength, Fat-Free Mass, or Lean Body Mass in Resistance-Trained Individuals: A Meta-analysis. Sports Med. 2016 Jan;46(1):125-37.

Devries MC, Phillips SM. Supplemental protein in support of muscle mass and health:

advantage whey. J Food Sci. 2015 Mar;80 Suppl 1:A8-A15.

Zhou LM, Xu JY, Rao CP, Han S, Wan Z, Qin LQ. Effect of whey supplementation on circulating C-reactive protein: a meta-analysis of randomized controlled trials. Nutrients. 2015 Feb 9;7(2):1131-43.

Bauer JM, Diekmann R. Protein supplementation with aging. Curr Opin Clin Nutr Metab Care. 2015 Jan;18(1):24-31.

Miller PE, Alexander DD, Perez V. Effects of whey protein and resistance exercise on body composition: a meta- analysis of randomized controlled trials. J Am Coll Nutr. 2014;33(2):163-75.

James L. Milk protein and the restoration of fluid balance after exercise. Med Sport Sci. 2012;59:120-6.

Josse AR, Phillips SM. Impact of milk consumption and resistance training on body composition of female athletes. Med Sport Sci. 2012;59:94-103.

Navarro M, Wood RJ. Plasma changes in micronutrients following a multivitamin and mineral supplement in healthy adults. J Am Coll Nutr. 2003 Apr;22(2):124-32.

Nimrouzi, M., Daneshfard, B., & Tafazoli, V. (2016). Avicenna's View on Optimal Daily Water Intake. Iranian Journal of Medical Sciences, 41(3 Suppl), S23.

Phillips SM, Tang JE, Moore DR. The role of milk- and soy-based protein in support of muscle protein synthesis and muscle protein accretion in young and elderly persons. J Am Coll Nutr. 2009 Aug;28(4):343-54. Review.

Zemel MB, Zhao F. [Role of whey protein and whey components in weight management and energy metabolism]. Wei Sheng Yan Jiu. 2009 Jan;38(1):114-7. Review. Chinese.

Luhovyy BL, Akhavan T, Anderson GH. Whey proteins in the regulation of food intake and satiety. J Am Coll Nutr. 2007 Dec;26(6):704S-12S. Review.

Popkin, B. M., D'Anci, K. E., & Rosenberg, I. H. (2010). Water, Hydration and Health. Nutrition Reviews, 68(8), 439–458.

Popkin, B. M., D'Anci, K. E., & Rosenberg, I. H. (2010). Water, Hydration and Health. Nutrition Reviews, 68(8), 439–458.

Qiao YL, Dawsey SM, Kamangar F, Fan JH, Abnet CC, Sun XD, Johnson LL, Gail MH, Dong ZW, Yu B, Mark SD, Taylor PR. Total and cancer mortality after supplementation with vitamins and minerals: follow-up of the Linxian General Population Nutrition Intervention Trial. J Natl Cancer Inst. 2009 Apr 1;101(7):507-18.

Rangel-Huerta OD, Aguilera CM, Mesa MD, Gil A. Omega-3 long-chain polyunsaturated fatty acids supplementation on inflammatory biomakers: a systematic review of randomised clinical trials. Br J Nutr. 2012 Jun;107 Suppl 2:S159-70.

Riebl, S. K., & Davy, B. M. (2013). The Hydration Equation: Update on Water Balance and Cognitive Performance. ACSM's Health & Fitness Journal, 17(6), 21–28.

Ruxton CH, Reed SC, Simpson MJ, Millington KJ. The health benefits of omega-3 polyunsaturated fatty acids: a review of the evidence. J Hum Nutr Diet. 2004 Oct;17(5):449-59. Review.

Salicio, V. M. M., Fett, C. A., Salicio, M. A., Brandäo, C. F. C. C. M., Stoppiglia, L. F., Fett, W. C. R., & Botelho, and. C. (2017). THE EFFECT OF CAFFEINE SUPPLEMENTATION ON TRAINED INDIVIDUALS SUBJECTED TO MAXIMAL TREADMILL TEST. African Journal of Traditional, Complementary, and Alternative Medicines, 14(1), 16–23.

Siddiqui RA, Shaikh SR, Sech LA, Yount HR, Stillwell W, Zaloga GP. Omega 3-fatty acids: health benefits and cellular mechanisms of action. Mini Rev Med Chem. 2004 Oct;4(8):859-71. Review.

Simopoulos AP. Omega-3 fatty acids in health and disease and in growth and development. Am J Clin Nutr. 1991 Sep;54(3):438-63. Review.

Smith, R. N., Agharkar, A. S., & Gonzales, E. B. (2014). A review of creatine supplementation in age-related diseases: more than a supplement for athletes. F1000Research, 3, 222.

Spriet, L. L. (2014). Exercise and Sport Performance with Low Doses of Caffeine. Sports Medicine (Auckland, N.z.), 44(Suppl 2), 175–184.

Stark, M., Lukaszuk, J., Prawitz, A., & Salacinski, A. (2012). Protein timing and its effects on muscular hypertrophy and strength in individuals engaged in weight- training. Journal of the International Society of Sports Nutrition, 9, 54.

Temple, J. L., Bernard, C., Lipshultz, S. E., Czachor, J. D., Westphal, J. A., & Mestre, M. A. (2017). The Safety of Ingested Caffeine: A Comprehensive Review. Frontiers in Psychiatry, 8, 80.

Trommelen, J., & van Loon, L. J. C. (2016). Pre-Sleep Protein Ingestion to Improve the Skeletal Muscle Adaptive Response to Exercise Training. Nutrients, 8(12), 763.

Tur JA, Bibiloni MM, Sureda A, Pons A. Dietary sources of omega 3 fatty acids: public health risks and benefits. Br J Nutr. 2012 Jun;107 Suppl 2:S23-52.

Villegas R, Takata Y, Murff H, Blot WJ. Fish, omega-3 long-chain fatty acids, and all-cause mortality in a low- income US population: Results from the Southern Community Cohort Study. Nutr Metab Cardiovasc Dis. 2015 Jul;25(7):651-8.

Ward E. Addressing nutritional gaps with multivitamin and mineral supplements. Nutr J. 2014 Jul 15;13:72. Review.

Wilborn, C. D., Taylor, L. W., Outlaw, J., Williams, L., Campbell, B., Foster, C. A., ... Hayward, S. (2013). The Effects of Pre- and Post-Exercise Whey vs. Casein Protein Consumption on Body Composition and Performance Measures in Collegiate Female Athletes. Journal of Sports Science & Medicine, 12(1), 74–79.

Yashodhara BM, Umakanth S, Pappachan JM, Bhat SK, Kamath R, Choo BH. Omega-3 fatty acids: a comprehensive review of their role in health and disease. Postgrad Med J. 2009 Feb;85(1000):84-90.

ZHANG, Jian-wei, Shu-fen HAN, and Li-qiang QIN. "Effects of whey protein supplement on body weight and body compositions in overweight and obese subjects: a meta-analysis of randomized controlled trials." Modern Preventive Medicine 13 (2014): 010.

Manninen, Anssi H. "Protein Hydrolysates in Sports Nutrition." Nutrition & Metabolism Nutr Metab (Lond): 38.

CHAPTER 7

Leung, A., Chan, R., Sea, M., & Woo, J. (2017). An Overview of Factors Associated with Adherence to Lifestyle Modification Programs for Weight Management in Adults. International journal of environmental research and public health, 14(8), 922.

Ogden J. The Psychology of Eating, From Healthy to Disordered Behavior. Wiley-Blackwell; 2010.

Rowland N, Splane EC. Psychology of Eating. Pearson College Division; 2013.

CHAPTER 8

Abramson EE, Stinson SG. Boredom and eating in obese and non-obese individuals. Addict Behav. 1977;2(4):181- 5.

Adams CE, Greenway FL, Brantley PJ. Lifestyle factors and ghrelin: critical review and implications for weight loss maintenance. Obes Rev. 2011 May;12(5):e211-8.

Alonso-Alonso, M., Woods, S. C., Pelchat, M., Grigson, P. S., Stice, E., Farooqi, S., ... Beauchamp, G. K. (2015).

Food reward system: current perspectives and future research needs. Nutrition Reviews, 73(5), 296–307.

Amin, T., & Mercer, J. G. (2016). Hunger and

Satiety Mechanisms and Their Potential Exploitation in the Regulation of Food Intake. Current Obesity Reports, 5, 106–112.

Appelhans, B. M., Woolf, K., Pagoto, S. L., Schneider, K. L., Whited, M. C., & Liebman, R. (2011). Inhibiting food reward: delay discounting, food reward sensitivity, and palatable food intake in overweight and obese women. Obesity (Silver Spring, Md.), 19(11), 2175–2182.

Astrup, A., Raben, A., & Geiker, N. (2015). The role of higher protein diets in weight control and obesity-related comorbidities. International Journal of Obesity (2005), 39(5), 721–726.

Barrington, W. E., Ceballos, R. M., Bishop, S. K., McGregor, B. A., & Beresford, S. A. A. (2012). Perceived Stress, Behavior, and Body Mass Index Among Adults Participating in a Worksite Obesity Prevention Program, Seattle, 2005–2007. Preventing Chronic Disease, 9, E152.

Beccuti, G., & Pannain, S. (2011). Sleep and obesity. Current Opinion in Clinical Nutrition and Metabolic Care, 14(4), 402–412.

Bendtsen, L. Q., Lorenzen, J. K., Bendsen, N. T., Rasmussen, C., & Astrup, A. (2013). Effect of Dairy Proteins on Appetite, Energy Expenditure, Body Weight, and Composition: a Review of the Evidence from Controlled Clinical Trials. Advances in Nutrition, 4(4), 418– 438.

Bendtsen, L. Q., Lorenzen, J. K., Bendsen, N. T., Rasmussen, C., & Astrup, A. (2013). Effect of Dairy Proteins on Appetite, Energy Expenditure, Body Weight, and Composition: a Review of the Evidence from Controlled Clinical Trials. Advances in Nutrition, 4(4), 418– 438.

Bergmann, N., Gyntelberg, F., & Faber, J. (2014). The appraisal of chronic stress and the development of the metabolic syndrome: a systematic review of prospective cohort studies. Endocrine Connections, 3(2), R55–R80.

Berthoud, H.-R., Lenard, N. R., & Shin, A. C. (2011). Food reward, hyperphagia, and obesity. American Journal of Physiology - Regulatory, Integrative and Comparative Physiology, 300(6), R1266–R1277.

Block, J. P., He, Y., Zaslavsky, A. M., Ding, L., & Ayanian, J. Z. (2009). Psychosocial Stress and Change in Weight Among US Adults. American Journal of Epidemiology, 170(2), 181–192.

Blundell JE, Burley VJ. Satiation, satiety and the action of fibre on food intake. Int J Obes. 1987;11 Suppl 1:9-25. Review.

Bose, M., Oliván, B., & Laferrère, B. (2009). Stress and obesity: the role of the hypothalamic–pituitary–adrenal axis in metabolic disease. Current Opinion in Endocrinology, Diabetes, and Obesity, 16(5), 340–346.

Cadegiani, F. A., & Kater, C. E. (2017). Hormonal aspects of overtraining syndrome: a systematic review. BMC Sports Science, Medicine and Rehabilitation, 9, 14.

Carreiro, A. L., Dhillon, J., Gordon, S., Jacobs, A. G., Higgins, K. A., McArthur, B. M., ... Mattes, R. D. (2016). The macronutrients, appetite and energy intake. Annual Review of Nutrition, 36, 73–103.

Chaput, J.-P., & Tremblay, A. (2012). Adequate sleep to improve the treatment of obesity. CMAJ : Canadian Medical Association Journal, 184(18), 1975–1976.

Clark MJ, Slavin JL. The effect of fiber on satiety and food intake: a systematic review. J Am Coll Nutr. 2013;32(3):200-11.

Coughlin JW, Smith MT. Sleep, obesity, and weight loss in adults: is there a rationale for providing sleep interventions in the treatment of obesity? Int Rev Psychiatry. 2014 Apr;26(2):177-88.

Cowan, D. C., & Livingston, E. (2012). Obstructive Sleep Apnoea Syndrome and Weight Loss: Review. Sleep Disorders, 2012, 163296.

Dahl WJ, Stewart ML. Position of the Academy of Nutrition and Dietetics: Health Implications of Dietary Fiber. J Acad Nutr Diet. 2015 Nov;115(11):1861-70.

Dallman, M. F., Pecoraro, N., Akana, S. F., la Fleur, S. E., Gomez, F., Houshyar, H., ... Manalo, S. (2003). Chronic stress and obesity: A new view of "comfort food." Proceedings of the National Academy of Sciences of the United States of America, 100(20), 11696–11701.

Daniels, M. C., & Popkin, B. M. (2010). The impact of water intake on energy intake and weight status: a systematic review. Nutrition Reviews, 68(9), 505–521.

DAVY, B. M., DENNIS, E. A., DENGO, A. L., WILSON, K. L., & DAVY, K. P. (2008). Water Consumption Reduces Energy Intake at a Breakfast Meal in Obese Older Adults. Journal of the American Dietetic Association, 108(7), 1236–1239.

Dhillon J, Craig BA, Leidy HJ, Amankwaah AF, Osei-Boadi Anguah K, Jacobs A, Jones BL, Jones JB, Keeler CL, Keller CE, McCrory MA, Rivera RL, Slebodnik M, Mattes RD, Tucker RM. The Effects of Increased Protein Intake on Fullness: A Meta-Analysis and Its Limitations. J Acad Nutr Diet. 2016 Jun;116(6):968-83.

Farias MM, Cuevas AM, Rodriguez F. Set-point theory and obesity. Metab Syndr Relat Disord. 2011 Apr;9(2):85- 9.

Fels R, Lohner S, Hollódy K, Erhardt É, Molnár D. Relationship between sleep duration and childhood obesity: Systematic review including the potential underlying mechanisms. Nutr Metab Cardiovasc Dis. 2017 Sep;27(9):751-761.

Ganley, R. M. (1989), Emotion and eating in obesity: A review of the literature. Int. J. Eat. Disord., 8: 343-361.

Geiker NRW, Astrup A, Hjorth MF, Sjödin A, Pijls L, Markus CR. Does stress influence sleep patterns, food intake, weight gain, abdominal obesity and weight loss interventions and vice versa? Obes Rev. 2018 Jan;19(1):81-97.

Greer, S. M., Goldstein, A. N., & Walker, M. P. (2013). The impact of sleep deprivation on food desire in the human brain. Nature Communications, 4, 2259.

Groesz, L., McCoy, S., Carl, J., Saslow, L., Stewart, J., Adler, N., ... Epel, E. (2012). What is eating you? Stress and the Drive to Eat. Appetite, 58(2), 717–721.

Guyenet SJ. The Hungry Brain, Outsmarting the Instincts That Make Us Overeat. Macmillan; 2017.

Hardy L. Psychological stress, performance, and injury in sport. Br Med Bull. 1992 Jul;48(3):615-29. Review.

Hargens, T. A., Kaleth, A. S., Edwards, E. S., & Butner, K.

L. (2013). Association between sleep disorders, obesity, and exercise: a review. Nature and Science of Sleep, 5, 27–35.

Hargens, T. A., Kaleth, A. S., Edwards, E. S., & Butner, K.

L. (2013). Association between sleep disorders, obesity, and exercise: a review. Nature and Science of Sleep, 5, 27–35.

Harpaz E, Tamir S, Weinstein A, Weinstein Y. The effect of caffeine on energy balance. J Basic Clin Physiol Pharmacol. 2017 Jan 1;28(1):1-10.

Harris RB. Role of set-point theory in regulation of body weight. FASEB J. 1990 Dec;4(15):3310-8. Review.

Hart, C. N., Cairns, A., & Jelalian, E. (2011). Sleep and Obesity in Children and Adolescents. Pediatric Clinics of North America, 58(3), 715–733.

Hill DC, Moss RH, Sykes-Muskett B, Conner M, O'Connor DB. Stress and eating behaviors in children and adolescents: Systematic review and meta-analysis.

Appetite. 2018 Apr 1;123:14-22.

Howarth NC, Saltzman E, Roberts SB. Dietary fiber and weight regulation. Nutr Rev. 2001 May;59(5):129-39.

Review.

Keesey RE, Hirvonen MD. Body weight set-points: determination and adjustment. J Nutr. 1997 Sep;127(9):1875S-1883S. Review.

Keijer, J., Hoevenaars, F. P. M., Nieuwenhuizen, A., & van Schothorst, E. M. (2014). Nutrigenomics of Body Weight Regulation: A Rationale for Careful Dissection of Individual Contributors. Nutrients, 6(10), 4531–4551.

Landis AM, Parker KP, Dunbar SB. Sleep, hunger, satiety, food cravings, and caloric intake in adolescents. J Nurs Scholarsh. 2009;41(2):115-23.

Lappalainen R, Mennen L, van Weert L, Mykkänen H. Drinking water with a meal: a simple method of coping with feelings of hunger, satiety and desire to eat. Eur J Clin Nutr. 1993 Nov;47(11):815-9.

Laugero, K. D., Falcon, L. M., & Tucker, K. L. (2011). Relationship between perceived stress and dietary and activity patterns in older adults participating in the Boston Puerto Rican Health Study,. Appetite, 56(1), 194–204.

Lepe M, Bacardí Gascón M, Jiménez Cruz A. Long-term efficacy of high-protein diets: a systematic review. Nutr Hosp. 2011 Nov-Dec; 26 (6): 1256-9.

Li L, Zhang S, Huang Y, Chen K. Sleep duration and obesity in children: A systematic review and meta-analysis of prospective cohort studies. J Paediatr Child Health. 2017 Apr;53(4):378-385.

Miller, A. L., Lumeng, J. C., & LeBourgeois, M. K. (2015). Sleep patterns and obesity in childhood. Current Opinion in Endocrinology, Diabetes, and Obesity, 22(1), 41–47.

Mitchell LJ, Davidson ZE, Bonham M, O'Driscoll DM, Hamilton GS, Truby H. Weight loss from lifestyle interventions and severity of sleep apnoea: a systematic review and meta-analysis. Sleep Med. 2014 Oct;15(10):1173-83.

Mollahosseini M, Shab-Bidar S, Rahimi MH, Djafarian K. Effect of whey protein supplementation on long and short term appetite: A meta-analysis of randomized controlled trials. Clin Nutr ESPEN. 2017 Aug;20:34-40.

Moore CJ, Cunningham SA. Social position, psychological stress, and obesity: a systematic review. J Acad Nutr Diet. 2012 Apr;112(4):518-26.

Mouchacca, J., Abbott, G. R., & Ball, K. (2013). Associations between psychological stress, eating, physical activity, sedentary behaviours and body weight among women: a longitudinal study. BMC Public Health, 13, 828.

Moynihan, A. B., van Tilburg, W. A. P., Igou, E. R., Wisman, A., Donnelly, A. E., & Mulcaire, J. B. (2015). Eaten up by boredom: consuming food to escape awareness of the bored self. Frontiers in Psychology, 6, 369.

Muckelbauer R, Barbosa CL, Mittag T, Burkhardt K, Mikelaishvili N, Müller-Nordhorn J. Association between water consumption and body weight outcomes in children and adolescents: a systematic review. Obesity (Silver Spring). 2014 Dec;22(12):2462-75.

Mudgil D, Barak S. Composition, properties and health benefits of indigestible carbohydrate polymers as dietary fiber: a review. Int J Biol Macromol. 2013 Oct;61:1-6.

Müller, M. J., Bosy-Westphal, A., & Heymsfield, S. B. (2010). Is there evidence for a set point that regulates human body weight? F1000 Medicine Reports, 2, 59.

Nguyen-Rodriguez, S. T., Chou, C.-P., Unger, J. B., & Spruijt-Metz, D. (2008). BMI as a Moderator of Perceived Stress and Emotional Eating in Adolescents. Eating Behaviors, 9(2), 238–246.

Paddon-Jones D, Westman E, Mattes RD, Wolfe RR, Astrup A, Westerterp-Plantenga M. Protein, weight management, and satiety. Am J Clin Nutr. 2008 May;87(5):1558S-1561S. Review.

Paddon-Jones D. Interplay of stress and physical inactivity on muscle loss: Nutritional countermeasures. J Nutr. 2006 Aug;136(8):2123-6. Review.

Patel, S. R., & Hu, F. B. (2008). Short sleep duration and weight gain: a systematic review. Obesity (Silver Spring, Md.), 16(3), 643–653.

Poornima, K. N., Karthick, N., & Sitalakshmi, R. (2014). Study of the Effect of Stress on Skeletal Muscle Function in Geriatrics. Journal of Clinical and Diagnostic Research: JCDR, 8(1), 8–9.

Poutanen KS, Dussort P, Erkner A, Fiszman S, Karnik K, Kristensen M, Marsaux CF, Miquel-Kergoat S, Pentikäinen SP, Putz P, Slavin JL, Steinert RE, Mela DJ. A review of the characteristics of dietary fibers relevant to appetite and energy intake outcomes in human intervention trials. Am J Clin Nutr. 2017 Sep;106(3):747-754.

Prinz, P. (2004). Sleep, Appetite, and Obesity— What Is the Link? PLoS Medicine, 1(3), e61.

Ravn, A.-M., Gregersen, N. T., Christensen, R., Rasmussen, L. G., Hels, O., Belza, A., ... Astrup, A. (2013). Thermic effect of a meal and appetite in adults: an individual participant data meta-analysis of meal-test trials. Food & Nutrition Research, 57, 10.3402/fnr.v57i0.19676.

Rebello, C. J., O'Neil, C. E., & Greenway, F. L. (2016). Dietary fiber and satiety: the effects of oats on satiety. Nutrition Reviews, 74(2), 131–147.

Schubert MM, Irwin C, Seay RF, Clarke HE, Allegro D, Desbrow B. Caffeine, coffee, and appetite control: a review. Int J Food Sci Nutr. 2017 Dec;68(8):901-912.

Schwarz, N. A., Rigby, B. R., La Bounty, P., Shelmadine, B., & Bowden, R. G. (2011). A

Review of Weight Control Strategies and Their Effects on the Regulation of Hormonal Balance. Journal of Nutrition and Metabolism, 2011, 237932.

Scott, K. A., Melhorn, S. J., & Sakai, R. R. (2012). Effects of Chronic Social Stress on Obesity. Current Obesity Reports, 1(1), 16–25.

Shimanoe C, Hara M, Nishida Y, Nanri H, Otsuka Y, Nakamura K, et al. (2015) Perceived Stress and Coping Strategies in Relation to Body Mass Index: Cross- Sectional Study of 12,045 Japanese Men and Women. PLoS ONE 10(2): e0118105

Singh, M. (2014). Mood, food, and obesity. Frontiers in Psychology, 5, 925.

Sinha, R., & Jastreboff, A. M. (2013). Stress as a common risk factor for obesity and addiction. Biological Psychiatry, 73(9), 827–835.

Slavin JL. Dietary fiber and body weight. Nutrition. 2005 Mar;21(3):411-8. Review.

Sominsky, L., & Spencer, S. J. (2014). Eating behavior and stress: a pathway to obesity. Frontiers in Psychology, 5, 434.

Speakman, J. R., Levitsky, D. A., Allison, D. B., Bray, M. S., de Castro, J. M., Clegg, D. J., ... Westerterp-Plantenga, M. S. (2011). Set points, settling points and some alternative models: theoretical options to understand how genes and environments combine to regulate body adiposity. Disease Models & Mechanisms, 4(6), 733–745.

Spivey, A. (2010). Lose Sleep, Gain Weight: Another Piece of the Obesity Puzzle. Environmental Health Perspectives, 118(1), A28–A33.

Stookey, J. J. D. (2016). Negative, Null and Beneficial Effects of Drinking Water on Energy Intake, Energy Expenditure, Fat Oxidation and Weight Change in Randomized Trials: A Qualitative Review. Nutrients, 8(1), 19.

Stults-Kolehmainen, M. A., & Sinha, R. (2014). The Effects of Stress on Physical Activity and Exercise. Sports Medicine (Auckland, N.Z.), 44(1), 81–121.

Tamashiro, K. L. K., Hegeman, M. A., Nguyen, M. M. N., Melhorn, S. J., Ma, L. Y., Woods, S. C., & Sakai, R. R. (2007). Dynamic body weight and body composition changes in response to subordination stress. Physiology & Behavior, 91(4), 440–448.

Temple, J. L., Bernard, C., Lipshultz, S. E., Czachor, J. D., Westphal, J. A., & Mestre, M. A. (2017). The Safety of Ingested Caffeine: A Comprehensive Review. Frontiers in psychiatry, 8, 80.

Thornton, S. N. (2016). Increased Hydration Can Be Associated with Weight Loss. Frontiers in Nutrition, 3, 18.

Van Cauter, E., & Knutson, K. L. (2008). Sleep and the epidemic of obesity in children and adults. European Journal of Endocrinology, 159(S1), S59–S66.

Wanders AJ, van den Borne JJ, de Graaf C, Hulshof T, Jonathan MC, Kristensen M, Mars M, Schols HA, Feskens EJ. Effects of dietary fibre on subjective appetite, energy intake and body weight: a systematic review of randomized controlled trials. Obes Rev. 2011 Sep;12(9):724-39.

Westerterp-Plantenga MS, Nieuwenhuizen A, Tomé D, Soenen S, Westerterp KR. Dietary protein, weight loss, and weight maintenance. Annu Rev Nutr. 2009;29:21-41.

Westerterp-Plantenga MS. The significance of protein in food intake and body weight regulation. Curr Opin Clin Nutr Metab Care. 2003 Nov;6(6):635-8. Review.

Wu, J., Wu, H., Wang, J., Guo, L., Deng, X., & Lu, C. (2015). Associations between Sleep Duration and Overweight/Obesity: Results from 66,817 Chinese Adolescents. Scientific Reports, 5, 16686.

Yau, Y. H. C., & Potenza, M. N. (2013). Stress and Eating Behaviors. Minerva Endocrinologica, 38(3), 255–267.

CHAPTER 9

Abd-Elfattah, H. M., Abdelazeim, F. H., & Elshennawy, S. (2015). Physical and cognitive consequences of fatigue: A review. Journal of Advanced Research, 6(3), 351–358.

Aune, D., Sen, A., Prasad, M., Norat, T., Janszky, I., Tonstad, S., ... Vatten, L. J. (2016). BMI and all cause mortality: systematic review and non-linear dose-response meta-analysis of 230 cohort studies with 3.74 million deaths among 30.3 million participants. The BMJ, 353, i2156.

Bouchard, C., Tchernof, A., & Tremblay, A. (2014). PREDICTORS OF BODY COMPOSITION AND BODY ENERGY CHANGES IN RESPONSE TO CHRONIC OVERFEEDING. International Journal of Obesity (2005), 38(2), 236–242.

Chaput, J.-P., & Tremblay, A. (2012). Adequate sleep to improve the treatment of obesity. CMAJ : Canadian Medical Association Journal, 184(18), 1975–1976.

Hargens, T. A., Kaleth, A. S., Edwards, E. S., & Butner, K.
L. (2013). Association between sleep disorders, obesity, and exercise: a review. Nature and Science of Sleep, 5, 27–35.

Cowan, D. C., & Livingston, E. (2012). Obstructive Sleep Apnoea Syndrome and Weight Loss: Review. Sleep Disorders, 2012, 163296.

Spivey, A. (2010). Lose Sleep, Gain Weight: Another Piece of the Obesity Puzzle. Environmental Health Perspectives, 118(1), A28–A33.

Beccuti, G., & Pannain, S. (2011). Sleep and obesity. Current Opinion in Clinical Nutrition and Metabolic Care, 14(4), 402–412.

Li L, Zhang S, Huang Y, Chen K. Sleep duration and obesity in children: A systematic review and meta-analysis of prospective cohort studies. J Paediatr Child Health. 2017 Apr;53(4):378-385.

Van Cauter, E., & Knutson, K. L. (2008). Sleep and the epidemic of obesity in children and adults. European Journal of Endocrinology, 159(S1), S59–S66.

Hargens, T. A., Kaleth, A. S., Edwards, E. S., & Butner, K. L. (2013). Association between sleep disorders, obesity, and exercise: a review. Nature and Science of Sleep, 5, 27–35.

Miller, A. L., Lumeng, J. C., & LeBourgeois, M. K. (2015). Sleep patterns and obesity in childhood. Current Opinion in Endocrinology, Diabetes, and Obesity, 22(1), 41–47.

Hart, C. N., Cairns, A., & Jelalian, E. (2011). Sleep and Obesity in Children and Adolescents. Pediatric Clinics of North America, 58(3), 715–733.

Fels R, Lohner S, Hollódy K, Erhardt É, Molnár D. Relationship between sleep duration and childhood obesity: Systematic review including the potential underlying mechanisms. Nutr Metab Cardiovasc Dis. 2017 Sep;27(9):751-761.

Wu, J., Wu, H., Wang, J., Guo, L., Deng, X., & Lu, C. (2015). Associations between Sleep Duration and Overweight/Obesity: Results from 66,817 Chinese Adolescents. Scientific Reports, 5, 16686.

Coughlin JW, Smith MT. Sleep, obesity, and weight loss in adults: is there a rationale for providing sleep interventions in the treatment of obesity? Int Rev Psychiatry. 2014 Apr;26(2):177-88.

Patel, S. R., & Hu, F. B. (2008). Short sleep duration and weight gain: a systematic review. Obesity (Silver Spring, Md.), 16(3), 643–653.

Mitchell LJ, Davidson ZE, Bonham M, O'Driscoll DM, Hamilton GS, Truby H. Weight loss from lifestyle interventions and severity of sleep apnoea: a systematic review and meta-analysis. Sleep Med. 2014 Oct;15(10):1173-83.

Cowley, J. C., Dingwell, J. B., & Gates, D. H. (2014). Effects of Local and Widespread Muscle Fatigue on Movement Timing. Experimental Brain Research, 232(12), 3939–3948.

Datla, Gowtami, Effects of Local Muscle Fatigue On Proprioception And Motor Learning (2016). Wayne State University Theses. 488.

Forbes GB. Body fat content influences the body composition response to nutrition and exercise. Ann N Y Acad Sci. 2000 May;904:359-65. Review.

Frank, S., Gonzalez, K., Lee-Ang, L., Young, M. C., Tamez, M., & Mattei, J. (2017). Diet and Sleep Physiology: Public Health and Clinical Implications. Frontiers in Neurology, 8, 393.

Hall, K. D. (2007). Body Fat and Fat-Free Mass Interrelationships: Forbes's Theory Revisited. The British Journal of Nutrition, 97(6), 1059–1063.

Helms, E. R., Aragon, A. A., & Fitschen, P. J. (2014). Evidence-based recommendations for natural bodybuilding contest preparation: nutrition and supplementation. Journal of the International Society of Sports Nutrition, 11, 20.

Heymsfield, S. B., Cristina Gonzalez, M. C., Shen, W., Redman, L., & Thomas, D. (2014). Weight Loss Composition is One-Fourth Fat-Free Mass: A Critical Review and Critique of This Widely Cited Rule. Obesity Reviews : An Official Journal of the International Association for the Study of Obesity, 15(4), 310–321.

Jeukendrup, A. E. (2017). Periodized Nutrition for Athletes. Sports Medicine (Auckland, N.z.), 47(Suppl 1), 51–63.

Jo, J., Gavrilova, O., Pack, S., Jou, W., Mullen, S., Sumner, A. E., ... Periwal, V. (2009). Hypertrophy and/or Hyperplasia: Dynamics of Adipose Tissue Growth. PLoS Computational Biology, 5(3), e1000324.

Klatsky, A. L., Zhang, J., Udaltsova, N., Li, Y., & Tran, H. N. (2017). Body Mass Index and Mortality in a Very Large Cohort: Is It Really Healthier to Be Overweight? The Permanente Journal, 21, 16–142.

Lee, M.-J., Wu, Y., & Fried, S. K. (2010). Adipose tissue remodeling in pathophysiology of obesity. Current Opinion in Clinical Nutrition and Metabolic Care, 13(4), 371–376.

Lorem, G. F., Schirmer, H., & Emaus, N. (2017). What is the impact of underweight on self-reported health trajectories and mortality rates: a cohort study. Health and Quality of Life Outcomes, 15, 191.

MacLean, P. S., Higgins, J. A., Giles, E. D., Sherk, V. D., & Jackman, M. R. (2015). The role for adipose tissue in weight regain after weight loss. Obesity Reviews, 16(Suppl 1), 45–54.

Nagai, M., Kuriyama, S., Kakizaki, M., Ohmori-Matsuda, K., Sone, T., Hozawa, A., ... Tsuji, I. (2012). Impact of obesity, overweight and underweight on life expectancy and lifetime medical expenditures: the Ohsaki Cohort Study. BMJ Open, 2(3), e000940.

Nakamura Y, Walker BR, Ikuta T. Systematic review and meta-analysis reveals acutely elevated plasma cortisol following fasting but not less severe calorie restriction. Stress. 2016;19(2):151-7.

Roh, L., Braun, J., Chiolero, A., Bopp, M., Rohrmann, S., & Faeh, D. (2014). Mortality risk associated with underweight: a census-linked cohort of 31,578 individuals with up to 32 years of follow-up. BMC Public Health, 14, 371.

Rutkowski, J. M., Stern, J. H., & Scherer, P. E. (2015). The cell biology of fat expansion. The Journal of Cell Biology, 208(5), 501–512.

St-Onge, M.-P., Mikic, A., & Pietrolungo, C. E. (2016). Effects of Diet on Sleep Quality. Advances in Nutrition, 7(5), 938–949.

Sun, K., Kusminski, C. M., & Scherer, P. E. (2011). Adipose tissue remodeling and obesity. The Journal of Clinical Investigation, 121(6), 2094–2101.

Tomiyama, A. J., Mann, T., Vinas, D., Hunger, J. M., DeJager, J., & Taylor, S. E. (2010). Low Calorie Dieting Increases Cortisol. Psychosomatic Medicine, 72(4), 357–364.

Trexler, E. T., Smith-Ryan, A. E., & Norton, L. E. (2014). Metabolic adaptation to weight loss: implications for the athlete. Journal of the International Society of Sports Nutrition, 11, 7.

Vafadar AK, Côté JN, Archambault PS. The effect of muscle fatigue on position sense in an upper limb multi- joint task. Motor Control. 2012 Apr;16(2):265-83. Epub 2012 Feb 16.

Wang, J.-B., Gu, M.-J., Shen, P., Huang, Q.-C., Bao, C.Z., Ye, Z.-H., ... Chen, K. (2016). Body Mass Index and Mortality: A 10-Year Prospective Study in China. Scientific Reports, 6, 31609.

CHAPTER 10

Economos CD, Bortz SS, Nelson ME. Nutritional practices of elite athletes. Practical recommendations. Sports Med. 1993 Dec;16(6):381-99. Review.

Gerrior, S., Juan, W., & Peter, B. (2006). An Easy Approach to Calculating Estimated Energy Requirements. Preventing Chronic Disease, 3(4), A129.

Heydenreich, J., Kayser, B., Schutz, Y., & Melzer, K. (2017). Total Energy Expenditure, Energy Intake, and Body Composition in Endurance Athletes Across the Training Season: A Systematic Review. Sports Medicine - Open, 3, 8.

Kreider, R. B., Wilborn, C. D., Taylor, L., Campbell, B., Almada, A. L., Collins, R., ... Antonio, J. (2010). ISSN exercise & sport nutrition review: research & recommendations. Journal of the International Society of Sports Nutrition, 7, 7.

Manore, M. M. (2015). Weight Management for Athletes and Active Individuals: A Brief Review. Sports Medicine (Auckland, N.z.), 45(Suppl 1), 83–92.

Mielgo-Ayuso J, Maroto-Sánchez B, Luzardo-Socorro R, Palacios G, Palacios Gil-Antuñano N, González-Gross M; EXERNET Study Group. Evaluation of nutritional status and energy expenditure in athletes. Nutr Hosp. 2015 Feb 26;31 Suppl 3:227-36.

Poehlman ET. A review: exercise and its influence on resting energy metabolism in man. Med Sci Sports Exerc. 1989 Oct;21(5):515-25. Review.

Pramuková, B., Szabadosová, V., & Šoltésová, A. (2011). Current knowledge about sports nutrition. The Australasian Medical Journal, 4(3), 107–110.

Purcell, L. K., & Canadian Paediatric Society, Paediatric Sports and Exercise Medicine Section. (2013). Sport nutrition for young athletes. Paediatrics & Child Health, 18(4), 200–202.

Westerterp KR. Control of Energy Expenditure in Humans. [Updated 2016 Nov 11]. In: De Groot LJ, Chrousos G, Dungan K, et al., editors. Endotext [Internet]. South Dartmouth (MA): MDText.com, Inc.; 2000.

Westerterp KR. Exercise, energy expenditure and energy balance, as measured with doubly labelled water. Proc Nutr Soc. 2018 Feb;77(1):4-10.

Westerterp, K. R. (2013). Physical activity and physical activity induced energy expenditure in humans: measurement, determinants, and effects. Frontiers in Physiology, 4, 90.

CHAPTER 12

Abernathy RP, Black DR. Healthy body weights: an alternative perspective. Am J Clin Nutr. 1996 Mar;63(3 Suppl):448S-451S. Review.

Ball SD, Altena TS. Comparison of the Bod Pod and dual energy x-ray absorptiometry in men. Physiol Meas. 2004 Jun;25(3):671-8.

Brodie D, Moscrip V, Hutcheon R. Body composition measurement: a review of hydrodensitometry, anthropometry, and impedance methods. Nutrition. 1998 Mar;14(3):296-310. Review.

Chen, K.-T., Chen, Y.-Y., Wang, C.-W., Chuang, C.-L., Chiang, L.-M., Lai, C.-L., ... Hsieh, K.-C. (2016). Comparison of Standing Posture Bioelectrical Impedance Analysis with DXA for Body Composition in a Large, Healthy Chinese Population. PLoS ONE, 11(7), e0160105.

Duren, D. L., Sherwood, R. J., Czerwinski, S. A., Lee, M., Choh, A. C., Siervogel, R. M., & Cameron

Chumlea, W. (2008). Body Composition Methods: Comparisons and Interpretation. Journal of Diabetes Science and Technology (Online), 2(6), 1139–1146.

Fields DA, Goran MI, McCrory MA. Body-composition assessment via air-displacement plethysmography in adults and children: a review. Am J Clin Nutr. 2002 Mar;75(3):453-67. Review.

Institute of Medicine (US) Committee on Military Nutrition Research; Marriott BM, Grumstrup-Scott J, editors. Body Composition and Physical Performance: Applications For the Military Services. Washington (DC): National Academies Press (US); 1990.

Institute of Medicine (US) Committee on Military Nutrition Research; Marriott BM, Grumstrup-Scott J, editors. Body Composition and Physical Performance: Applications

For the Military Services. Washington (DC): National Academies Press (US); 1990. 14, Body Composition Measurement: Accuracy, Validity, and Comparability.

Jensen NS, Camargo TF, Bergamaschi DP. Comparison of methods to measure body fat in 7-to-10-year-old children: a systematic review. Public Health. 2016 Apr;133:3-13.

Laskey MA. Dual-energy X-ray absorptiometry and body composition. Nutrition. 1996 Jan;12(1):45-51. Review.

Lee, S. Y., & Gallagher, D. (2008). Assessment methods in human body composition. Current Opinion in Clinical Nutrition and Metabolic Care, 11(5), 566–572.

Lopez, Ygnacio III; Mama, Scherezade; Wilson, Penny; and Lee, Rebecca E. (2009) "Body composition assessment methods: A systematic review and recommendations," International Journal of Exercise Science: Conference Proceedings: Vol. 3 : Iss. 1 , Article 9.

Lorenzini, A. (2014). How Much Should We Weigh for a Long and Healthy Life Span? The Need to Reconcile Caloric Restriction versus Longevity with Body Mass Index versus Mortality Data. Frontiers in Endocrinology, 5, 121.

Lukaski HC. Methods for the assessment of human body composition: traditional and new. Am J Clin Nutr. 1987 Oct;46(4):537-56. Review.

Mazi S, Lazovi B, Deli M, Lazi JS, A imovi T, Brki P. Body composition assessment in athletes: a systematic review. Med Pregl. 2014 Jul-Aug;67(7-8):255-60. Review.

Nuttall, F. Q. (2015). Body Mass Index: Obesity, BMI, and Health: A Critical Review. Nutrition Today, 50(3), 117–128.

Pasco, J. A., Holloway, K. L., Dobbins, A. G.,

Kotowicz, M. A., Williams, L. J., & Brennan, S. L. (2014). Body mass index and measures of body fat for defining obesity and underweight: a cross-sectional, population-based study. BMC Obesity, 1, 9.

Reilly, J. J., Wilson, J., & Durnin, J. V. (1995). Determination of body composition from skinfold thickness: a validation study. Archives of Disease in Childhood, 73(4), 305–310.

Santos, D. A., Dawson, J. A., Matias, C. N., Rocha, P. M., Minderico, C. S., Allison, D. B., ... Silva, A. M. (2014). Reference Values for Body Composition and Anthropometric Measurements in Athletes. PLoS ONE, 9(5), e97846.

Santos, D. A., Silva, A. M., Matias, C. N., Fields, D. A., Heymsfield, S. B., & Sardinha, L. B. (2010). Accuracy of DXA in estimating body composition changes in elite athletes using a four compartment model as the reference method. Nutrition & Metabolism, 7, 22.

Vigotsky, A. D., Schoenfeld, B. J., Than, C., & Brown, J.M. (2018). Methods matter: the relationship between strength and hypertrophy depends on methods of measurement and analysis. PeerJ, 6, e5071.

Wagner DR, Heyward VH. Techniques of body composition assessment: a review of laboratory and field methods. Res Q Exerc Sport. 1999 Jun;70(2):135-49. Review.

Wang J, Thornton JC, Kolesnik S, Pierson RN Jr. Anthropometry in body composition. An overview. Ann N Y Acad Sci. 2000 May;904:317-26. Review.

Wells, J. C. K., & Fewtrell, M. S. (2006). Measuring body composition. Archives of Disease in Childhood, 91(7), 612–617.

CHAPTER 13

American Dietetic Association; Dietitians of Canada. Position of the American Dietetic Association and Dietitians of Canada: Vegetarian diets. J Am Diet Assoc. 2003 Jun;103(6):748-65.

Barr SI, Rideout CA. Nutritional considerations for vegetarian athletes. Nutrition. 2004 Jul-Aug;20(7-8):696- 703. Review.

Berning, J. R. (2013). The Vegetarian Athlete. In The Encyclopaedia of Sports Medicine, R. J. Maughan (Ed.).

Borge, T. C., Aase, H., Brantsæter, A. L., & Biele, G. (2017). The importance of maternal diet quality during pregnancy on cognitive and behavioural outcomes in children: a systematic review and meta-analysis. BMJ Open, 7(9), e016777.

Bravi F, Wiens F, Decarli A, Dal Pont A, Agostoni C, Ferraroni M. Impact of maternal nutrition on breast-milk composition: a systematic review. Am J Clin Nutr. 2016 Sep;104(3):646-62.

Clifton, P. (2017). Assessing the evidence for weight loss strategies in people with and without type 2 diabetes. World Journal of Diabetes, 8(10), 440–454.

Cotunga N, Vickery CE, McBee S. Sports nutrition for young athletes. J Sch Nurs. 2005 Dec;21(6):323-8. Review.

Craig WJ, Mangels AR; American Dietetic Association. Position of the American Dietetic Association: vegetarian diets. J Am Diet Assoc. 2009 Jul;109(7):1266-82.

Craig WJ. Health effects of vegan diets. Am J Clin Nutr. 2009 May;89(5):1627S-1633S.

Craig WJ. Health effects of vegan diets. Am J Clin Nutr. 2009 May;89(5):1627S-1633S.

Dagnelie PC. [Nutrition and health–potential health benefits and risks of vegetarianism and limited consumption of meat in the Netherlands]. Ned TijdschrGeneeskd. 2003 Jul 5;147(27):1308-13. Review. Dutch.

Danielewicz, H., Myszczyszyn, G., D bi ska, A., Myszkal, A., Bozna ski, A., & Hirnle, L. (2017). Diet in pregnancy– more than food. European Journal of Pediatrics, 176(12), 1573–1579.

Davis SR, Castelo-Branco C, Chedraui P, Lumsden MA, Nappi RE, Shah D, Villaseca P; Writing Group of the International Menopause Society for World Menopause Day 2012. Understanding weight gain at menopause. Climacteric. 2012 Oct;15(5):419-29.

Dean, S. V., Lassi, Z. S., Imam, A. M., & Bhutta, Z. A. (2014). Preconception care: nutritional risks and interventions. Reproductive Health, 11(Suppl 3), S3.

Douglas, C. C., Gower, B. A., Darnell, B. E., Ovalle, F., Oster, R. A., & Azziz, R. (2006). Role of diet in the treatment of polycystic ovary syndrome. Fertility and Sterility, 85(3), 679–688.

Evert, A. B., Boucher, J. L., Cypress, M., Dunbar, S. A., Franz, M. J., Mayer-Davis, E. J., ... Yancy, W. S. (2013). Nutrition Therapy Recommendations for the Management of Adults With Diabetes. Diabetes Care, 36(11), 3821– 3842.

Faghfoori Z, Fazelian S, Shadnoush M, Goodarzi R. Nutritional management in women with polycystic ovary syndrome: A review study. Diabetes Metab Syndr. 2017 Nov;11 Suppl 1:S429-S432.

Farrar, D., Simmonds, M., Bryant, M., Sheldon, T. A., Tuffnell, D., Golder, S., & Lawlor, D. A. (2017). Treatments for gestational diabetes: a systematic review and meta- analysis. BMJ open, 7(6), e015557.

Farshchi H, Rane A, Love A, Kennedy RL. Diet and nutrition in polycystic ovary syndrome (PCOS): pointers for nutritional management. J Obstet Gynaecol. 2007 Nov;27(8):762-73. Review.

Forsum, E., Brantsæter, A. L., Olafsdottir, A.-S., Olsen, S. F., & Thorsdottir, I. (2013). Weight loss before conception: A systematic literature review. Food & Nutrition Research, 57, 10.3402/fnr.v57i0.20522.

Franz MJ, Boucher JL, Rutten-Ramos S, VanWormer JJ. Lifestyle weight-loss intervention outcomes in overweight and obese adults with type 2 diabetes: a systematic review and meta-analysis of randomized clinical trials. J Acad Nutr Diet. 2015 Sep;115(9):1447-63.

Franz MJ, Powers MA, Leontos C, Holzmeister LA, Kulkarni K, Monk A, Wedel N, Gradwell E. The evidence for medical nutrition therapy for type 1 and type 2 diabetes in adults. J Am Diet Assoc. 2010 Dec;110(12):1852-89.

Franz MJ. Diabetes Nutrition Therapy: Effectiveness, Macronutrients, Eating Patterns and Weight Management. Am J Med Sci. 2016 Apr;351(4):374-9.

Franz MJ. Evidence-based medical nutrition therapy for diabetes. Nutr Clin Pract. 2004 Apr;19(2):137-44.

Franz, M. J., Boucher, J. L., & Evert, A. B. (2014). Evidence-based diabetes nutrition therapy recommendations are effective: the key is individualization. Diabetes, Metabolic Syndrome and Obesity: Targets and Therapy, 7, 65–72.

Freeland-Graves J. Mineral adequacy of vegetarian diets. Am J Clin Nutr. 1988 Sep;48(3 Suppl):859-62. Review.

Fuhrman, J., & Ferreri, D. M. (2010). Fueling the Vegetarian (Vegan) Athlete. Current Sports Medicine Reports, 9(4), 233–241.

Galanti, G., Stefani, L., Scacciati, I., Mascherini, G., Buti, G., & Maffulli, N. (2015). Eating and nutrition habits in young competitive athletes: a comparison between soccer players and cyclists. Translational Medicine @ UniSa, 11, 44–47.

Gaskins AJ, Chavarro JE. Diet and fertility: a review. Am J Obstet Gynecol. 2018 Apr; 218 (4): 379-389.

Geraghty, A. A., Lindsay, K. L., Alberdi, G., McAuliffe, F. M., & Gibney, E. R. (2015). Nutrition During Pregnancy Impacts Offspring's Epigenetic Status—Evidence from Human and Animal Studies. Nutrition and Metabolic Insights, 8(Suppl 1), 41–47.

Grieger, J. A., & Clifton, V. L. (2015). A Review of the Impact of Dietary Intakes in Human Pregnancy on Infant Birthweight. Nutrients, 7(1), 153–178.

Haider LM, Schwingshackl L, Hoffmann G, Ekmekcioglu C. The effect of vegetarian diets on iron status in adults: A systematic review and meta-analysis. Crit Rev Food Sci Nutr. 2016 Nov 23:1-16.

Hamdy O, Barakatun-Nisak MY. Nutrition in Diabetes. Endocrinol Metab Clin North Am. 2016 Dec;45(4):799-817.

Hamilton-Reeves, J. M., Vazquez, G., Duval, S. J., Phipps, W. R., Kurzer, M. S., & Messina, M. J. (2010). Clinical studies show no effects of soy protein or isoflavones on reproductive hormones in men: results of a meta-analysis. Fertility and Sterility, 94(3), 997–1007.

Hever, J. (2016). Plant-Based Diets: A Physician's Guide. The Permanente Journal, 20(3), 93–101.

Hillier SE, Olander EK. Women's dietary changes before and during pregnancy: A systematic review. Midwifery. 2017 Jun;49:19-31.

Hoffman, J. R., & Falvo, M. J. (2004). Protein - Which is Best?. Journal of sports science & medicine, 3(3), 118-30.

Hunt JR. Bioavailability of iron, zinc, and other trace minerals from vegetarian diets. Am J Clin Nutr. 2003 Sep;78(3 Suppl):633S-639S. Review.

Jackson AA, Robinson SM. Dietary guidelines for pregnancy: a review of current evidence. Public Health Nutr. 2001 Apr;4(2B):625-30. Review.

Jebeile H, Mijatovic J, Louie JCY, Prvan T, Brand-Miller JC. A systematic review and metaanalysis of energy intake and weight gain in pregnancy. Am J Obstet Gynecol. 2016 Apr;214(4):465-483.

Jonklaas, J., Bianco, A. C., Bauer, A. J., Burman, K. D., Cappola, A. R., Celi, F. S., … Sawka, A. M. (2014). Guidelines for the Treatment of Hypothyroidism: Prepared by the American Thyroid Association Task Force on Thyroid Hormone Replacement. Thyroid, 24(12), 1670–1751.

Jull, J., Stacey, D., Beach, S., Dumas, A., Strychar, I., Ufholz, L.-A., … Prud'homme, D. (2014). Lifestyle Interventions Targeting Body Weight Changes during the Menopause Transition: A Systematic Review. Journal of Obesity, 2014, 824310.

Kampmann, U., Madsen, L. R., Skajaa, G. O., Iversen, D. S., Moeller, N., & Ovesen, P. (2015). Gestational diabetes: A clinical update. World journal of diabetes, 6(8), 1065-72.

Kataoka, J., Tassone, E. C., Misso, M., Joham, A. E., Stener-Victorin, E., Teede, H., & Moran, L. J. (2017). Weight Management Interventions in Women with and without PCOS: A Systematic Review. Nutrients, 9(9), 996.

Key TJ, Appleby PN, Rosell MS. Health effects of vegetarian and vegan diets. Proc Nutr Soc. 2006 Feb;65(1):35-41. Review.

Kim, D. (2017). The Role of Vitamin D in Thyroid Diseases. International Journal of Molecular Sciences, 18(9), 1949.

Kominiarek, M. A., & Rajan, P. (2016). Nutrition Recommendations in Pregnancy and Lactation. The Medical Clinics of North America, 100(6), 1199–1215.

Kramer MS, Kakuma R. Energy and protein intake in pregnancy. Cochrane Database Syst Rev. 2003;(4):CD000032. Review. Update in: Cochrane Database Syst Rev. 2012;9:CD000032.

Lecerf JM. Fatty acids and cardiovascular disease. Nutr Rev. 2009 May;67(5):273-83.

Li Y, Nishihara E, Kakudo K. Hashimoto's thyroiditis: old concepts and new insights. Curr Opin Rheumatol. 2011 Jan;23(1):102-7.

Liontiris MI, Mazokopakis EE. A concise review of Hashimoto thyroiditis (HT) and the importance of iodine, selenium, vitamin D and gluten on the autoimmunity and dietary management of HT patients.Points that need more investigation. Hell J Nucl Med. 2017 Jan-Apr;20(1):51-56.

López-Fernández G, Barrios M, Goberna-Tricas J, Gómez-Benito J. Breastfeeding during pregnancy: A systematic review. Women Birth. 2017 Dec;30(6):e292- e300.

Marangoni, F., Cetin, I., Verduci, E., Canzone, G., Giovannini, M., Scollo, P., ... Poli, A. (2016). Maternal Diet and Nutrient Requirements in Pregnancy and Breastfeeding. An Italian Consensus Document. Nutrients, 8(10), 629.

Marsh K, Brand-Miller J. The optimal diet for women with polycystic ovary syndrome? Br J Nutr. 2005 Aug;94(2):154-65. Review.

McEvoy CT, Temple N, Woodside JV. Vegetarian diets, low-meat diets and health: a review. Public Health Nutr. 2012 Dec;15(12):2287-94.

McEvoy CT, Temple N, Woodside JV. Vegetarian diets, low-meat diets and health: a review. Public Health Nutr. 2012 Dec;15(12):2287-94.

Meyer F, O'Connor H, Shirreffs SM; International Association of Athletics Federations. Nutrition for the young athlete. J Sports Sci. 2007;25 Suppl 1:S73-82. Review. Erratum in: J Sports Sci. 2009 Apr;27(6):667.

Monte, S., Valenti, O., Giorgio, E., Renda, E., Hyseni, E., Faraci, M., ... Di Prima, F. A. F. (2011). Maternal weight gain during pregnancy and neonatal birth weight: a review of the literature. Journal of Prenatal Medicine, 5(2), 27–30.

Moran LJ, Ko H, Misso M, Marsh K, Noakes M, Talbot M, Frearson M, Thondan M, Stepto N, Teede HJ. Dietary composition in the treatment of polycystic ovary syndrome: a systematic review to inform evidence-based guidelines. J Acad Nutr Diet. 2013 Apr;113(4):520-45.

Morrison, J. L., & Regnault, T. R. H. (2016). Nutrition in Pregnancy: Optimising Maternal Diet and Fetal Adaptations to Altered Nutrient Supply. Nutrients, 8(6), 342.

Mottalib, A., Kasetty, M., Mar, J. Y., Elseaidy, T., Ashrafzadeh, S., & Hamdy, O. (2017). Weight Management in Patients with Type 1 Diabetes and Obesity. Current Diabetes Reports, 17(10), 92.

Muktabhant, B., Lumbiganon, P., Ngamjarus, C., & Dowswell, T. (2012). Interventions for preventing excessive weight gain during pregnancy. The Cochrane Database of Systematic Reviews, 4, CD007145.

Obersby D, Chappell DC, Dunnett A, Tsiami AA. Plasma total homocysteine status of vegetarians compared with omnivores: a systematic review and meta-analysis. Br J Nutr. 2013 Mar 14;109(5):785-94.

Pawlak R. Is vitamin B12 deficiency a risk factor for cardiovascular disease in vegetarians? Am J Prev Med. 2015 Jun;48(6):e11-26.

Purcell, L. K., & Canadian Paediatric Society, Paediatric Sports and Exercise Medicine Section. (2013). Sport nutrition for young athletes. Paediatrics & Child Health, 18(4), 200–202.

Rizzo, G., Laganà, A. S., Rapisarda, A. M. C., La Ferrera, G. M. G., Buscema, M., Rossetti, P., ... Vitale, S. G. (2016). Vitamin B12 among Vegetarians: Status, Assessment and Supplementation. Nutrients, 8(12), 767.

Rogerson, D. (2017). Vegan diets: practical advice for athletes and exercisers. Journal of the International Society of Sports Nutrition, 14, 36.

Sabato, T. M., Walch, T. J., & Caine, D. J. (2016). The elite young athlete: strategies to ensure physical and emotional health. Open Access Journal of Sports Medicine, 7, 99–113.

Sami, W., Ansari, T., Butt, N. S., & Hamid, M. R. A. (2017). Effect of diet on type 2 diabetes mellitus: A review. International Journal of Health Sciences, 11(2), 65–71.

Sharma R, Bharti S, Kumar KH. Diet and thyroid - myths and facts. J Med Nutr Nutraceut 2014;3:60-5

Smith, J. W., Holmes, M. E., & McAllister, M. J. (2015). Nutritional Considerations for Performance in Young Athletes. Journal of Sports Medicine, 2015, 734649.

Sutnick MR. Vegetarian diets. Prim Care. 1975 Jun;2(2):309-15.

Tuso, P. J., Ismail, M. H., Ha, B. P., & Bartolotto, C. (2013). Nutritional Update for Physicians: Plant-Based Diets. The Permanente Journal, 17(2), 61–66.

Vetter ML, Amaro A, Volger S. Nutritional management of type 2 diabetes mellitus and obesity and pharmacologic therapies to facilitate weight loss. Postgrad Med. 2014 Jan;126(1):139-52.

Khazrai YM, Defeudis G, Pozzilli P. Effect of diet on type 2 diabetes mellitus: a review. Diabetes Metab Res Rev. 2014 Mar;30 Suppl 1:24-33.

Ajala O, English P, Pinkney J. Systematic review and meta-analysis of different dietary approaches to the management of type 2 diabetes. Am J Clin Nutr. 2013 Mar;97(3):505-16.

Li R, Zhang P, Barker LE, Chowdhury FM, Zhang X. Cost- effectiveness of interventions to prevent and control diabetes mellitus: a systematic review. Diabetes Care. 2010 Aug;33(8):1872-94.

Choudhary P. Review of dietary recommendations for diabetes mellitus. Diabetes Res Clin Pract. 2004 Sep;65 Suppl 1:S9-S15. Review.

Aucott L, Poobalan A, Smith WC, Avenell A, Jung R, Broom J, Grant AM. Weight loss in obese diabetic and non-diabetic individuals and long-term diabetes outcomes—a systematic review. Diabetes Obes Metab. 2004 Mar;6(2):85-94. Review.

Anderson JW, Kendall CW, Jenkins DJ. Importance of weight management in type 2 diabetes: review with meta- analysis of clinical studies. J Am Coll Nutr. 2003 Oct;22(5):331-9. Review.

Wang S, Wu Y, Zuo Z, Zhao Y, Wang K. The effect of vitamin D supplementation on thyroid autoantibody levels in the treatment of autoimmune thyroiditis: a systematic review and a meta-analysis. Endocrine. 2018 Mar;59(3):499-505.

Wang, J., Lv, S., Chen, G., Gao, C., He, J., Zhong, H., & Xu, Y. (2015). Meta-Analysis of the Association between Vitamin D and Autoimmune Thyroid Disease. Nutrients, 7(4), 2485–2498.

Woo, K. S., Kwok, T. C. Y., & Celermajer, D. S. (2014). Vegan Diet, Subnormal Vitamin B-12 Status and Cardiovascular Health. Nutrients, 6(8), 3259–3273.

CHAPTER 14

Backes, T., & Fitzgerald, K. (2016). Fluid consumption, exercise, and cognitive performance. Biology of Sport, 33(3), 291–296.

Barr SI. Effects of dehydration on exercise performance. Can J Appl Physiol. 1999 Apr;24(2):164-72. Review.

Burke LM, Hawley JA, Wong SH, Jeukendrup AE. Carbohydrates for training and competition. J Sports Sci. 2011;29 Suppl 1:S17-27.

Burke LM, Millet G, Tarnopolsky MA; International Association of Athletics Federations. Nutrition for distance events. J Sports Sci. 2007;25 Suppl 1:S29-38. Review. Erratum in: J Sports Sci. 2009 Apr;27(6):667.

Burke LM, Millet G, Tarnopolsky MA; International Association of Athletics Federations. Nutrition for distance events. J Sports Sci. 2007;25 Suppl 1:S29-38. Review. Erratum in: J Sports Sci. 2009 Apr;27(6):667.

Burke LM. Nutrition strategies for the marathon : fuel for training and racing. Sports Med. 2007;37(4-5):344-7.

Burke LM. Nutrition strategies for the marathon : fuel for training and racing. Sports Med. 2007;37(4-5):344-7.

Cheuvront SN, Kenefick RW. Dehydration: physiology, assessment, and performance effects. Compr Physiol. 2014 Jan;4(1):257-85.

Fogelholm M. Effects of bodyweight reduction on sports performance. Sports Med. 1994 Oct;18(4):249-67. Review.

Franchini et al.: Weight loss in combat sports: physiological, psychological and performance effects. Journal of the International Society of Sports Nutrition 2012 9:52

Gentil, P. (2015). A nutrition and conditioning intervention for natural bodybuilding contest preparation: observations and suggestions. Journal of the International Society of Sports Nutrition, 12, 50.

Goulet ED. Effect of exercise-induced dehydration on endurance performance: evaluating the impact of exercise protocols on outcomes using a meta-analytic procedure. Br J Sports Med. 2013 Jul;47(11):679-86.

Helms, E. R., Aragon, A. A., & Fitschen, P. J. (2014). Evidence-based recommendations for natural bodybuilding contest preparation: nutrition and supplementation. Journal of the International Society of Sports Nutrition, 11, 20.

Judelson DA, Maresh CM, Anderson JM, Armstrong LE, Casa DJ, Kraemer WJ, Volek JS. Hydration and muscular performance: does fluid balance affect strength, power and high-intensity endurance? Sports Med. 2007;37(10):907-21. Review.

Khodaee M, Olewinski L, Shadgan B, Kiningham RR. Rapid Weight Loss in Sports with Weight Classes. Curr Sports Med Rep. 2015 Nov-Dec;14(6):435-41.

Kiens B. Diet and training in the week before competition. Can J Appl Physiol. 2001;26 Suppl:S56-63. Review.

Kiens B. Diet and training in the week before competition. Can J Appl Physiol. 2001;26 Suppl:S56-63. Review.

Kraft JA, Green JM, Bishop PA, Richardson MT, Neggers YH, Leeper JD. The influence of hydration on anaerobic performance: a review. Res Q Exerc Sport. 2012 Jun;83(2):282-92. Review.

Kreider, R. B., Wilborn, C. D., Taylor, L., Campbell, B., Almada, A. L., Collins, R., ... Antonio, J. (2010). ISSN exercise & sport nutrition review: research & recommendations. Journal of the International Society of Sports Nutrition, 7, 7.

Lambert CP, Frank LL, Evans WJ. Macronutrient considerations for the sport of bodybuilding. Sports Med. 2004;34(5):317-27. Review.

Maughan RJ, Shirreffs SM. Dehydration and rehydration in competative sport. Scand J Med Sci Sports. 2010 Oct;20 Suppl 3:40-7.

McCartney, D., Desbrow, B., & Irwin, C. (2017). The Effect of Fluid Intake Following Dehydration on Subsequent Athletic and Cognitive Performance: a Systematic Review and Meta-analysis. Sports Medicine - Open, 3, 13.

Mitchell L, Hackett D, Gifford J, Estermann F, O'Connor H. Do Bodybuilders Use Evidence-Based Nutrition Strategies to Manipulate Physique? Sports. 2017; 5(4):76.

Nuccio, R. P., Barnes, K. A., Carter, J. M., & Baker, L. B. (2017). Fluid Balance in Team Sport Athletes and the Effect of Hypohydration on Cognitive, Technical, and Physical Performance. Sports Medicine (Auckland, N.z.), 47(10), 1951–1982.

Pettersson, S., Ekström, M. P., & Berg, C. M. (2013). Practices of Weight Regulation Among Elite Athletes in Combat Sports: A Matter of Mental Advantage? Journal of Athletic Training, 48(1), 99–108.

Popkin, B. M., D'Anci, K. E., & Rosenberg, I. H. (2010). Water, Hydration and Health. Nutrition Reviews, 68(8), 439–458.

Reale R, Slater G, Burke LM. Acute-Weight-Loss Strategies for Combat Sports and Applications to Olympic Success. Int J Sports Physiol Perform. 2017 Feb;12(2):142-151.

Reale R, Slater G, Burke LM. Individualised dietary strategies for Olympic combat sports: Acute weight loss, recovery and competition nutrition. Eur J Sport Sci. 2017 Jul;17(6):727-740.

Sawka, M. N., Cheuvront, S. N., & Kenefick, R. W. (2015). Hypohydration and Human Performance: Impact of Environment and Physiological Mechanisms. Sports Medicine (Auckland, N.z.), 45(Suppl 1), 51–60.

Sherman WM, Costill DL. The marathon: dietary manipulation to optimize performance. Am J Sports Med. 1984 Jan-Feb;12(1):44-51. Review.

Sherman WM, Costill DL. The marathon: dietary manipulation to optimize performance. Am J Sports Med. 1984 Jan-Feb;12(1):44-51. Review.

Shirreffs SM. The importance of good hydration

for work and exercise performance. Nutr Rev. 2005 Jun;63(6 Pt 2):S14-21. Review.

Slater G, Phillips SM. Nutrition guidelines for strength sports: sprinting, weightlifting, throwing events, and bodybuilding. J Sports Sci. 2011;29 Suppl 1:S67-77.

Sundgot-Borgen J, Garthe I. Elite athletes in aesthetic and Olympic weight-class sports and the challenge of body weight and body compositions. J Sports Sci. 2011;29 Suppl 1:S101-14.

Turocy, P. S., DePalma, B. F., Horswill, C. A., Laquale, K. M., Martin, T. J., Perry, A. C., … Utter, A. C. (2011). National Athletic Trainers' Association Position Statement: Safe Weight Loss and Maintenance Practices in Sport and Exercise. Journal of Athletic Training, 46(3), 322–336.

Walberg-Rankin, J. A review of nutritional practices and needs of bodybuilders. J. Strength and Cond. Res. 9(2):116-124. 1995

CHAPTER 15

Bibbo, S., Ianiro, G., Giorgio, V., Scaldaferri, F., Masucci, L., Gasbarrini, A., & Cammarota, G. (2016). The role of diet on gut microbiota composition. European Review for Medical and Pharmacological Sciences, 20(22), 4742–4749.

Bonder, M. J., Tigchelaar, E. F., Cai, X., Trynka, G., Cenit, M. C., Hrdlickova, B., … Zhernakova, A. (2016). The influence of a short-term gluten-free diet on the human gut microbiome. Genome Medicine, 8(1), 1–11.

Brahe, L. K., Astrup, A., & Larsen, L. H. (2016). Can We Prevent Obesity-Related Metabolic Diseases by Dietary Modulation of the Gut Microbiota? Advances in Nutrition (Bethesda, Md.), 7(1), 90–101.

Bressa, C., Bailén-Andrino, M., Pérez-Santiago, J., González-Soltero, R., Pérez, M., Montalvo-Lominchar, M. G., … Larrosa, M. (2017). Differences in gut microbiota profile between women with active lifestyle and sedentary women. PLoS ONE, 12(2), 1–20.

Byrne, C. S., Chambers, E. S., Morrison, D. J., & Frost, G. (2015). The role of short chain fatty acids in appetite regulation and energy homeostasis. International Journal of Obesity, 39(9), 1331–1338.

Campbell, S. C., & Wisniewski, P. J. (2017). Exercise is a Novel Promoter of Intestinal Health and Microbial Diversity. Exercise and Sport Sciences Reviews, 45(1), 41–47.

Campbell, S. C., Wisniewski, P. J., Noji, M., McGuinness, L. R., Häggblom, M. M., Lightfoot, S. A., … Kerkhof, L. J. (2016). The effect of diet and exercise on intestinal integrity and microbial diversity in mice. PLoS ONE, 11(3), 1–17.

Cani, P. D., Amar, J., Iglesias, M. A., Poggi, M., Knauf, C., Bastelica, D., … Burcelin, R. (2007). Metabolic Endotoxemia Initiates Obesity and Insulin Resistance. Diabetes, 56(7). Retrieved from

Cerdá, B., Pérez, M., Pérez-Santiago, J. D., Tornero- Aguilera, J. F., González-Soltero, R., & Larrosa, M. (2016). Gut microbiota modification: Another piece in the puzzle of the benefits of physical exercise in health? Frontiers in Physiology, 7(FEB), 1–11.

Chung, W. S. F., Walker, A. W., Louis, P., Parkhill, J., Vermeiren, J., Bosscher, D., … Flint, H. J. (2016). Modulation of the human gut microbiota by dietary fibres occurs at the species level. BMC Biology, 14(1), 1–14.

Clarke, S. F., Murphy, E. F., O'Sullivan, O., Lucey, A. J., Humphreys, M., Hogan, A., … Cotter, P. D. (2014). Exercise and associated dietary extremes impact on gut microbial diversity. Gut.

Cronin, O., Barton, W., Skuse, P., Penney, N. C., Garcia- Perez, I., Murphy, E. F., … Shanahan, F. (2018). A Prospective Metagenomic and Metabolomic Analysis of the Impact of Exercise and/or Whey Protein Supplementation on the Gut Microbiome of Sedentary Adults. MSystems, 3(3), e00044-18.

Cronin, O., Molloy, M. G., & Shanahan, F. (2016). Exercise, fitness, and the gut. Current Opinion in Gastroenterology, 32(2), 67–73.

Cronin, O., O'Sullivan, O., Barton, W., Cotter, P. D., Molloy, M. G., & Shanahan, F. (2017). Gut microbiota: Implications for sports and exercise medicine. British Journal of Sports Medicine, 51(9), 700–701.

de Almada, C. N., Nunes de Almada, C., Martinez, R. C. R., & Sant'Ana, A. de S. (2015). Characterization of the intestinal microbiota and its interaction with probiotics and health impacts. Applied Microbiology and Biotechnology, 99(10), 4175–4199.

Diamanti, A., Capriati, T., Basso, M. S., Panetta, F., Laurora, V. M. D. C., Bellucci, F., ... Francavilla, R. (2014). Celiac disease and overweight in children: An update. Nutrients, 6(1), 207–220.

Effects, M., & Sweeteners, O. F. N. (2016). HHS Public Access, 152(0 0), 450–455.

Estaki, M., Pither, J., Baumeister, P., Little, J. P., Gill, S. K., Ghosh, S., ... Gibson, D. L. (2016). Cardiorespiratory fitness as a predictor of intestinal microbial diversity and distinct metagenomic functions. Microbiome, 4, 1–13.

Frei, R., Akdis, M., & O'mahony, L. (2015). Prebiotics, probiotics, synbiotics, and the immune system: Experimental data and clinical evidence. Current Opinion in Gastroenterology, 31(2), 153–158.

Galipeau, H. J., & Verdu, E. F. (2015). Gut microbes and adverse food reactions: Focus on gluten related disorders. Gut Microbes, 5(5), 594–605.

Gorvitovskaia, A., Holmes, S. P., & Huse, S. M. (2016). Interpreting prevotella and bacteroides as biomarkers of diet and lifestyle. Microbiome, 4, 1–12.

Harvie, R. M., Chisholm, A. W., Bisanz, J. E., Burton, J. P., Herbison, P., Schultz, K., & Schultz, M. (2017). Long- term irritable bowel syndrome symptom control with reintroduction of selected FODMAPs. World Journal of Gastroenterology, 23(25), 4632–4643.

Hsu, Y. J., Chiu, C. C., Li, Y. P., Huang, W. C., Huang, Y. Te, Huang, C. C., & Chuang, H.

L. (2015). Effect of intestinal microbiota on exercise performance in mice. Journal of Strength and Conditioning Research, 29(2), 552–558.

Hulston, C. J., Churnside, A. A., & Venables, M. C. (2015). Probiotic supplementation prevents high-fat, overfeeding- induced insulin resistance in human subjects. The British Journal of Nutrition, 113(4), 596–602.

Kabbani, T. A., Goldberg, A., Kelly, C. P., Pallav, K., Tariq, S., Peer, A., ... Leffler, D. A. (2012). Body mass index and the risk of obesity in coeliac disease treated with the gluten-free diet. Alimentary Pharmacology and Therapeutics, 35(6), 723–729.

Karl, J. P., Meydani, M., Barnett, J. B., Vanegas, S. M., Goldin, B., Kane, A., ... Roberts, S. B. (2017). Substituting whole grains for refined grains in a 6-week randomized trial favorably affects energy balance parameters in healthy men and post-menopausal women. The American Journal of Clinical Nutrition, ajcn139683.

Lai, H.-C., Young, J., Lin, C.-S., Chang, C.-J., Lu, C.-C., Martel, J., ... Ko, Y.-F. (2014). Impact of the gut microbiota, prebiotics, and probiotics on human health and disease. Biomedical Journal, 37(5), 259.

Lam, Y. Y., Maguire, S., Palacios, T., & Caterson, I. D. (2017). Are the gut bacteria telling us to eat or not to eat? Reviewing the role of gut microbiota in the etiology, disease progression and treatment of eating disorders. Nutrients, 9(6).

Lamoureux, E. V., Grandy, S. A., & Langille, M. G. I. (2017). Moderate Exercise Has Limited but Distinguishable Effects on the Mouse Microbiome. MSystems, 2(4), e00006-17.

Linares, D. M., Ross, P., & Stanton, C. (2016). Beneficial Microbes: The pharmacy in the gut. Bioengineered, 7(1), 11–20.

Lyte, J. M., Gabler, N. K., & Hollis, J. H. (2016). Postprandial serum endotoxin in healthy humans is modulated by dietary fat in a randomized, controlled, cross-over study. Lipids in Health and Disease, 15(1), 1– 10.

Mach, N., & Fuster-Botella, D. (2017). Endurance exercise and gut microbiota: A review. Journal of Sport and Health Science, 6(2), 179–197.

Managing irritable bowel syndrome: The low-FODMAP diet. (n.d.). https://doi.org/10.3949/ccjm.83a.14159

Marone, P. A., Lau, F. C., Gupta, R. C., Bagchi, M., Bagchi, D., Shamie, A. N., & Udani, J. K. (2010). Safety and toxicological evaluation of undenatured type II collagen. Toxicology Mechanisms and Methods, 20(4), 175–189.

Monda, V., Villano, I., Messina, A., Valenzano, A., Esposito, T., Moscatelli, F., ... Messina, G. (2017). Exercise Modifies the Gut Microbiota with Positive Health Effects. Oxidative Medicine and Cellular Longevity, 2017, 3831972.

Moshfegh, A. J., Friday, J. E., Goldman, J. P., & Ahuja, J.K. (1999). Presence of inulin and oligofructose in the diets of Americans. The Journal of Nutrition, 129(7 Suppl), 1407S–11S. Retrieved from O'Sullivan, O., Cronin, O., Clarke, S. F., Murphy, E. F., Molloy, M. G., Shanahan, F., & Cotter, P. D. (2015). Exercise and the microbiota. Gut Microbes, 6(2), 131–136.

Osterberg, K. L., Boutagy, N. E., McMillan, R. P., Stevens, J. R., Frisard, M. I., Kavanaugh, J. W., ... Hulver, M. W. (2015). Probiotic supplementation attenuates increases in body mass and fat mass during high-fat diet in healthy young adults. Obesity, 23(12), 2364–2370.

Pereira, M. A. (2014). Sugar-Sweetened and Arti fi cially- Sweetened Beverages in Relation to Obesity Risk. Advances in Nutrition, 5, 797–808.

Petersen, L. M., Bautista, E. J., Nguyen, H., Hanson, B. M., Chen, L., Lek, S. H., ... Weinstock, G. M. (2017). Community characteristics of the gut microbiomes of competitive cyclists. Microbiome, 5(1), 1–13.

Portune, K. J., Benítez-Páez, A., Del Pulgar, E. M. G., Cerrudo, V., & Sanz, Y. (2017). Gut microbiota, diet, and obesity-related disorders— The good, the bad, and the future challenges. Molecular Nutrition and

Roberts, J. D., Suckling, C. A., Peedle, G. Y., Murphy, J. A., Dawkins, T. G., & Roberts, M. G. (2016). An exploratory investigation of endotoxin levels in novice long distance triathletes, and the effects of a multi-strain probiotic/prebiotic, antioxidant intervention. Nutrients, 8(11), 1–18.

Sanchez, B., Delgado, S., Blanco-Mïguez, A., Lourenzo, A., Gueimonde, M., & Margolles, A. (2017). Probiotics, gut microbiota, and their influence on host health and disease. Molecular Nutrition and Food Research, 61(1), 1–16.

Sanz, Y. (2015). Microbiome and Gluten. Annals of Nutrition & Metabolism, 67(suppl 2), 28–41.

Schiffman, S. S., & Rother, K. I. (2013). Sucralose, a synthetic organochlorine sweetener: Overview of biological issues. Journal of Toxicology and Environmental Health - Part B: Critical Reviews, 16(7), 399–451.

Simpson, H. L., & Campbell, B. J. (2015). Review article: Dietary fibre-microbiota interactions. Alimentary Pharmacology and Therapeutics, 42(2), 158–179.

Successful Low-FODMAP Living – Experts Discuss Meal- Planning Strategies to Help IBS Clients Better Control GI Distress. (n.d.). Retrieved August 10, 2018, from http://www.todaysdietitian.com/newarchives/030612p36.shtml

Suez, J., Korem, T., Zilberman-Schapira, G., Segal, E., & Elinav, E. (2015). Non-caloric artificial sweeteners and the microbiome: Findings and challenges. Gut Microbes, 6(2), 149–155.

The Low FODMAP Diet (FODMAP = Fermentable Oligosaccharides, Disaccharides, Monosaccharides and Polyols). (n.d.). Retrieved from www.uwhealth.org/nutrition

Thursby, E., & Juge, N. (2017). Introduction to the human gut microbiota, 0, 1823–1837.

U.S. Department of Health and Human Services and U.S. Department of Agriculture. 2015–2020 Dietary Guidelines for Americans. 8th Edition. December 2015. Available at http://health.gov/dietaryguidelines/2015/guidelines/

Venkataraman, A., Sieber, J. R., Schmidt, A. W., Waldron, C., Theis, K. R., & Schmidt, T. M. (2016). Variable responses of human microbiomes to dietary supplementation with resistant starch. Microbiome, 4, 1–9.

Yang, Y., Shi, Y., Wiklund, P., Tan, X., Wu, N., Zhang, X.,... Cheng, S. (2017). The association between cardiorespiratory fitness and gut microbiota composition in premenopausal women. Nutrients, 9(8), 1–11.

Zhao, X., Zhang, Z., Hu, B., Huang, W., Yuan, C., & Zou, (2018). Response of gut microbiota to metabolite changes induced by endurance exercise. Frontiers in Microbiology, 9(APR), 1–11.

CHAPTER 16

Barnes MJ. Alcohol: impact on sports performance and recovery in male athletes. Sports Med. 2014 Jul;44(7):909-19.

El-Sayed MS, Ali N, El-Sayed Ali Z. Interaction between alcohol and exercise: physiological and haematological implications. Sports Med. 2005;35(3):257-69. Review.

Gutgesell M, Canterbury R. Alcohol usage in sport and exercise. Addict Biol. 1999 Oct;4(4):373-83.

Lemon J. Alcoholic hangover and performance: a review. Drug Alcohol Rev. 1993;12(3):299-314.

National Institute on Alcohol Abuse and Alcoholism. What Is A Standard Drink?: https://www.niaaa.nih.gov/alcohol- health/overview-alcohol-consumption/what-standard-drink

O'Brien CP, Lyons F. Alcohol and the athlete. Sports Med. 2000 May;29(5):295-300. Review.

Shirreffs SM, Maughan RJ. The effect of alcohol on athletic performance. Curr Sports Med Rep. 2006 Jun;5(4):192-6. Review.

Shirreffs SM, Maughan RJ. The effect of alcohol on athletic performance. Curr Sports Med Rep. 2006 Jun;5(4):192-6. Review.

Suter PM, Schutz Y. The effect of exercise, alcohol or both combined on health and physical performance. Int J Obes (Lond). 2008 Dec;32 Suppl 6:S48-52.

U.S. Department of Health and Human Services and U.S. Department of Agriculture. 2015–2020 Dietary Guidelines for Americans. 8th Edition. December 2015. Available at http://health.gov/dietaryguidelines/2015/guidelines/

Vella, L. D., & Cameron-Smith, D. (2010). Alcohol, Athletic Performance and Recovery. Nutrients, 2(8), 781–789.

Vella, L. D., & Cameron-Smith, D. (2010). Alcohol, Athletic Performance and Recovery. Nutrients, 2(8), 781–789.

CHAPTER 17

Butter/Fats Added to Coffee

Engel, S., & Tholstrup, T. (2015). Butter increased total and LDL cholesterol compared with olive oil but resulted in higher HDL cholesterol compared with a habitual diet. The American Journal of Clinical Nutrition, 102(2), 309–315.

Huth, P. J., & Park, K. M. (2012). Influence of dairy product and milk fat consumption on cardiovascular disease risk: a review of the evidence. Advances in nutrition (Bethesda, Md.), 3(3), 266-85.

Markus, R. (2000). Effects of food on cortisol and mood in vulnerable subjects under controllable and uncontrollable stress. Physiology & Behavior, 70(3-4), 333–342.

Intermittent Fasting

Collier, R. (2013). Intermittent fasting: the next big weight loss fad. CMAJ : Canadian Medical Association Journal, 185(8), E321–E322.

Harris L, Hamilton S, Azevedo LB, Olajide J, De Brún C, Waller G, Whittaker V, Sharp T, Lean M, Hankey C, Ells L. Intermittent fasting interventions for treatment of overweight and obesity in adults: a systematic review and meta-analysis. JBI Database System Rev Implement Rep. 2018 Feb;16(2):507-547.

Harvie, M., & Howell, A. (2017). Potential Benefits and Harms of Intermittent Energy Restriction and Intermittent Fasting Amongst Obese, Overweight and Normal Weight Subjects—A Narrative Review of Human and Animal Evidence. Behavioral Sciences, 7(1), 4.

Headland, M., Clifton, P. M., Carter, S., & Keogh, J. B. (2016). Weight-Loss Outcomes: A Systematic Review and Meta-Analysis of

Intermittent Energy Restriction Trials Lasting a Minimum of 6 Months. Nutrients, 8(6), 354.

Tinsley GM, La Bounty PM. Effects of intermittent fasting on body composition and clinical health markers in humans. Nutr Rev. 2015 Oct;73(10):661-74.

Carb Backloading

Markus, R. (2000). Effects of food on cortisol and mood in vulnerable subjects under controllable and uncontrollable stress. Physiology & Behavior, 70(3-4), 333–342.

Van Cauter, E., Blackman, J. D., Roland, D., Spire, J. P., Refetoff, S., & Polonsky, K. S. (1991). Modulation of glucose regulation and insulin secretion by circadian rhythmicity and sleep. The Journal of clinical investigation, 88(3), 934-42.

Cleanses and Detoxes

Acosta RD, Cash BD. Clinical effects of colonic cleansing for general health promotion: a systematic review. Am J Gastroenterol. 2009 Nov;104(11):2830-6; quiz 2837. Epub 2009 Sep 1. Review. Erratum in: Am J Gastroenterol. 2010 May;105(5):1214.

Kesavarapu, K., Kang, M., Shin, J. J., & Rothstein, K. (2017). Yogi Detox Tea: A Potential Cause of Acute Liver Failure. Case Reports in Gastrointestinal Medicine, 2017, 3540756.

Klein AV, Kiat H. Detox diets for toxin elimination and weight management: a critical review of the evidence. J Hum Nutr Diet. 2015 Dec;28(6):675-86.

Makkapati S, D'Agati VD, Balsam L. "Green Smoothie Cleanse" Causing Acute Oxalate Nephropathy. Am J Kidney Dis. 2018 Feb;71(2):281-286.

Alkaline/Acidic Diets

Fenton CJ, Fenton TR, Huang T. Further Evidence of No Association between Dietary Acid Load and Disease. J Nutr. 2017 Feb;147(2):272.

Fenton, T. R., & Huang, T. (2016). Systematic review of the association between dietary acid load, alkaline water and cancer. BMJ Open, 6(6), e010438.

Schwalfenberg, G. K. (2012). The Alkaline Diet: Is There Evidence That an Alkaline pH Diet Benefits Health? Journal of Environmental and Public Health, 2012, 727630.

Inflammation

Beavers, K. M., Brinkley, T. E., & Nicklas, B. J. (2010). Effect of exercise training on chronic inflammation. Clinica chimica acta; international journal of clinical chemistry, 411(11-12), 785-93.

Ertek, S., & Cicero, A. (2012). Impact of physical activity on inflammation: effects on cardiovascular disease risk and other inflammatory conditions. Archives of medical science : AMS, 8(5), 794-804.

Flynn, M. G., McFarlin, B. K., & Markofski, M. M. (2007). The Anti-Inflammatory Actions of Exercise Training. American journal of lifestyle medicine, 1(3), 220- 235.

Forsythe LK, Wallace JM, Livingstone MB. Obesity and inflammation: the effects of weight loss. Nutr Res Rev. 2008 Dec;21(2):117-33. Review.

Monteiro, R., & Azevedo, I. (2010). Chronic inflammation in obesity and the metabolic syndrome. Mediators of inflammation, 2010, 289645.

Peake JM, Neubauer O, Della Gatta PA, Nosaka K. Muscle damage and inflammation during recovery from exercise. J Appl Physiol (1985). 2017 Mar 1;122(3):559-570.

Pedersen BK. The anti-inflammatory effect of exercise: its role in diabetes and cardiovascular disease control. Essays Biochem. 2006;42:105-17. Review.

You T, Nicklas BJ. Chronic inflammation: role of adipose tissue and modulation by weight loss. Curr Diabetes Rev. 2006 Feb;2(1):29-37. Review.

Hormones as Causes of Weight Gain

Davis RB, Turner LW. A review of current weight management: research and recommendations.

J Am Acad Nurse Pract. 2001 Jan;13(1):15-9; quiz 20-1. Review.

Hall KD. A review of the carbohydrate-insulin model of obesity. Eur J Clin Nutr. 2017 Mar;71(3):323-326. Epub 2017 Jan 11. Review.

Hill, J. O., Wyatt, H. R., & Peters, J. C. (2012). Energy balance and obesity. Circulation, 126(1), 126-32.

Steinbeck K. Obesity: the science behind the management. Intern Med J. 2002 May-Jun;32(5-6):237-41. Review.

Coconut Oil

Boateng, L., Ansong, R., Owusu, W. B., & Steiner-Asiedu, (2016). Coconut oil and palm oil's role in nutrition, health and national development: A review. Ghana Medical Journal, 50(3), 189–196.

Clifton PM, Keogh JB. A systematic review of the effect of dietary saturated and polyunsaturated fat on heart disease. Nutr Metab Cardiovasc Dis. 2017 Dec;27(12):1060-1080.

Cox C, Mann J, Sutherland W, Chisholm A, Skeaff M. Effects of coconut oil, butter, and safflower oil on lipids and lipoproteins in persons with moderately elevated cholesterol levels.J Lipid Res.

Eyres L, Eyres MF, Chisholm A, Brown RC. Coconut oil consumption and cardiovascular risk factors in humans.Nutr Rev. 2016;74:267–280.

Eyres, L., Eyres, M. F., Chisholm, A., & Brown, R. C. (2016). Coconut oil consumption and cardiovascular risk factors in humans. Nutrition Reviews, 74(4), 267–280.

Nettleton, J. A., Brouwer, I. A., Geleijnse, J. M., & Hornstra, G. (2017). Saturated Fat Consumption and Risk of Coronary Heart Disease and Ischemic Stroke: A Science Update. Annals of Nutrition & Metabolism, 70(1), 26–33.

St-Onge, M.-P., Bosarge, A., Goree, L. L. T., & Darnell, B. (2008). Medium Chain Triglyceride Oil Consumption as Part of a Weight Loss Diet Does Not Lead to an Adverse Metabolic Profile When Compared to Olive Oil. Journal of the American College of Nutrition, 27(5), 547–552.

Natural Is Better

Appeal to nature. (n.d.). In RationalWiki. Retrieved December 6, 2018, from https://rationalwiki.org/wiki/Appeal_to_nature

Tanner, J. (2006). The naturalistic fallacy. The Richmond Journal of Philosophy, 13, 1–6.

Processed Food

Martínez Steele, E., Popkin, B. M., Swinburn, B., & Monteiro, C. A. (2017). The share of ultra-processed foods and the overall nutritional quality of diets in the US: evidence from a nationally representative cross-sectional study. Population health metrics, 15(1), 6.

Patel S. (2015). Emerging trends in nutraceutical applications of whey protein and its derivatives. Journal of food science and technology, 52(11), 6847-58.

Jargin S. V. (2014). Soy and phytoestrogens: possible side effects. German medical science : GMS e-journal, 12, Doc18.

Non-Genetically Modified Food (Non-GMO)

Azevedo JL, Araujo WL. Genetically modified crops: environmental and human health concerns. Mutat Res. 2003 Nov;544(2-3):223-33. Review.

Bawa, A. S., & Anilakumar, K. R. (2013). Genetically modified foods: safety, risks and public concerns—a review. Journal of Food Science and Technology, 50(6), 1035–1046.

Domingo JL, Giné Bordonaba J. A literature review on the safety assessment of genetically modified plants. Environ Int. 2011 May;37(4):734-42.

Domingo JL. Safety assessment of GM plants: An updated review of the scientific literature. Food Chem Toxicol. 2016 Sep;95:12-8.

EFSA GMO Panel Working Group on Animal Feeding Trials. Safety and nutritional assessment of GM plants and derived food and feed: the role of animal feeding trials. Food Chem Toxicol. 2008 Mar;46 Suppl 1:S2-70.

Hielscher, S., Pies, I., Valentinov, V., & Chatalova, L. (2016). Rationalizing the GMO Debate: The Ordonomic Approach to Addressing Agricultural Myths. International Journal of Environmental Research and Public Health, 13(5), 476.

Hug K. Genetically modified organisms: do the benefits outweigh the risks? Medicina (Kaunas). 2008;44(2):87-99. Review.

Jones, L. (1999). Genetically modified foods. BMJ : British Medical Journal, 318(7183), 581–584.

Key, S., Ma, J. K.-C., & Drake, P. M. (2008). Genetically modified plants and human health. Journal of the Royal Society of Medicine, 101(6), 290–298.

Klümper, W., & Qaim, M. (2014). A Meta-Analysis of the Impacts of Genetically Modified Crops. PLoS ONE, 9(11), e111629.

Martinelli, L., Karbarz, M., & Siipi, H. (2013). Science, safety, and trust: the case of transgenic food. Croatian Medical Journal, 54(1), 91–96.

Ramessar K, Peremarti A, Gómez-Galera S, Naqvi S, Moralejo M, Muñoz P, Capell T, Christou P. Biosafety and risk assessment framework for selectable marker genes in transgenic crop plants: a case of the science not supporting the politics. Transgenic Res. 2007 Jun;16(3):261-80. Epub 2007 Apr 14. Review.

Shelton AM, Zhao JZ, Roush RT. Economic, ecological, food safety, and social consequences of the deployment of bt transgenic plants. Annu Rev Entomol. 2002;47:845-81. Review.

Snell C, Bernheim A, Bergé JB, Kuntz M, Pascal G, Paris A, Ricroch AE. Assessment of the health impact of GM plant diets in long-term and multigenerational animal feeding trials: a literature review. Food Chem Toxicol. 2012 Mar;50(3-4):1134-48.

Uzogara SG. The impact of genetic modification of human foods in the 21st century: a review. Biotechnol Adv. 2000 May;18(3):179-206.

Weil JH. Are genetically modified plants useful and safe? IUBMB Life. 2005 Apr-May;57(4-5):311-4. Review.

Organic Foods

Mie A, Andersen HR, Gunnarsson S, Kahl J, Kesse-Guyot E, Rembiałkowska E, Quaglio G, Grandjean P. Human health implications of organic food and organic agriculture: a comprehensive review. Environ Health. 2017 Oct 27;16(1):111.

rednicka-Tober D, Bara ski M, Seal C, Sanderson R, Benbrook C, Steinshamn H, Gromadzka-Ostrowska J, Rembiałkowska E, Skwarło-So ta K, Eyre M, Cozzi G, Krogh Larsen M, Jordon T, Niggli U, Sakowski T, Calder PC, Burdge GC, Sotiraki S, Stefanakis A, Yolcu H, Stergiadis S, Chatzidimitriou E, Butler G, Stewart G, Leifert C. Composition differences between organic and conventional meat: a systematic literature review and meta-analysis. Br J Nutr. 2016 Mar 28;115(6):994-1011.

Forman J, Silverstein J; Committee on Nutrition; Council on Environmental Health; American Academy of Pediatrics. Organic foods: health and environmental advantages and disadvantages. Pediatrics. 2012 Nov;130(5):e1406-15.

Smith-Spangler C, Brandeau ML, Hunter GE, Bavinger JC, Pearson M, Eschbach PJ, Sundaram V, Liu H, Schirmer P, Stave C, Olkin I, Bravata DM. Are organic foods safer or healthier than conventional alternatives?: a systematic review. Ann Intern Med. 2012 Sep 4;157(5):348-66.

Bahlai CA, Xue Y, McCreary CM, Schaafsma AW, Hallett RH. Choosing organic pesticides over synthetic pesticides may not effectively mitigate environmental risk in soybeans. PLoS One. 2010 Jun 22;5(6):e11250.

Dangour AD, Lock K, Hayter A, Aikenhead A, Allen E, Uauy R. Nutrition-related health effects of organic foods: a systematic review. Am J Clin Nutr. 2010 Jul;92(1):203-10.

Dangour AD, Dodhia SK, Hayter A, Allen E, Lock K, Uauy R. Nutritional quality of organic foods: a systematic review. Am J Clin Nutr. 2009 Sep;90(3):680-5.

Magkos F, Arvaniti F, Zampelas A. Putting the safety of organic food into perspective. Nutr Res Rev. 2003 Dec;16(2):211-22.

Rosen, J. D. (2010), A Review of the Nutrition Claims Made by Proponents of Organic Food. Comprehensive Reviews in Food Science and Food Safety, 9: 270-277.

Eating at Night Makes You Fat

Kinsey, A. W., & Ormsbee, M. J. (2015). The Health Impact of Nighttime Eating: Old and New Perspectives. Nutrients, 7(4), 2648–2662.

Schoenfeld BJ, Aragon AA, Krieger JW. Effects of meal frequency on weight loss and body composition: a meta- analysis. Nutr Rev. 2015 Feb;73(2):69-82.

Breakfast Is the Most Important Meal of the Day

Betts, J. A., Richardson, J. D., Chowdhury, E. A., Holman, G. D., Tsintzas, K., & Thompson, D. (2014). The causal role of breakfast in energy balance and health: a randomized controlled trial in lean adults. The American Journal of Clinical Nutrition, 100(2), 539–547.

Jakubowicz D, Wainstein J, Ahren B, Landau Z, Bar- Dayan Y, Froy O. Fasting until noon triggers increased postprandial hyperglycemia and impaired insulin response after lunch and dinner in individuals with type 2 diabetes: a randomized clinical trial. Diabetes Care. 2015 Oct;38(10):1820-6.

Farshchi HR, Taylor MA, Macdonald IA. Deleterious effects of omitting breakfast on insulin sensitivity and fasting lipid profiles in healthy lean women. Am J Clin Nutr. 2005 Feb;81(2):388-96.

LeCheminant GM, LeCheminant JD, Tucker LA, Bailey BW. A randomized controlled trial to study the effects of breakfast on energy intake, physical activity, and body fat in women who are nonhabitual breakfast eaters. Appetite. 2017 May 1;112:44-51.

Geliebter, A., Astbury, N. M., Aviram-Friedman, R., Yahav, E., & Hashim, S. (2014). Skipping breakfast leads to weight loss but also elevated cholesterol compared with consuming daily breakfasts of oat porridge or frosted cornflakes in overweight individuals: a randomised controlled trial. Journal of Nutritional Science, 3, e56.

Nonino-Borges CB, Martins Borges R, Bavaresco M, Suen VM, Moreira AC, Marchini JS. Influence of meal time on salivary circadian cortisol rhythms and weight loss in obese women. Nutrition. 2007 May;23(5):385-91.

Reeves S, Huber JW, Halsey LG, Horabady-Farahani Y, Ijadi M, Smith T. Experimental manipulation of breakfast in normal and overweight/obese participants is associated with changes to nutrient and energy intake consumption patterns. Physiol Behav. 2014 Jun 22;133:130-5.

Schlundt DG, Hill JO, Sbrocco T, Pope-Cordle J, Sharp T. The role of breakfast in the treatment of obesity: a randomized clinical trial. Am J Clin Nutr. 1992 Mar;55(3):645-51.

Sensi S, Capani F. Chronobiological aspects of weight loss in obesity: effects of different meal timing regimens. Chronobiol Int. 1987;4(2):251-61.

Sofer S, Eliraz A, Kaplan S, Voet H, Fink G, Kima T, Madar Z. Greater weight loss and hormonal changes after 6 months diet with carbohydrates eaten mostly at dinner. Obesity (Silver Spring). 2011 Oct;19(10):2006-14.

Hormones in Food

Hartmann, S., M. Lacorn and H. Steinhart. 1998. Natural occurrence of steroid hormones in food. Food Chemistry 62:7-20.

Hoffmann, B. and Evers, P., 1986. Anabolic agents with sex hormone-like activities: problems of residues. In: A.G. Rico (Editor), Drug Residues in Animals. Academic Press, Orlando, FL, pp. 111-146.

Shore, L. S., and M. Shemesh. 2003. Naturally produced steroid hormones and their release into the environment. Pure Appl. Chem. 75:1859-71.

Smith, G., Heaton, K., Sofos, J., Tatum, J., Aaronson, M., & Clayton, R. Residues Of Antibiotics, Hormones And Pesticides In Conventional, Natural And Organic Beef. Journal of Muscle Foods, 157-172.

Stephany RW. Hormones in meat: different approaches in the EU and in the USA. APMIS Suppl. 2001;(103):S357- 63; discussion S363-4. Review.

U.S. Department of Agriculture, Agricultural Research Service. 2002. USDA-Iowa State University Database on the Isofl avone Content of Foods, Release 1.3 - 2002. Nutrient Data Laboratory website: http://www.nal.usda.gov/fnic/foodcomp/Data/isofl av/isofl av.html

Antibiotics in Food

Dodsworth, T., & Ball, C. A report on the treatment of beef cattle with tranquilisers and antibiotics. Animal Production Anim. Prod., 315-319.

Smith, G., Heaton, K., Sofos, J., Tatum, J., Aaronson, M., & Clayton, R. Residues Of Antibiotics, Hormones And Pesticides In Conventional, Natural And Organic Beef. Journal of Muscle Foods, 157-172.

Chemicals in Food

AGENTS CLASSIFIED BY THE IARC MONOGRAPHS, VOLUMES 1–123 (2018)

Ames, B. N., Profet, M., & Gold, L. S. (1990). Dietary pesticides (99.99% all natural). Proceedings of the National Academy of Sciences of the United States of America, 87(19), 7777-81.

Artificial Sweeteners

Brown, R. J., De Banate, M. A., & Rother, K. I. (2010). Artificial Sweeteners: A systematic review of metabolic effects in youth. International Journal of Pediatric Obesity : IJPO : An Official Journal of the International Association for the Study of Obesity, 5(4), 305–312.

Miller, P. E., & Perez, V. (2014). Low-calorie sweeteners and body weight and composition: a meta-analysis of randomized controlled trials and prospective cohort studies. The American Journal of Clinical Nutrition, 100(3), 765–777.

Rogers, P. J., Hogenkamp, P. S., de Graaf, C., Higgs, S., Lluch, A., Ness, A. R., ... Mela, D. J. (2016). Does low- energy sweetener consumption affect energy intake and body weight? A systematic review, including meta-analyses, of the evidence from human and animal studies. International Journal of Obesity (2005), 40(3), 381–394.

Stanhope, K. L., Goran, M. I., Bosy- Westphal, A., King, J. C., Schmidt, L. A., Schwarz, J.- M., Stice, E., Sylvetsky,A.C., Turnbaugh, P. J., Bray, G. A., Gardner, C. D., Havel, P. J., Malik, V., Mason, A. E., Ravussin, E., Rosenbaum, M., Welsh, J. A., Allister- Price, C., Sigala, D. M., Greenwood, M. R. C., Astrup, A., and Krauss, R. M. (2018) Pathways and mechanisms linking dietary components to cardiometabolic disease: thinking beyond calories. Obesity Reviews, 19: 1205–1235.

Sylvetsky AC, Rother KI. Nonnutritive Sweeteners in Weight Management and Chronic Disease: A Review. Obesity (Silver Spring). 2018 Apr;26(4):635-640.

Rogers PJ, Hogenkamp PS, de Graaf C, Higgs S, Lluch A, Ness AR, Penfold C, Perry R, Putz P, Yeomans MR, Mela DJ. Does low-energy sweetener consumption affect energy intake and body weight? A systematic review, including meta-analyses, of the evidence from human and animal studies. Int J Obes (Lond). 2016 Mar;40(3):381-94.

Bellisle F. Intense Sweeteners, Appetite for the Sweet Taste, and Relationship to Weight Management. Curr Obes Rep. 2015 Mar;4(1):106-10.

Marinovich M, Galli CL, Bosetti C, Gallus S, La Vecchia C. Aspartame, low-calorie sweeteners and disease: regulatory safety and epidemiological issues. Food Chem Toxicol. 2013 Oct;60:109-15.

Grotz VL, Munro IC. An overview of the safety of sucralose. Regul Toxicol Pharmacol. 2009 Oct;55(1):1-5. doi: 10.1016/j.yrtph.2009.05.011. Epub 2009 May 21. Review.

Magnuson BA, Burdock GA, Doull J, Kroes RM, Marsh GM, Pariza MW, Spencer PS, Waddell WJ, Walker R, Williams GM. Aspartame: a safety evaluation based on current use

levels, regulations, and toxicological and epidemiological studies. Crit Rev Toxicol. 2007;37(8):629- 727. Review.

Lim U, Subar AF, Mouw T, Hartge P, Morton LM, Stolzenberg-Solomon R, Campbell D, Hollenbeck AR, Schatzkin A. Consumption of aspartame-containing beverages and incidence of hematopoietic and brain malignancies. Cancer Epidemiol Biomarkers Prev. 2006 Sep;15(9):1654-9.

Weihrauch MR, Diehl V. Artificial sweeteners– do they bear a carcinogenic risk? Ann Oncol. 2004 Oct;15(10):1460-5. Review.

Butchko HH, Stargel WW, Comer CP, Mayhew DA, Benninger C, Blackburn GL, de Sonneville LM, Geha RS, Hertelendy Z, Koestner A, Leon AS, Liepa GU, McMartin KE, Mendenhall CL, Munro IC, Novotny EJ, Renwick AG, Schiffman SS, Schomer DL, Shaywitz BA, Spiers PA, Tephly TR, Thomas JA, Trefz FK. Aspartame: review of safety. Regul Toxicol Pharmacol. 2002 Apr;35(2 Pt 2):S1-93. Review.

Butchko HH, Stargel WW. Aspartame: scientific evaluation in the postmarketing period. Regul Toxicol Pharmacol. 2001 Dec;34(3):221-33.

Baird IM, Shephard NW, Merritt RJ, Hildick-Smith G. Repeated dose study of sucralose tolerance in human subjects. Food Chem Toxicol. 2000;38 Suppl 2:S123-9.

Renwick AG. Acceptable daily intake and the regulation of intense sweeteners. Food Addit Contam. 1990 Jul- Aug;7(4):463-75. Review.

Yost DA. Clinical safety of aspartame. Am Fam Physician. 1989 Feb;39(2):201-6. Review. PubMed

Aspartame. Review of safety issues. Council on Scientific Affairs. JAMA. 1985 Jul 19;254(3):400-2.

Tandel, K. R. (2011). Sugar substitutes: Health controversy over perceived benefits. Journal of Pharmacology & Pharmacotherapeutics, 2(4), 236–243.

Juicing

Hyson, D. A. (2015). A Review and Critical Analysis of the Scientific Literature Related to 100% Fruit Juice and Human Health. Advances in Nutrition, 6(1), 37–51.

Klein AV, Kiat H. Detox diets for toxin elimination and weight management: a critical review of the evidence. J Hum Nutr Diet. 2015 Dec;28(6):675-86.

Obert J, Pearlman M, Obert L, Chapin S. Popular Weight Loss Strategies: a Review of Four Weight Loss Techniques. Curr Gastroenterol Rep. 2017 Nov 9;19(12):61.

Zheng, J., Zhou, Y., Li, S., Zhang, P., Zhou, T., Xu, D.-P., & Li, H.-B. (2017). Effects and Mechanisms of Fruit and Vegetable Juices on Cardiovascular Diseases. International Journal of Molecular Sciences, 18(3), 555.

Mistaking Thirst for Hunger

Corney RA, Sunderland C, James LJ. The effect of hydration status on appetite and energy intake. J Sports Sci. 2015;33(8):761-8.

McKiernan, F., Hollis, J. H., McCabe, G., & Mattes, R. D. (2009). Thirst-drinking, hunger-eating; tight coupling? Journal of the American Dietetic Association, 109(3), 486– 490.

Hyperhydration Extremism

Cotter, J. D., Thornton, S. N., Lee, J. K., & Laursen, P. B. (2014). Are we being drowned in hydration advice? Thirsty for more? Extreme Physiology & Medicine, 3, 18.

El-Sharkawy AM, Sahota O, Lobo DN. Acute and chronic effects of hydration status on health. Nutr Rev. 2015 Sep;73 Suppl 2:97-109.

Malisova, O., Athanasatou, A., Pepa, A., Husemann, M., Domnik, K., Braun, H., ... Kapsokefalou, M. (2016). Water Intake and Hydration Indices in Healthy European Adults: The European Hydration Research Study (EHRS). Nutrients, 8(4), 204.

Popkin, B. M., D'Anci, K. E., & Rosenberg, I. H. (2010). Water, Hydration and Health. Nutrition Reviews, 68(8), 439–458.

Gaining Weight From Undereating

Buhl KM, Gallagher D, Hoy K, Matthews DE, Heymsfield SB. Unexplained disturbance in body weight regulation: diagnostic outcome assessed by doubly labeled water and body composition analyses in obese patients reporting low energy intakes. J Am Diet Assoc. 1995 Dec;95(12):1393- 400; quiz 1401-2.

Heitmann, B. L., & Lissner, L. (1995). Dietary underreporting by obese individuals--is it specific or non-specific? BMJ : British Medical Journal, 311(7011), 986– 989.

Johannsen, D. L., Knuth, N. D., Huizenga, R., Rood, J. C., Ravussin, E., & Hall, K. D. (2012). Metabolic Slowing with Massive Weight Loss despite Preservation of Fat-Free Mass. The Journal of Clinical Endocrinology and Metabolism, 97(7), 2489–2496.

Knuth, N. D., Johannsen, D. L., Tamboli, R. A., Marks- Shulman, P. A., Huizenga, R., Chen, K. Y., ... Hall, K. D. (2014). Metabolic adaptation following massive weight loss is related to the degree of energy imbalance and changes in circulating leptin. Obesity (Silver Spring, Md.), 22(12), 2563–2569.

Lichtman SW, Pisarska K, Berman ER, Pestone M, Dowling H, Offenbacher E, Weisel H, Heshka S, Matthews DE, Heymsfield SB. Discrepancy between self-reported and actual caloric intake and exercise in obese subjects. N Engl J Med. 1992 Dec 31;327(27):1893-8.

Müller MJ, Enderle J, Pourhassan M, Braun W, Eggeling B, Lagerpusch M, Glüer CC, Kehayias JJ, Kiosz D, Bosy- Westphal A. Metabolic adaptation to caloric restriction and subsequent refeeding: the Minnesota Starvation Experiment revisited. Am J Clin Nutr. 2015 Oct;102(4):807-19.

Dietary Versus Serum Cholesterol

Baigent, C., Blackwell, L., Emberson, J., Holland, L. E., Reith, C., Bhala, N., Peto, R., Barnes, E. H., Keech, A., Simes, J., ... Collins, R. (2010). Efficacy and safety of more intensive lowering of LDL cholesterol: a meta- analysis of data from 170,000 participants in 26 randomised trials. Lancet (London, England), 376(9753), 1670-81.

Djoussé, L., & Michael Gaziano, J. (2009). Dietary cholesterol and coronary artery disease: A systematic review. Current Atherosclerosis Reports, 11(6), 418–422.

Griffin, J. D., & Lichtenstein, A. H. (2013). Dietary Cholesterol and Plasma Lipoprotein Profiles: Randomized- Controlled Trials. Current nutrition reports, 2(4), 274-282.

Lecerf, J.-M., & de Lorgeril, M. (2011). Dietary cholesterol: from physiology to cardiovascular risk. British Journal of Nutrition, 106(01), 6–14.

Veganism as the Only Way to Health

Craig WJ, Mangels AR; American Dietetic Association. Position of the American Dietetic Association: vegetarian diets. J Am Diet Assoc. 2009 Jul;109(7):1266-82.

Craig WJ. Health effects of vegan diets. Am J Clin Nutr. 2009 May;89(5):1627S-1633S. doi: 10.3945/ajcn.2009.26736N. Epub 2009 Mar 11. Review.

Freeland-Graves J. Mineral adequacy of vegetarian diets. Am J Clin Nutr. 1988 Sep;48(3 Suppl):859-62. Review.

Hever, J. (2016). Plant-Based Diets: A Physician's Guide. The Permanente Journal, 20(3), 93–101.

Key TJ, Appleby PN, Rosell MS. Health effects of vegetarian and vegan diets. Proc Nutr Soc. 2006 Feb;65(1):35-41. Review.

McEvoy CT, Temple N, Woodside JV. Vegetarian diets, low-meat diets and health: a review. Public Health Nutr. 2012 Dec;15(12):2287-94.

Tuso, P. J., Ismail, M. H., Ha, B. P., & Bartolotto, C. (2013). Nutritional Update for Physicians: Plant-Based Diets. The Permanente Journal, 17(2), 61–66.

Excess Protein Concerns

Clase, C. M., & Smyth, A. (2015). Chronic kidney disease: diet. BMJ Clinical Evidence, 2015, 2004.

Excess protein concerns: Mathur, M. and N.C. Nayak. "Effect of low protein diet on low dose chronic aflatoxin B1 induced hepatic injury in rhesus monkeys." Toxin Reviews. 1989;8(1-2):265-273.

Junshi C., et al. Life-style and Mortality in China: A Study of the Characteristics of 65 Chinese Counties. Oxford: Oxford University Press, 1990.

Kamper AL, Strandgaard S. Long-Term Effects of High- Protein Diets on Renal Function. Annu Rev Nutr. 2017 Aug 21;37:347-369.

Ko GJ, Obi Y, Tortorici AR, Kalantar-Zadeh K. Dietary protein intake and chronic kidney disease. Curr Opin Clin Nutr Metab Care. 2017 Jan;20(1):77-85. Review.

Aparicio M. Protein intake and chronic kidney disease: literature review, 2003 to 2008. J Ren Nutr. 2009 Sep;19(5 Suppl):S5-8.

Friedman AN. High-protein diets: potential effects on the kidney in renal health and disease. Am J Kidney Dis. 2004 Dec;44(6):950-62. Review.

Martin, W. F., Armstrong, L. E., & Rodriguez, N. R. (2005). Dietary protein intake and renal function. Nutrition & Metabolism, 2, 25.

Pedersen, A. N., Kondrup, J., & Børsheim, E. (2013). Health effects of protein intake in healthy adults: a systematic literature review. Food & Nutrition Research, 57, 10.3402/fnr. v57i0.21245.

Schwingshackl, L., & Hoffmann, G. (2014). Comparison of High vs. Normal/Low Protein Diets on Renal Function in Subjects without Chronic Kidney Disease: A Systematic Review and Meta-Analysis. PLoS ONE, 9(5), e97656.

Keto/Anti-Carb Diets

Burke, L. M. (2015). Re-Examining High-Fat Diets for Sports Performance: Did We Call the "Nail in the Coffin" Too Soon? Sports Medicine (Auckland, N.z.), 45(Suppl 1), 33–49.

Hall KD. A review of the carbohydrate-insulin model of obesity. Eur J Clin Nutr. 2017 Mar;71(3):323-326.Epub 2017 Jan 11. Review. Erratum in: Eur J Clin Nutr. 2017 May;71(5):679.

Karl, J. P., & Saltzman, E. (2012). The Role of Whole Grains in Body Weight Regulation. Advances in Nutrition, 3(5), 697–707.

Kiens B, Astrup A. Ketogenic Diets for Fat Loss and Exercise Performance: Benefits and Safety? Exerc Sport Sci Rev. 2015 Jul;43(3):109.

Phinney, S. D. (2004). Ketogenic diets and physical performance. Nutrition & Metabolism, 1, 2.

Pinckaers, P. J. M., Churchward-Venne, T. A., Bailey, D., & van Loon, L. J. C. (2017). Ketone Bodies and Exercise Performance: The Next Magic Bullet or Merely Hype? Sports Medicine (Auckland, N.z.), 47(3), 383–391.

Pol K, Christensen R, Bartels EM, Raben A, Tetens I, Kristensen M. Whole grain and body weight changes in apparently healthy adults: a systematic review and meta- analysis of randomized controlled studies. Am J Clin Nutr. 2013 Oct;98(4):872-84.

Zajac, A., Poprzecki, S., Maszczyk, A., Czuba, M., Michalczyk, M., & Zydek, G. (2014). The Effects of a Ketogenic Diet on Exercise Metabolism and Physical Performance in Off-Road Cyclists. Nutrients, 6(7), 2493– 2508.

Low-Fat Diets

de Souza RJ, Mente A, Maroleanu A, Cozma AI, Ha V, Kishibe T, Uleryk E, Budylowski P, Schünemann H, Beyene J, Anand SS. Intake of saturated and trans unsaturated fatty acids and risk of all cause mortality, cardiovascular disease, and type 2 diabetes: systematic review and meta-analysis of observational studies. BMJ. 2015 Aug 11;351:h3978.

Nettleton, J. A., Brouwer, I. A., Geleijnse, J. M., & Hornstra, G. (2017). Saturated Fat Consumption and Risk of Coronary Heart Disease and Ischemic Stroke: A Science Update. Annals of Nutrition & Metabolism, 70(1), 26–33.

Lawrence, G. D. (2013). Dietary Fats and Health: Dietary Recommendations in the Context of Scientific Evidence. Advances in Nutrition, 4(3), 294–302.

Clifton PM, Keogh JB. A systematic review of the effect of dietary saturated and polyunsaturated fat on heart disease. Nutr Metab Cardiovasc Dis. 2017 Dec;27(12):1060-1080.

Briggs, M. A., Petersen, K. S., & Kris-Etherton, P. M. (2017). Saturated Fatty Acids and Cardiovascular Disease: Replacements for Saturated Fat to Reduce Cardiovascular Risk. Healthcare, 5(2), 29.

Astrup, A., Dyerberg, J., Elwood, P., Hermansen, K., Hu, F. B., Jakobsen, M. U., ... Willett, W. C. (2011). The role of reducing intakes of saturated fat in the prevention of cardiovascular disease: where does the evidence stand in 2010? The American Journal of Clinical Nutrition, 93(4), 684–688.

Hooper L, Martin N, Abdelhamid A, Davey Smith G. Reduction in saturated fat intake for cardiovascular disease. Cochrane Database Syst Rev. 2015 Jun 10;(6):CD011737.

Gluten-Free/Anti-Grain Diets

Bardella MT, Elli L, Ferretti F. Non Celiac Gluten Sensitivity. Curr Gastroenterol Rep. 2016 Dec;18(12):63. Review.

Karl, J. P., & Saltzman, E. (2012). The Role of Whole Grains in Body Weight Regulation. Advances in Nutrition, 3(5), 697–707

Lebwohl, B., Ludvigsson, J. F., & Green, P. H. R. (2015). Celiac disease and non-celiac gluten sensitivity. The BMJ, 351, h4347.

Leonard MM, Sapone A, Catassi C, Fasano A. Celiac Disease and Nonceliac Gluten Sensitivity: A Review. JAMA. 2017 Aug 15;318(7):647-656.

Lionetti, E., Pulvirenti, A., Vallorani, M., Catassi, G., Verma, A. K., Gatti, S., & Catassi, C. (2017). Re-challenge Studies in Non-celiac Gluten Sensitivity: A Systematic Review and Meta-Analysis. Frontiers in Physiology, 8, 621.
Molina-Infante J, Santolaria S, Sanders DS, Fernández- Bañares F. Systematic review: noncoeliac gluten sensitivity. Aliment Pharmacol Ther. 2015 May;41(9):807- 20.

Pol K, Christensen R, Bartels EM, Raben A, Tetens I, Kristensen M. Whole grain and body weight changes in apparently healthy adults: a systematic review and meta- analysis of randomized controlled studies. Am J Clin Nutr. 2013 Oct;98(4):872-84.
Vici G, Belli L, Biondi M, Polzonetti V. Gluten free diet and nutrient deficiencies: A review. Clin Nutr. 2016 Dec;35(6):1236-1241.

Anti-Dairy

Astrup, A., Rice Bradley, B. H., Brenna, J. T., Delplanque, B., Ferry, M., & Torres-Gonzalez, M. (2016). Regular-Fat Dairy and Human Health: A Synopsis of Symposia Presented in Europe and North America (2014–2015). Nutrients, 8(8), 463.
Brown-Riggs, C. (2016). Nutrition and Health Disparities: The Role of Dairy in Improving Minority Health Outcomes. International Journal of Environmental Research and Public Health, 13(1), 28.
Chen, G.-C., Szeto, I. M. Y., Chen, L.-H., Han, S.-F., Li, Y.-J., van Hekezen, R., & Qin, L.-Q. (2015). Dairy products consumption and metabolic syndrome in adults: systematic review and meta-analysis of observational studies. Scientific Reports, 5, 14606.
Davoodi, S. H., Shahbazi, R., Esmaeili, S., Sohrabvandi, S., Mortazavian, A., Jazayeri, S., & Taslimi, A. (2016). Health-Related Aspects of Milk Proteins. Iranian Journal of Pharmaceutical Research : IJPR, 15(3), 573–591.
Ebringer L, Ferencík M, Krajcovic J. Beneficial health effects of milk and fermented dairy products--review. Folia Microbiol (Praha). 2008;53(5):378-94.
Elwood, P. C., Pickering, J. E., Givens, D. I., & Gallacher, J. E. (2010). The Consumption of Milk and Dairy Foods and the Incidence of Vascular Disease and Diabetes: An Overview of the Evidence. Lipids, 45(10), 925–939.
Haug, A., Høstmark, A. T., & Harstad, O. M. (2007). Bovine milk in human nutrition – a review. Lipids in Health and Disease, 6, 25.
Juhl, C. R., Bergholdt, H., Miller, I. M., Jemec, G., Kanters, J. K., & Ellervik, C. (2018). Dairy Intake and Acne Vulgaris: A Systematic Review and Meta-Analysis of 78,529 Children, Adolescents, and Young Adults. Nutrients, 10(8), 1049.
Rozenberg, S., Body, J.-J., Bruyère, O., Bergmann, P., Brandi, M. L., Cooper, C., ... Reginster, J.-Y. (2016). Effects of Dairy Products Consumption on Health: Benefits and Beliefs—A Commentary from the Belgian Bone Club and the European Society for Clinical and Economic Aspects of Osteoporosis, Osteoarthritis and Musculoskeletal Diseases. Calcified Tissue International, 98, 1–17.
Thorning, T. K., Raben, A., Tholstrup, T., Soedamah- Muthu, S. S., Givens, I., & Astrup, A. (2016). Milk and dairy products: good or bad for human health? An assessment of the totality of scientific evidence. Food & Nutrition Research, 60, 10.3402/fnr.v60.32527.
Visioli, F., & Strata, A. (2014). Milk, Dairy Products, and Their Functional Effects in Humans: A Narrative Review of Recent Evidence. Advances in Nutrition, 5(2), 131–143.

Genetic Diets

Görman, U., Mathers, J. C., Grimaldi, K. A., Ahlgren, J., & Nordström, K. (2013). Do we know enough? A scientific and ethical analysis of the basis for genetic-based personalized nutrition. Genes & nutrition, 8(4), 373-81.

Sales, N. M., Pelegrini, P. B., & Goersch, M. C. (2014). Nutrigenomics: definitions and advances of this new science. Journal of nutrition and metabolism, 2014, 202759.
Blood-Type Dieting

Cusack L, De Buck E, Compernolle V, Vandekerckhove P. Blood type diets lack supporting evidence: a systematic review. Am J Clin Nutr. 2013 Jul;98(1):99-104.

Wang J, Jamnik J, García-Bailo B, Nielsen DE, Jenkins DJA, El-Sohemy A. ABO Genotype Does Not Modify the Association between the "Blood-Type" Diet and Biomarkers of Cardiometabolic Disease in Overweight Adults. J Nutr. 2018 Apr 1;148(4):518-525.

Elimination Diets

Baker B. Weight loss and diet plans. Am J Nurs. 2006 Jun;106(6):52-9; quiz 60. Review.

Berg, A. C., Johnson, K. B., Straight, C. R., Reed, R. A., O'Connor, P. J., Evans, E. M., & Johnson, M. A. (2018). Flexible Eating Behavior Predicts Greater Weight Loss Following a Diet and Exercise Intervention in Older Women. Journal of Nutrition in Gerontology and Geriatrics, 37(1), 14–29.

Energy balance, body composition, sedentariness and appetite regulation: pathways to obesity. Clin Sci (Lond). 2016 Sep 1;130(18):1615-28.

Hall K. D. (2018). Did the Food Environment Cause the Obesity Epidemic? Obesity (Silver Spring, Md.), 26(1), 11-13.

Macronutrient Content of the Diet: What Do We Know About Energy Balance and Weight Maintenance? Curr Obes Rep. 2016 Jun;5(2):208-13.

Malik VS, Hu FB. Popular weight-loss diets: from evidence to practice. Nat Clin Pract Cardiovasc Med. 2007 Jan;4(1):34-41. Review.

Schaumberg, K., Anderson, D. A., Anderson, L. M., Reilly, E. E., & Gorrell, S. (2016). Dietary restraint: what's the harm? A review of the relationship between dietary restraint, weight trajectory and the development of eating pathology. Clinical Obesity, 6(2), 89–100.

Smith, C. F., Williamson, D. A., Bray, G. A., & Ryan, D. H. (1999). Flexible vs. Rigid Dieting Strategies: Relationship with Adverse Behavioral Outcomes. Appetite, 32(3), 295–305.

Tangney CC, Gustashaw KA, Stefan TM, Sullivan C, Ventrelle J, Filipowski CA, Heffernan AD, Hankins J; Clinical Nutrition Department at Rush University Medical Center. A review: which dietary plan is best for your patients seeking weight loss and sustained weight management? Dis Mon. 2005 May;51(5):284-316. Review.

Intuitive Eating

Guyenet, S. (2017). Hungry Brain: Why We Overeat and What We Can Do about It. Flatiron Books.

Hall K. D. (2018). Did the Food Environment Cause the Obesity Epidemic?. Obesity (Silver Spring, Md.), 26(1), 11-13.

Fast Weight Loss for the Very Obese

Astrup A, Rössner S. Lessons from obesity management programmes: greater initial weight loss improves long-term maintenance. Obes Rev. 2000 May;1(1):17-9. Review.

Avenell A, Brown TJ, McGee MA, Campbell MK, Grant AM, Broom J, Jung RT, Smith WC. What are the long-term benefits of weight reducing diets in adults? A systematic review of randomized controlled trials. J Hum Nutr Diet. 2004 Aug;17(4):317-35. Review.

Elfhag K, Rössner S. Who succeeds in maintaining weight loss? A conceptual review of factors associated with weight loss maintenance and weight regain. Obes Rev. 2005 Feb;6(1):67-85. Review.

Henry RR, Gumbiner B. Benefits and limitations of very-low-calorie diet therapy in obese NIDDM. Diabetes Care. 1991 Sep;14(9):802-23. Review.

Monnier L, Colette C, Percheron C, Boniface H. [Very-low- calorie-diets: is there a place for them in the management of the obese diabetic?]. Diabetes Metab. 2000 Jun;26 Suppl 3:46-51. Review. French.

Saris WH. Very-low-calorie diets and sustained weight loss. Obes Res. 2001 Nov;9 Suppl 4:295S-301S. Review.

Thomas JG, Bond DS, Phelan S, Hill JO, Wing RR. Weight-loss maintenance for 10 years in the National Weight Control Registry. Am J Prev Med. 2014 Jan;46(1):17-23.

Tsai AG, Wadden TA. The evolution of very-low-calorie diets: an update and meta-analysis. Obesity (Silver Spring). 2006 Aug;14(8):1283-93. Review.

Testosterone Boosters

Willoughby, D. S., Spillane, M., & Schwarz, N. (2014). Heavy Resistance Training and Supplementation With the Alleged Testosterone Booster Nmda has No Effect on Body Composition, Muscle Performance, and Serum Hormones Associated With the Hypothalamo-Pituitary- Gonadal Axis in Resistance-Trained Males. Journal of Sports Science & Medicine, 13(1), 192–199.

Brown GA, Vukovich M, King DS. Testosterone prohormone supplements. Med Sci Sports Exerc. 2006 Aug;38(8):1451-61. Review.

Rogerson S, Riches CJ, Jennings C, Weatherby RP, Meir RA, Marshall-Gradisnik SM. The effect of five weeks of Tribulus terrestris supplementation on muscle strength and body composition during preseason training in elite rugby league players. J Strength Cond Res. 2007

About the Authors

Dr. Mike Israetel holds a PhD in Sport Physiology and is currently the head science consultant for Renaissance Periodization. Mike was formerly a professor of Exercise and Sport Science in the School of Public Health at Temple University in Philadelphia, where he taught several courses, including Nutrition for Public Health, Advanced Sports Nutrition and Exercise, and Nutrition and Behavior. He has worked as a consultant on sports nutrition to the U.S. Olympic Training Site in Johnson City, TN, and has been an invited speaker at numerous scientific and performance and health conferences, including nutritional seminars at the U.S. Olympic Training Center in Lake Placid, NY. A co-founder of Renaissance Periodization, Mike has coached numerous athletes and busy professionals in both diet and weight training. Originally from Moscow, Russia, Mike is a competitive bodybuilder and Brazilian Jiu Jitsu grappler.

Dr. Melissa Davis holds a PhD in Neurobiology and Behavior and is a consultant for Renaissance Periodization. She has 10 years of research experience studying somatosensory-based disease intervention, cortical plasticity, and brain development at UC Irvine. Her work has been featured in *Scientific American,* published in high-impact, peer-reviewed journals, and recognized by faculty of 1,000. Melissa has earned awards for teaching, scholarship, and excellence in research. She has also been involved in science outreach activities for over a decade. Melissa is currently a Brazilian Jiu Jitsu black belt under Giva Santana at One Jiu Jitsu in Irvine, CA. She is a repeat IBJJF Master World Champion and has also represented the United States twice for her division in the international Abu Dhabi World Pro Competition.

Dr. Jen Case holds a PhD in Human Nutrition, with an emphasis in Nutrition and Performance. She is also a Registered Dietitian (RD) and Certified Strength and Conditioning Specialist (CSCS). She was formerly a professor of Exercise Science at the University of Central Missouri, where she taught Advanced Exercise Metabolism, Exercise Prescription, Functional Anatomy, and other Kinesiology and Nutrition courses. Jen holds two black belts in two different martial arts: She is both a Hawiian Kempo black belt under Steve Twemlow at SOMMA, in Topeka, KS and a Brazilian Jiu Jitsu black belt under Jason Bircher at KCBJJ, a Renato Tavares Affiliate, in Kansas

City, KS. She is also a former Mixed Martial Arts (MMA) fighter. In Jiu Jitsu, Jen is a repeat IBJJF Masters World Champion and IBJJF Pan Am champion.

Dr. James Hoffmann holds a PhD in Sport Physiology and is a consultant for Renaissance Periodization. He is the former program director of the Exercise and Sport Science program and the women's rugby team coach at Temple University in Philadelphia, PA. While at Temple, James taught courses in Strength and Conditioning Theory, Strength and Conditioning Practice, Exercise Physiology, and Biochemistry. James earned his PhD under Dr. Mike Stone at ETSU, where he focused on the application of sled pushing to sport performance enhancement in rugby players. As the team's assistant coach and Head Sport Scientist, James has coached numerous Rugby players at ETSU, where he was also the head strength and conditioning coach and weight room manager. Originally from Chicago, IL, James is a lifelong athlete, who has achieved high ranks in competitive rugby, American football, and wrestling and is currently pursuing Thai boxing.

GUEST AUTHORS

Dr. Gabrielle Fundaro, PhD – Human Nutrition, Foods, and Exercise, Virginia Tech; Certified Health Coach, American Council on Exercise, Certified Sports Nutritionist, International Society of Sports Nutrition

Dr. Alex Harrison, PhD – Sport Physiology and Performance, East Tennessee State University; Elite Coach, Throwing Events (IAAF/USATF), Level 2 Coach, All other disciplines (USATF), Level 1 Coach (USA Triathlon) Certified Strength and Conditioning Specialist (NSCA), Weightlifting Coach, Level 1, (USAW)

Paul Salter, MS, RD – Former Nutrition Editor for Bodybuilding.com and former Sports Dietitian for IMG Academy

A SPECIAL THANKS TO OUR EDITOR

Stephen Dvorak holds an MFA in Creative Writing from University of Miami and is currently a Research Study Assistant at Northwestern University's Feinberg School of Medicine.

Credits

Cover & interior design: Annika Naas

Layout: Zerosoft

Cover & interior photos: © AdobeStock, unless otherwise noted

Illustrations: © Renaissance Periodization

Managing editor: Elizabeth Evans